Basic Principles of Applied Medical Statistics

Jos W. R. Twisk

Basic Principles of Applied Medical Statistics

A Practical Guide

Springer

Jos W. R. Twisk
Department of Epidemiology and Data Science
Amsterdam UMC
Amsterdam, The Netherlands

ISBN 978-3-031-86277-9 ISBN 978-3-031-86278-6 (eBook)
https://doi.org/10.1007/978-3-031-86278-6

This Springer imprint is published by the registered company Springer Nature Switzerland AG
The registered company address is: Gewerbestrasse 11, 6330 Cham, Switzerland

Preface

Although many books have been written about (the basic principles of) medical statistics, this book is different than usual. In the first place, the starting point for the explanation of the statistical methods is the research question. After all, statistics is no more than a tool to get an answer to a research question. Secondly, this book is specifically written for the user. This means that mathematics is kept to a minimum and that the emphasis lies on the interpretation of the results of the statistical analyses. That is why the word applied appears in the title of this book. Thirdly, each analysis performed in this book is accompanied by general computer output. Besides that, specific computer output of the examples generated by SPSS, STATA and R will be available on request.

Amsterdam, The Netherlands Jos W. R. Twisk

Competing Interests

The author has no competing interests to declare that are relevant to the content of this manuscript.

Contents

Chapter 1
Introduction

1.1 Study Designs in Medical Research

Although this book is not about setting up and performing medical research, it is important to discuss the different study designs that are used within medical research. This is mainly due to the fact that the use of an effect estimate (and sometimes also the use of a statistical method) depends on the study design. Basically, medical studies can be divided into observational studies and intervention studies. In an observational study the researcher only observes, i.e. measurements are made on the subject without influencing the subject. The different measurements are then related to each other. In an intervention study, the subject is not only observed, but there is also some kind of intervention performed. In fact, the intervention is the most important part of the study, because the aim of the study is to investigate the effect of the intervention.

Observational studies can be divided into two main groups; cohort studies and case control studies. Cohort actually means group, so any observational study in which a group of subjects is observed is an observational cohort study. Within observational cohort studies, retrospective, cross-sectional and prospective studies can be distinguished. This distinction is based on the time frame of the study. In a retrospective cohort study, information is collected retrospectively (looking back in time), while in a cross-sectional cohort study, the information is collected at the time the study is performed. In a prospective cohort study, the cohort of subjects is followed over time. The differences between the three types of observational cohort studies are probably best illustrated by an example. Suppose researchers are interested in the relationship between systolic blood pressure and smoking in medical students. As a cohort, for example, the group of first-year medical students in Amsterdam is used. In this cohort, the researchers measure the systolic blood pressure of all students and make an inventory of which students smoke and which do not smoke. When they then relate systolic blood pressure to smoking, this study is a cross-sectional observational cohort study. When they ask this group

J. W. R. Twisk, *Basic Principles of Applied Medical Statistics*,
https://doi.org/10.1007/978-3-031-86278-6_1

of students when they started smoking and then relate the starting date of smoking to the systolic blood pressure just measured, it is a retrospective cohort study. For a prospective cohort study, the researchers must follow the cohort for a while, for example to answer the question whether starting or quitting smoking is related to systolic blood pressure.

In a case control study, a group of subjects with a certain disease (the cases) is compared to a group of control subjects. The control subjects are generally more or less similar to the cases (e.g. according to age and gender), but do not have the disease in question. The groups are then compared regarding possible causes of the disease. Because these causes have occurred in the past (otherwise they cannot be causes), this type of research is retrospective.

As has been mentioned before, an intervention study differs from an observational study because an intervention is performed on the subjects. It is important to realize that an intervention study is always a prospective cohort study. The best example of an intervention study is a randomized controlled trial (RCT). In an RCT, a group of subjects is randomly divided into an intervention group and a control group. The intervention group receives the intervention of interest (e.g. a new medication), while the control group receives for example usual care or a placebo medication. After a certain amount of time, the two groups are measured in order to investigate the effect of the intervention.

Figure 1.1 shows an overview of the different study designs within medical research. A detailed description of the different designs can be found in epidemiology books such as Rothman (2002).

1.2 Terminology

In statistics, the terminology is of great importance. In this book, the term outcome variable will be frequently used. The outcome variable is the most important variable in a study. When an intervention study is performed to investigate the effect of a new weight loss program, body weight is the outcome variable. When an observational study is performed to investigate the relationship between systolic blood pressure and smoking, systolic blood pressure is the outcome variable. In statistical terminology, the outcome variable is also known as the dependent variable. The other variables (for example, smoking behaviour in the last example, or the variable that defines the intervention group and the control group in an intervention study) are the independent variables. For independent variables, many synonyms are used, such as determinants, explanatory variables, predictors or covariates.

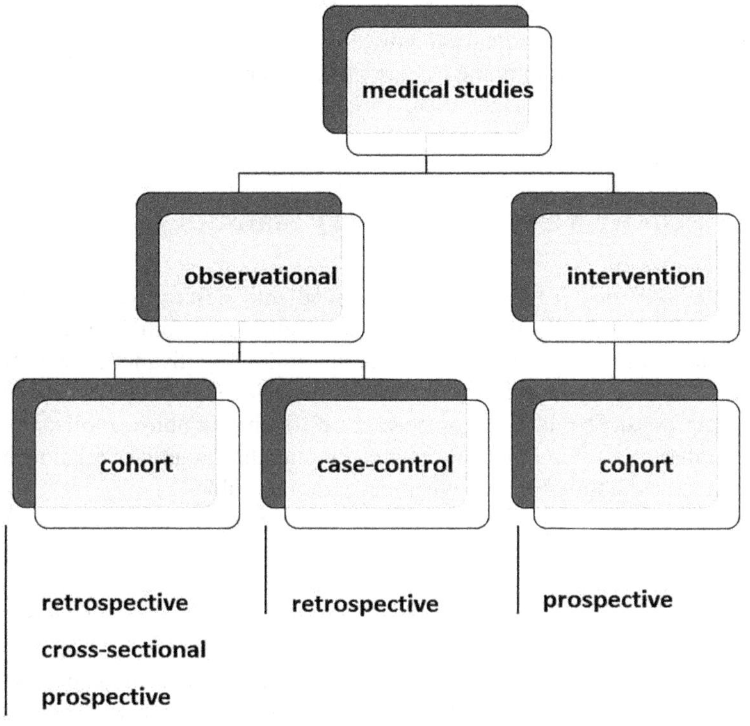

Fig. 1.1 Overview of different study designs in medical research

1.3 Variables

In order to choose the appropriate statistical method, not only the study design is important. The characteristic of the outcome variable of the study is perhaps even more important. The outcome variable of a medical study is usually continuous, dichotomous or categorical. Continuous variables are variables that, in theory, can have an infinite number of values. This seems rather abstract, but it involves variables such as body weight, cholesterol or systolic blood pressure. Although these variables theoretically can have an infinite number of values, in practice this is of course not the case. In practice this depends, for example, on the population used. In an adult population, for example, body weight probably ranges between 60 and 120 kilograms, while in a population of baby's the observed body weights will be much lower. Dichotomous variables can only take two values: yes or no. The subject is either sick or not sick, is either recovered or not recovered, is either dead or alive. It should be clear that dichotomous variables occur frequently in medical research. When the variable consists of more than two groups, then the variable is categorical. Body weight, for example, is a categorical variable when a distinction is made between normal weight, overweight and obesity. Because there is a certain order in this type of categorical variable, it is known as an ordinal categorical variable.

Another kind of categorical variable is a nominal categorical variable. The difference between a nominal and an ordinal categorical variable is that in a nominal categorical variable there is no ordering in the categories. The variable occupation, for example, is an example of a nominal categorical variable.

1.4 Descriptive Versus Explanatory Statistics

In principle, statistical analysis can be divided into descriptive and explanatory statistics. Although the distinction is clear in itself, the terminology is not always correctly used in the literature. In this book the following distinction will be made: descriptive statistics is basically used to summarize the research data, without investigating possible relationships between different variables. Explanatory (also known as inferential) statistics deals with estimating the strength of relationships, the reliability of these estimates and, when necessary, p-values.

1.5 Structure of the Book

The first two chapters of the book contain some general information about statistical analysis: In Chap. 2 descriptive statistics is discussed, while Chap. 3 introduces the underlying principles of explanatory statistics. In Chaps. 4, 5 and 6 the statistical analysis of a continuous outcome variable, a dichotomous outcome variable and survival data is explained. In Chap. 7 multiple regression analysis is discussed and in Chap. 8 machine learning is briefly introduced. Chapter 9 contains the analysis of other outcome variables, such as a categorical outcome variable, a count outcome variable, an outcome variable with floor or ceiling effects, and correlated outcome variables. In Chap. 10, missing data is discussed, while Chap. 11 deals with pitfalls in (multiple) regression analysis, such as collinearity and mediation analysis. Chapter 12 contains a discussion about sample size calculations en about the reliability of measurements. In Chap. 13 an overview is given of the different statistical methods that can be used to analyse the different outcome variables and in which situations they can be used and finally, Chap. 14 contains an overview of the example datasets used in the book.

1.6 Software and Data

The results of all analyses performed in this book are shown by general computer output. Besides that, specific computer output of the examples generated by SPSS, STATA and R will be available on request (jwr.twisk@amsterdamumc.nl). The same holds for all example datasets. It should be realized that the presentation of the general computer output sometimes depends on the statistical software used and on the version of the statistical software. It is, therefore, possible that the general output presented in the book is slightly different from the output generated by particular statistical software.

1.7 Position of Applied Statistics Within Medical Research

Before reading this book, it is important to understand the position of applied statistics within medical research. Medical research is carried out to answer a (medical) research question. That is always the starting point of the analysis. Usually the answer to the question can be obtained directly from the data, without using complicated statistical methods. The statistical analysis is then used to refine the answer to the research question. This refining is mainly related to quantifying the reliability of the observed result in the generalization from the study population to the population for which the study is intended (i.e. the source population). The next step is to answer the question to what extent the observed result is clinically relevant. That question can only be answered by content experts. In this step, statistical analysis does not play a leading role, although some statisticians often claim otherwise. The clinical relevance of a study result is very important, but since this book is about applied medical statistics, the clinical relevance of the observed results will hardly be discussed.

Chapter 2
Descriptive Statistics

Abstract Descriptive statistics are used to describe a study population. In this chapter it is shown that different statistics are used for continuous variables and for dichotomous or categorical variables. Furthermore, a distinction can be made between numerical descriptives and graphical descriptives. Numerical descriptives are, for example, the mean, median and measures to describe the spread in the data, such as the standard deviation. Graphical descriptives are, for example, a histogram and a stem-and-leaf plot.

2.1 Introduction

As has been mentioned in Chap. 1, the aim of descriptive statistics is to summarise research data. This can be either graphical or numerical. The choice between the two usually has to do with the purpose of the summary. When the data are summarized in an oral presentation at a conference or something similar, a graphical method is mostly used. When the data are presented in a scientific paper, it is often not allowed to use many figures and then it is more common to present the data numerically. The different methods that can be used for descriptive statistics are illustrated using Example 2.1, which contains data from an observational cross-sectional cohort study among 100 subjects. The aim of the study is to analyse the relationship between the outcome variable cholesterol and a number of independent variables such as age, smoking and alcohol consumption. In the example, the outcome variable cholesterol and the independent variable age are continuous. The independent variable smoking (non-smoker/smoker) is dichotomous and the independent variable alcohol consumption is an ordinal categorical variable (non-drinker, moderate drinker, heavy drinker).

J. W. R. Twisk, *Basic Principles of Applied Medical Statistics*,
https://doi.org/10.1007/978-3-031-86278-6_2

2.2 Graphical Presentation of Research Data

A continuous variable can be graphically displayed using a histogram. Figure 2.1 shows the histogram of cholesterol. In Fig. 2.1, the number of subjects are displayed on the y-axis, while the x-axis shows the values of cholesterol, which are divided into different classes (i.e. classes of 0.5 mmol/l). The histogram shows that most subjects in the example dataset have a cholesterol concentration between 4 mmol/l and 5.5 mmol/l.

An alternative way to graphically display a continuous variable is using a stem and leaf-plot. Figure 2.2 shows the stem and leaf-plot of age.

Although the stem and leaf-plot in Fig. 2.2 seems a bit primitive, some researchers find this plot particularly informative. In the stem the tens are presented and the leaf shows the units. In this example, the first two subjects are 19 years old. In the second line of the plot, it can be seen that two subjects are 21 years old, three subjects 22 years old, one subject 23 years old and three subjects 24 years old, and so on.

Dichotomous and categorical (both ordinal and nominal) variables can be graphically displayed using a bar chart or a pie chart. Figure 2.3 shows the bar chart for the dichotomous variable smoking and the categorical variable alcohol consumption.

In Fig. 2.3, it can be seen that the example dataset contains about 75 non-smokers and about 25 smokers. Regarding alcohol consumption it can be seen that most subjects do not drink (i.e. 40 subjects). Next, it can be seen that slightly fewer subjects are moderate drinkers and the least amount of subjects are heavy drinkers.

Figure 2.4 shows the pie charts for smoking and alcohol consumption. From the pie chart it is not possible to directly obtain the numbers, but it can be seen that the

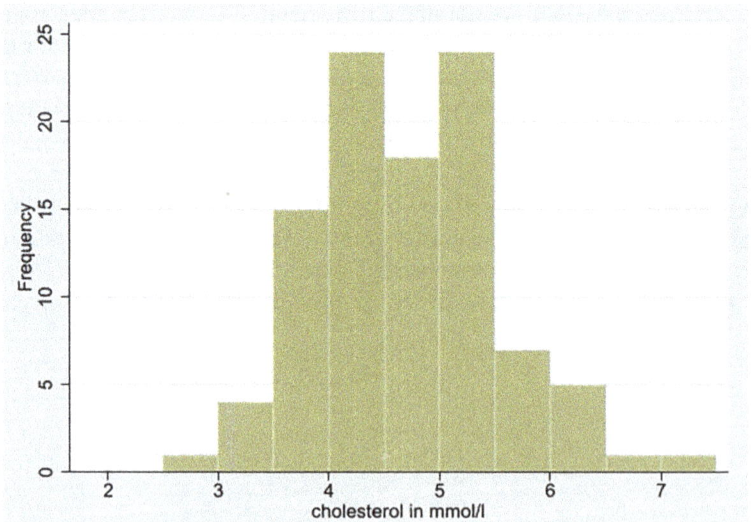

Fig. 2.1 Histogram of cholesterol

```
1. | 99
2* | 112223444
2. | 5566778888999999
3* | 0011122333344
3. | 66667788899
4* | 001233444
4. | 5557788
5* | 00122333444
5. | 56667778899
6* | 22234
6. | 578
7* | 2
7. |
8* | 02
```

Fig. 2.2 Stem and leaf-plot of age

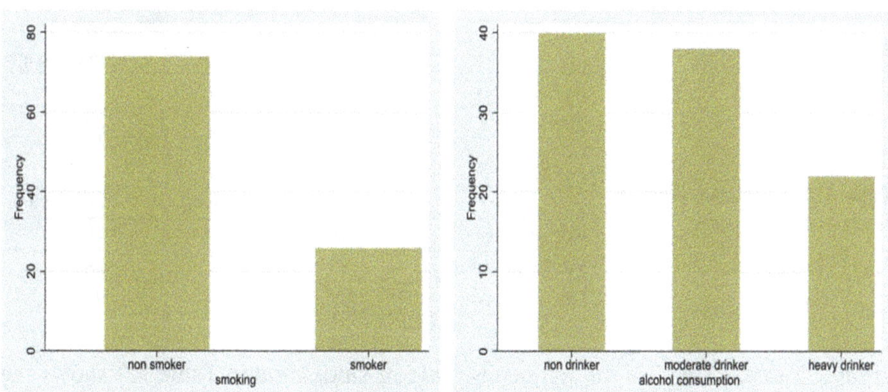

Fig. 2.3 Bar charts of smoking and alcohol consumption

example dataset contains about 75% non-smokers and about 25% smokers and that the number of non-drinkers is less than half of the total number of subjects and that there are more moderate drinkers than heavy drinkers.

2.3 Numerical Presentation of Research Data

As for the graphical presentation of research data, the characteristic of the particular variable also plays a role in the numerical presentation of research data. It is common to present dichotomous and categorical variables using a frequency table. A frequency table shows both the number of subjects and the percentages in the different

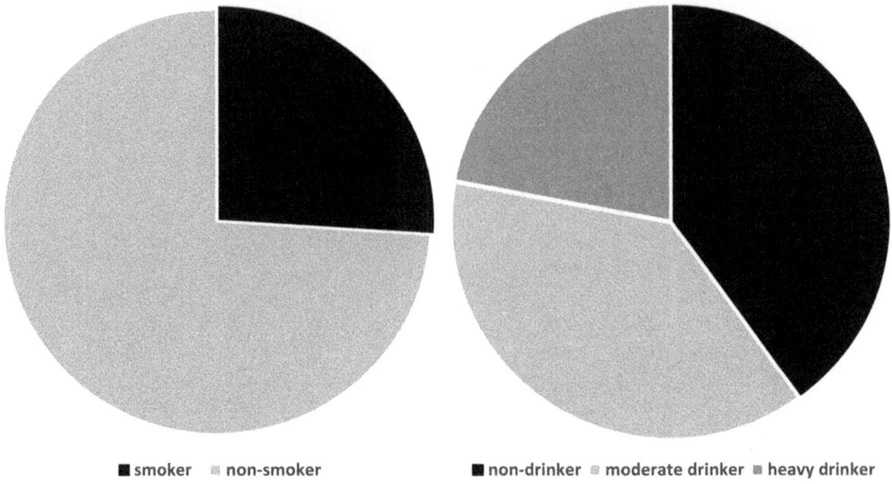

Fig. 2.4 Pie charts of smoking and alcohol consumption

Table 2.1 Frequency table of smoking

	Number of subjects	Percentage
Non-smoker	74	74%
Smoker	26	26%

Table 2.2 Frequency table of alcohol consumption

	Number of subjects	Percentage
Non-drinker	40	40%
Moderate drinker	38	38%
Heavy drinker	22	22%

groups. Table 2.1 shows the frequency table of smoking and Table 2.2 shows the frequency table of alcohol consumption.

In Table 2.1 it can be seen that the example dataset contains 74 non-smokers and 26 smokers. In Table 2.2 it can be seen that 40 subjects are non-drinkers, that 38 subjects are moderate drinkers and that 22 subjects are heavy drinkers.

For continuous variables, a frequency table is not informative, because there are too many possible values, all of which occur at most a few times. That is why so-called summary measures are used to describe continuous variables. The most commonly used summary measure is the mean, which can be calculated by adding up all the values together and then dividing that number by the number of subjects in the study population (see Eq. 2.1).

$$\overline{y} = \frac{\sum_{i=1}^{n} y_i}{n} \tag{2.1}$$

where $\bar{y}$ = mean value; n = number of subjects in the study population; y_i = value of variable y for subject i.

In addition to the mean, it is also important to indicate the spread of the observations. In the following chapters it will be shown that this spread plays an important role in statistical analysis. The spread of the observations is usually represented by the standard deviation. The magnitude of the standard deviation can be interpreted as the mean difference between the individual observations and the overall mean. It should be realized that some values are greater than the mean and some values are smaller than the mean. The mean difference between the individual observations and the overall mean is therefore not informative, because that value is always 0. That is why the differences between the observations and the overall mean are first squared and then the square root of the sum of these squared differences is taken. The mean of the squared differences is called the variance, and the square root of the variance is the standard deviation (see Eqs. 2.2a and 2.2b).

$$variance = \frac{\sum_{i=1}^{n} (y_i - \bar{y})^2}{n-1} \tag{2.2a}$$

$$sd = \sqrt{variance} \tag{2.2b}$$

where $\bar{y}$ = mean value; n = number of subjects in the study population; y_i= value of variable y for subject i and sd = standard deviation.

Suppose there are 5 subjects in a dataset with ages 41, 42, 43, 44 and 45 years. The mean age is then equal to (41 + 42 + 43 + 44 + 45) /5 = 43 years. The corresponding variance is equal to $[(41–43)^2 + (42–43)^2 + (43–43)^2 + (44–43)^2 + (45–43)^2]$ /4 = 10/4 = 2.5. The standard deviation is then $\sqrt{2.5}$= 1.58.

Surprisingly, the sum of the squared differences is divided by n − 1 and not by n. This has a mathematical background and because it is not very important, this will not be explained further (for an explanation see for example Kirkwood & Sterne, 2003).

The example dataset contains two continuous variables, i.e. cholesterol and age. Table 2.3 shows the descriptive information of these two variables.

Table 2.3 shows that the mean cholesterol in the example dataset is 4.71 mmol/l and the corresponding standard deviation is 0.81 mmol/l. For age, the mean and standard deviation are 41.7 years and 14.6 years, respectively. Table 2.3 also shows the lowest and highest values that occur in the example dataset for cholesterol and age. In scientific papers, mostly only the mean and standard deviation are reported.

Table 2.3 Descriptive information of cholesterol and age

	Number of subjects	Mean	sd	Minimum	Maximum
Cholesterol	100	4.71	0.81	2.96	7.06
Age	100	41.7	14.6	19	82

sd standard deviation

Table 2.4 Percentiles of cholesterol and age

	Median	25th percentile	75th percentile
Cholesterol	4.58	4.12	5.27
Age	39.0	29.0	53.5

In addition to the mean and standard deviation, there are a number of other summary measures, which are mostly based on so-called percentile points. The mostly used summary measure, which is based on percentile points, is the median. The median is the value, for which 50% of the observations (ordered from low to high) are below this value and 50% of the observations are above this value. For the five subjects with ages 41, 42, 43, 44 and 45 years, the median of these observations is 43 years, because 50% of the observations are lower than 43 years and 50% of the observations are higher than 43 years. Like the mean, the median is therefore an indication of the middle of the observations. The extent to which the median has the same value as the mean has to do with the symmetry of the distribution of the observations. In the example above, the mean is exactly the same as the median, because the distribution of the observations is perfectly symmetric (41 and 42 differ in absolute terms exactly as much from 43 as 44 and 45). In addition to the median, there are a number of other summary measures based on percentile points. In practice, the 25th and 75th percentile points are mostly used. The 25th percentile point is the value for which 25% of the observations are below that value, the 75th percentile point is the value of the observations for which 75% of the observations are below that value (or 25% of the observations are above that value). Table 2.4 shows the median and the 25th and 75th percentile points of cholesterol and age.

When the means for both variables are compared to the medians it can be seen that for cholesterol the mean is 4.71 mmol/l and the median is 4.58 mmol/l. For age, the mean is 41.7 years and the median is 39.0 years. So, for both variables the median is slightly lower than the mean and that indicates that the distribution of the observations is not completely symmetric. In Chap. 3 the importance of the distribution of the observations will be discussed in detail.

There is another way to summarize data from a continuous variable and that is the box plot. The box plot is a combination of a graphical and a numerical presentation. Graphical because it is a figure and numerical because certain summary measures are incorporated into the figure. Figure 2.5 shows the box plots of cholesterol and age.

The box plot contains two parts: First, the box, whose boundaries are the 25th and 75th percentile points. The line in the middle of the box is the median. Secondly, there are two lines at the top and bottom of the box. Depending on the statistical software used, these lines usually are the minimum and maximum values (or the 5th and 95th percentile points). In the box plot of cholesterol, there is also one outlier (shown as a dot above the box plot). Outliers are defined as values that deviate more than one and a half times the box height from the upper or lower limit of the box.

The nice part of a box plot is that it is possible to see at a glance whether there is a symmetric distribution of the observations. In Fig. 2.5 it can be seen that the distribution of cholesterol is fairly symmetric, while the distribution of age is not so symmetric (the part below the box is much smaller than the part above it). The

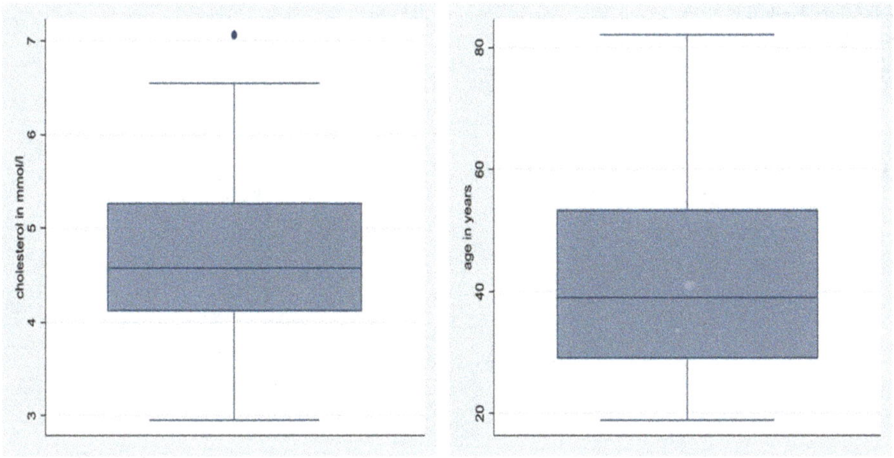

Fig. 2.5 Box plots of cholesterol and age

parts below and above the box are also called the whiskers of the box and therefore a box plot is also known as a box and whisker plot.

2.4 The Normal Distribution

One of the purposes of descriptive statistics of a continuous variable (both graphical and numerical) is to evaluate whether the variable has a so-called normal distribution. This is important because all statistical methods that can be used to analyze a continuous outcome variable assume that the outcome variable is more or less normally distributed. One of the first steps in the analysis is, therefore, to evaluate whether the outcome variable is normally distributed or not. It should be noted that later in this book, it will be shown that it is not the normal distribution of the outcome variable itself which is the key issue, but the normal distribution of the residuals (see Sect. 4.4.7). Figure 2.6 shows an example of a continuous variable that is (more or less) normally distributed. With a perfect normal distribution, the observations are distributed symmetric around the mean. Basically, the distribution of the observations is a sort of mountain, with a top which indicates the mean value. The fact that the distribution of the observations is symmetric around the mean directly implies that the median must be equal to the mean. Regarding the shape of the mountain, in a perfect normal distribution, 95% of the observations are between the mean $\pm$ 2 times the standard deviation.

To evaluate whether a continuous variable is more or less normally distributed, it can be evaluated whether the median and the mean are equal. When this is the case, then the distribution of the observations is at least symmetric. The property that 95% of observations are between the mean $\pm$ 2 times the standard deviation can only be

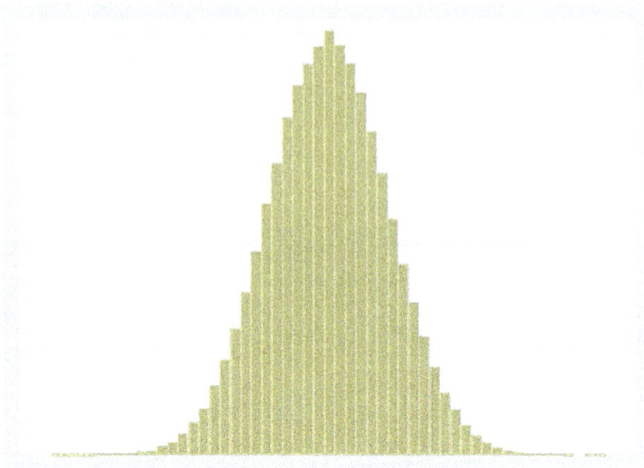

Fig. 2.6 Example of a continuous variable that is (more or less) normally distributed

used to evaluate whether a continuous variable is more or less normally distributed when the continuous variable can only have positive values. Suppose that a certain blood parameter has a mean value of 10 and a standard deviation of 10. When this variable would have been normally distributed, it means that 95% of the observations are between the mean 10 $\pm$ 2 times the standard deviation. This suggests that 95% of the observations are between -10 and +30, an impossible situation with a variable that can only have positive values. In other words, a continuous variable that can only have positive values, where the mean and standard deviation are more or less equal, cannot be normally distributed. Many different possibilities are mentioned in the literature to evaluate whether a certain variable is normally distributed or not (see also Sect. 4.4.7), but the most obvious methods are (1) observing the histogram, (2) comparing the mean and median and (3) comparing the mean and standard deviation. The latter, of course, only for continuous variables that can only have positive values.

The most common non-normal distribution of observations is a distribution that is skewed to the right. This distribution is characterized by the fact that the majority of the subjects has more or less normal values, but part of the subjects have (extremely) high values. Figure 2.7 shows a histogram of a skewed to the right distribution.

Skewed to the right (also known as positively skewed) distributions are very common in medical research. Blood parameters, for example, often have a skewed to the right distribution. In Sects. 4.2.1 and 4.4.7 the analysis of a skewed to the right outcome variable will be discussed. Besides skewed to the right distributions, there are also skewed to the left (or negatively skewed) distributions (see Fig. 2.8). Skewed to the left distributed variables are much less common than skewed to the right distributed variables; they often have to do with a certain length of time, such as gestational age.

So, for a continuous variable multiple summary measures are available, i.e. the mean with the standard deviation and the median with the 25th and 75th percentile points. It is unusual to report both summary measures; the choice depends on whether or not the variable is (more or less) normally distributed. For example, when the distribution of a continuous variable is skewed to the right, then the mean is

Fig. 2.7 Example of a continuous variable with a skewed to the right distribution

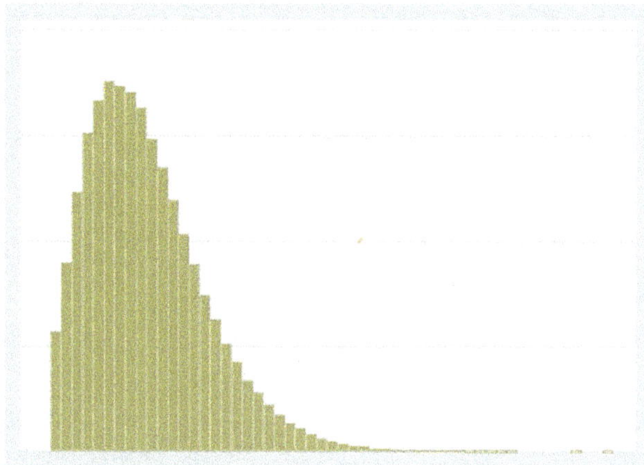

Fig. 2.8 Example of a continuous variable with a skewed to the left distribution

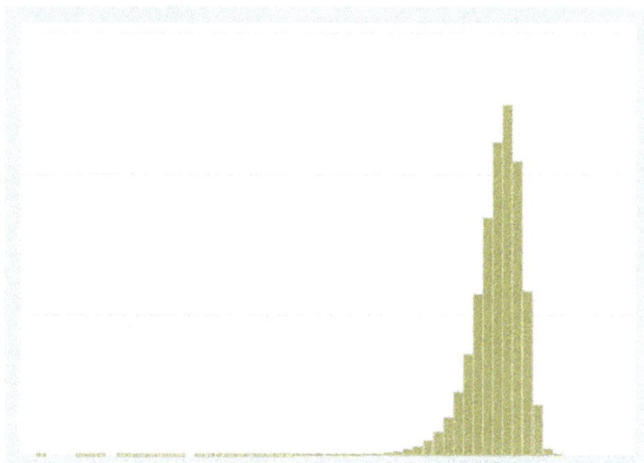

not a good indicator of the middle of the observations. The mean will be influenced too much by the (extremely) high values. A characteristic of a skewed to the right distribution is that the mean is (much) higher than the median. Because the standard deviation is directly related to the mean (see Eqs. 2.2a and 2.2b), reporting the standard deviation of a continuous variable with a skewed to the right distribution is also incorrect. In the case of a skewed to the right distribution, it is therefore common to report the median and the 25th and 75th percentile points. In principle, the same applies to a skewed to the left distribution; only the mean will be influenced too much by the (extremely) low values and will therefore be pulled to the left. Therefore, when a variable has a skewed to the left distribution the mean is (much) lower than the median. Also in this situation the median and the 25th and 75th percentile points are reported. So, the mean and standard deviation are only reported when there is a (more or less) normal distribution. In all other cases, the median and the 25th and 75th percentile points are reported.

Chapter 3
Basic Principles of Explanatory Statistics

Abstract In this chapter, first of all, the difference between effect estimation and statistical testing is discussed and it is shown that effect estimation is more important than statistical testing. Furthermore, It is shown that probabilities and probability distributions play a crucial role in the estimation of the confidence intervals around effect estimates and in statistical testing. Furthermore, the t-distribution is introduced as an alternative for the standard normal distribution. Besides that, it is also shown that the binomial probability distribution can be used for dichotomous variables.

3.1 Introduction

Suppose a study is being performed to estimate the effect of a new medication for pain reduction in 100 patients. These 100 patients are randomly taken from a very large group of patients with pain complaints (i.e. the source population). In these 100 patients, pain is measured prior to the start of the new medication (i.e. the pre-measurement) and then all 100 patients receive the new medication. At the end of the study, the pain is measured again (i.e. the post-measurement). The question of the study is whether pain has changed between the pre-measurement and the post-measurement. The result of the study can be obtained by calculating the change in pain between the two measurements for all patients. Table 3.1 shows part of the dataset of this study and Table 3.2 shows the final result of this study.

Table 3.2 shows the mean value of pain of the 100 patients at the pre-measurement (75.8), the corresponding standard deviation (8.8), the mean value of pain of the 100 patients at the post-measurement (65.8), the corresponding standard deviation (10.1), the mean of the individual changes (−10.0) and the standard deviation of the individual changes (6.8). The result of the study is that the mean change in pain between the pre-measurement and the post-measurement is 10 points.

This is in fact the answer to the research question; an answer obtained without using a (complicated) statistical analysis. The problem with this result, however, is that it is obtained from a group of 100 patients (i.e. the sample or study population) who were randomly selected from the source population which is a much larger

J. W. R. Twisk, *Basic Principles of Applied Medical Statistics*,
https://doi.org/10.1007/978-3-031-86278-6_3

Table 3.1 Part of the example dataset

Id	Pre-measurement	Post-measurement	Change
1	60	55	−5
2	70	55	−15
3	50	40	−10
4	60	61	1
5	80	60	−20
.			
100	55	55	0

Table 3.2 Result of the study based on the example dataset shown in Table 3.1

	Pre-measurement	Post-measurement	Change
Medication	75.8 (8.8)	65.8 (10.1)	−10 (6.8)

group of patients. So, the study is performed in a sample of the source population. Actually, the real source population is not even known, because the source population also includes future patients with pain complaints. Since the result relates to the study population, it has to be evaluated to what extent it also applies to the entire source population. In other words: to what extent can this result be generalized to all other patients with pain complaints and to what extent can it be generalized to all future patients with pain complaints? To answer this question, explanatory statistics should be used.

Two principles play a major role in explanatory statistics: effect estimation and statistical testing. With effect estimation, first, of course, the effect is estimated, but secondly the uncertainty of the effect is estimated. This uncertainty indicates to what extent the observed result can be generalized to the source population. Statistical testing has to do with the calculation of a probability (see Sect. 3.3), which is also related to the uncertainty. So, for both effect estimation and statistical testing, the uncertainty of the observed result in the generalization to the source population plays a major role.

Two aspects of the performed study are important in the estimation of the uncertainty. First, the number of subjects in the study population is important. The more subjects in the study population, the less uncertain the observed result will be. In other words, the larger the study population, the better the observed result can be generalized to the source population. Second, the spread of the observations in the study population is important. In the example, a mean pain reduction of 10 points is observed. When each patient in the study population has a pain reduction of 10 points, then it is obvious that for all other patients in the source population a pain reduction of about 10 points will also be observed. However, when there are large differences between the patients in the study population (e.g. one patient has a pain reduction of 30 points, while another patient has a pain increase of 20 points), it is much less likely that a pain reduction of about 10 points will be observed in the other patients in the source population. The spread of the observations in the study population is represented by the standard deviation. The higher the standard deviation, the more uncertain the observed result will be, i.e. it will be more difficult to generalize the observed result to the source population. The other way around is, of course, also true; the generalization of the observed result to the source population will be better when the standard deviation is small. These two aspects of the uncertainty of the observed result are combined in the so-called standard error of the mean. The standard error of the mean is calculated by dividing the standard deviation by the square root of the number of subjects in the study population (see Eq. 3.1).

$$sem = \frac{sd}{\sqrt{n}} \tag{3.1}$$

where *sem* = standard error of the mean, *sd* = standard deviation in the study population and n = number of subjects in the study population.

To understand how the standard error of the mean is used in explanatory statistics, it is necessary to discuss probabilities and the related probability distributions.

3.2 Probabilities and Probability Distributions

The concept of probability plays an important role in explanatory statistics. The probability of a particular outcome can be defined as: 1 divided by the number of possible outcomes. When flipping a coin, there are two possible outcomes (head or tail) and the probability of either is 0.5 (1 divided by 2). When rolling a die, there are six possible outcomes and the probability of getting 6, for example, is 1/6 = 0.167. The probability of 6 or 5 can be calculated by adding up the individual probabilities: 1/6 + 1/6 = 1/3 = 0.33.

3.2.1 Binomial Probability Distribution

Within explanatory statistics, the concept of a probability distribution is frequently used. A probability distribution can be seen as the theoretical probability of different outcomes. This rather abstract definition becomes more understandable with a simple example. Suppose a coin is flipped twice and there is interest in the number of times the coin shows tail. For the number of times tail, a probability distribution can be made (see Table 3.3).

In Table 3.3 it can be seen that the probability of getting tail twice is 0.25, that the probability of one time tail is 0.5 (there are two combinations where tail is flipped once) and the probability of zero times tail is 0.25. This probability distribution for the number of times tail can be graphically displayed in a bar chart (see Fig. 3.1).

Table 3.3 Probability distribution for the number of times tail when a coin is flipped twice

1ᵉ flip	2ᵉ flip	Number of time tail	Probability
Tail	Tail	2	0.25
Tail	Head	1	0.25
Head	Tail	1	0.25
Head	Head	0	0.25

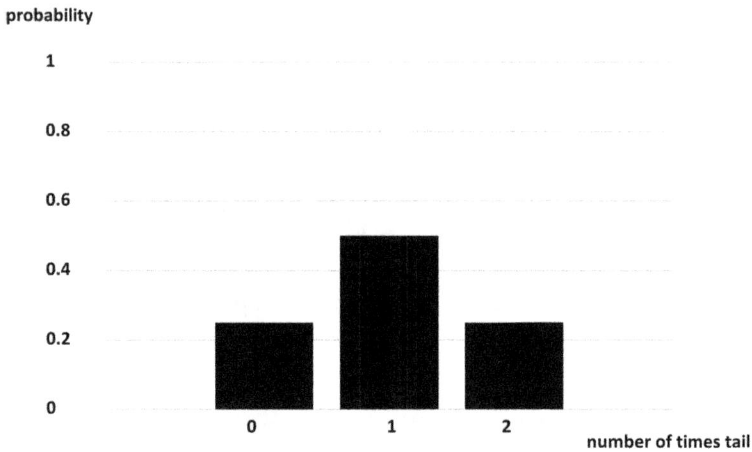

Fig. 3.1 Probability distribution for the number of times tail when a coin is flipped twice

Table 3.4 Probability distribution for the number of times 6 when a die is rolled twice

1ᵉ role	2ᵉ role	Number of time 6	Probability
6	6	2	$1/6 \times 1/6 = 1/36$
6	No 6	1	$1/6 \times 5/6 = 5/36$
No 6	6	1	$5/6 \times 1/6 = 5/36$
No 6	No 6	0	$5/6 \times 5/6 = 25/36$

The probability distribution associated with a situation where there are only two possibilities (i.e. head or tail), is known as a binomial probability distribution. Another example of a binomial probability distribution is the probability distribution when rolling a die. Suppose a die is rolled twice and the interest is in the number of times 6. Also in this situation, there are two possibilities (6 or no 6), and also for this situation a probability distribution can be made (see Table 3.4 and Fig. 3.2).

The probability distribution for the number of times tail when a coin is flipped twice, or for the number of times 6 when a die is rolled twice, is easy to calculate. With more experiments, it quickly becomes difficult to calculate the different probabilities. To determine the probability distribution in this type of situation, a general equation can be used (see Eqs. 3.2a and 3.2b).

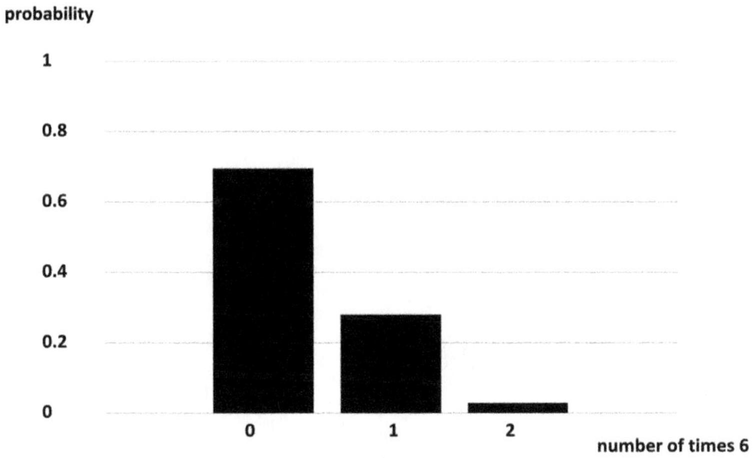

Fig. 3.2 Probability distribution for the number of times 6 when a die is rolled twice

$$p(r) = \frac{n!}{r!(n-r)!} p^r (1-p)^{n-r} \tag{3.2a}$$

$$n! = 1 \times 2 \times 3 \times \ldots \times n \tag{3.2b}$$

where p = probability of the outcome of interest, r = number of the outcome of interest, n = number of experiments and $n!$ = n faculty.

For example, when the probability has to be calculated for one 6 when a die is rolled twice, the equation looks like this:

$$p(r) = \frac{2!}{1!(2-1)!} 0.167^1 (1-0.167)^{2-1}$$

$$p(r) = \frac{1 \times 2}{1 \times 1} 0.167 \times 0.833 = 0.278$$

The probability of one 6 when a die is rolled twice is therefore 0.278 and that corresponds of course to 10/36, which was already seen in Table 3.2. Table 3.2 and Fig. 3.2 showed the probability distribution for the number of times 6 when a die is rolled twice. Based on Eqs. 3.2a and 3.2b, a probability distribution can also be made for the number of times 6 when a die is rolled 10 times or when a die is rolled 100 times. Figures 3.3 and 3.4 show both probability distributions.

Based on the probability distribution, a statement can be made about the so-called expected value. The expected value can be determined by multiplying the probability of a certain outcome (e.g. the probability of 6) by the number of times the die is rolled. In the last example when a die is rolled 100 times, the expected value for the number of times 6 is equal to 100 × 0.167 = 16.7. So, it is most likely that 6 will be rolled 16 or 17 times when the die is rolled 100 times. The expected value 16.7 can be seen as a kind of mean value of the probability distribution. When a mean value

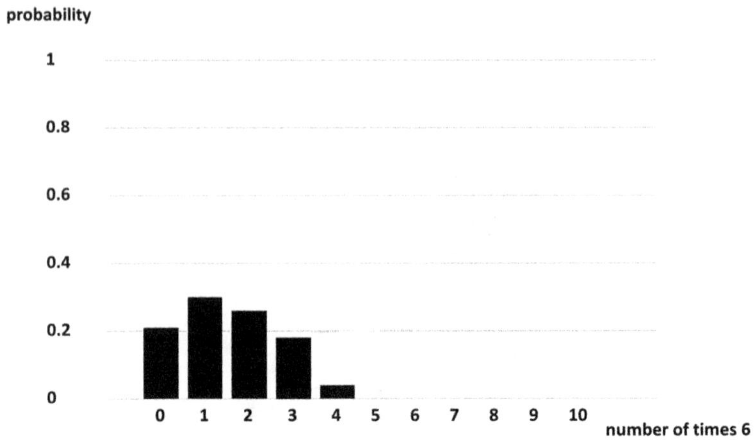

Fig. 3.3 Probability distribution for the number of times 6 when a die is rolled 10 times

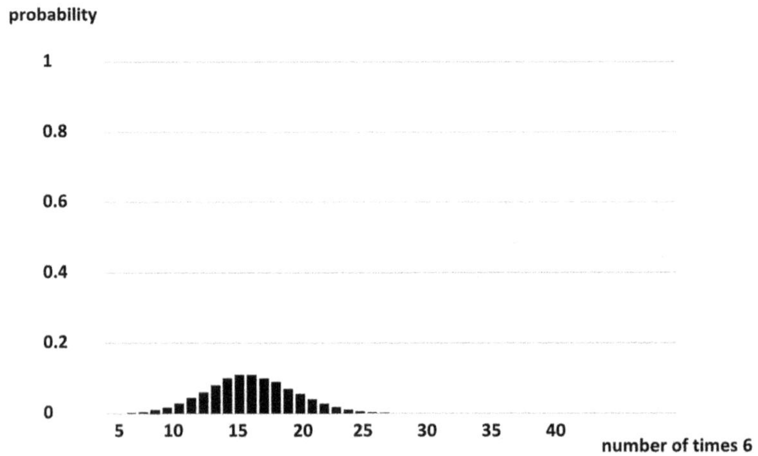

Fig. 3.4 Probability distribution for the number of times 6 when a die is rolled 100 times

can be calculated, then a standard deviation can also be calculated. Equation 3.3 shows how to calculate the standard deviation of a binomial probability distribution.

$$sd = \sqrt{n \times p \times (1 - p)} \tag{3.3}$$

where sd = standard deviation of the binomial probability distribution, n = number of experiments and p = probability of the outcome of interest.

The standard deviation in the situation where a die is rolled 100 times is therefore 3.7.

$$sd = \sqrt{100 \times 0.167 \times (1 - 0.167)} = 3.7$$

3.2.2 Normal Probability Distribution

The binomial probability distribution is suitable for a dichotomous variable. Within a binomial probability distribution, the probabilities of certain outcomes can be calculated exactly. However, the situation is different for a continuous variable. Suppose a study in which body mass index of 500 subjects is measured. The body mass index is a widely used measure for overweight and is defined as weight (in kg) divided by height (in meters) squared. Suppose the question is about the probability of finding a subject with a body mass index of 30. Because a continuous variable can theoretically have an infinite number of values, the probability of a given outcome (i.e. a body mass index of 30) is by definition 0. The probability is defined as 1 divided by the number of possibilities, or $1/\infty = 0$. There will be undoubtedly a subject with a body mass index of 30 in the study population, but not someone with a body mass index of 30.000…. With continuous variables, therefore, no exact probabilities can be calculated, but instead, so-called probability densities are calculated. A probability density represents the probability that something is equal to or greater than a certain value, or that something is equal to or less than a certain value. In the example, for instance, the probability that a subject in the population has a body mass index ≥30 can be calculated. For a dichotomous variable the binomial probability distribution is used, for continuous variables the so-called normal probability distribution is used. Table 3.5 shows the characteristics of the normal probability distribution.

The basic idea behind calculating probabilities based on the normal probability distribution is that the value of interest (in the example, a body mass index of 30) is located in the normal probability distribution, which can be created with the mean and the standard deviation of the observed values. Suppose that in the example the mean body mass index of the 500 subjects is 27 and the standard deviation is 4. Based on these data, a normal probability distribution can be made (see Fig. 3.5).

After locating the value of interest in in this probability distribution (i.e. 30), the area of the probability distribution to the right of this value has to be calculated; right

Table 3.5 Characteristics of the normal probability distribution

The distribution is symmetric
The distribution has one top
Range x-axis = [−∞ to +∞]
y-axis shows not the probability but the probability density
Probability of an exact value = 0.
Total are under the curve = 1 (i.e. 100%)
Characterized by 2 parameters: Expected value (mean value) and the standard deviation

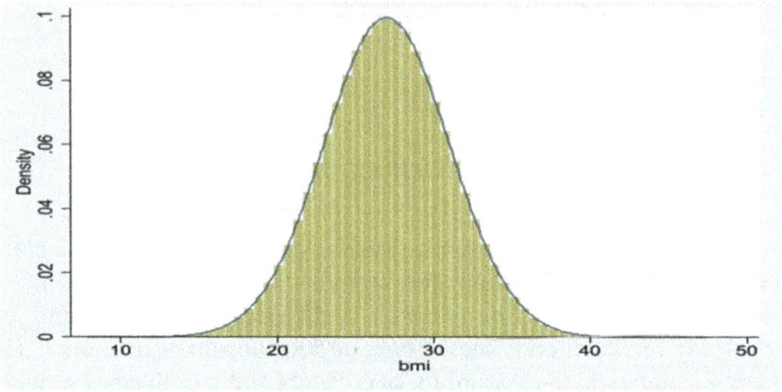

Fig. 3.5 Normal probability distribution for body mass index with a mean of 27 and a standard deviation of 4

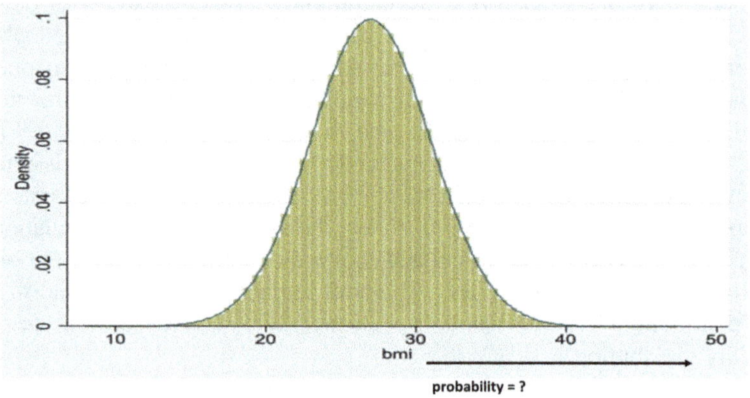

Fig. 3.6 Normal probability distribution for body mass index with a mean of 27 and a standard deviation of 4; probability (body mass index ≥30) = ?

because the question is about the probability that a subject has a body mass index ≥30 (see Fig. 3.6).

Because this area (i.e. the probability) cannot be calculated directly, an intermediate step is needed. In this intermediate step, the value of interest has to be standardized. This standardization is done in two steps. In the first step the mean value is subtracted from the value of interest and in the second step this difference is divided by the standard deviation. The result is that the difference between the value of interest and the mean value is expressed in standard deviation units. The probability distribution that then arises is known as the standard normal probability distribution or z-distribution. The z-distribution has the property that the mean is 0 and the standard deviation is 1. To standardize the value of interest in the example (i.e. 30), the mean and standard deviation of the study population are needed. In the

Table 3.6 Probabilities (p-value) for different values of the standard normal probability distribution (z-value)

z-value	p-value
0.00	0.500
0.25	0.411
0.50	0.309
0.75	0.227
1.00	0.159
1.25	0.106
1.50	0.067
1.75	0.040
2.00	0.023
2.25	0.012
2.50	0.006
2.75	0.003
3.00	0.001

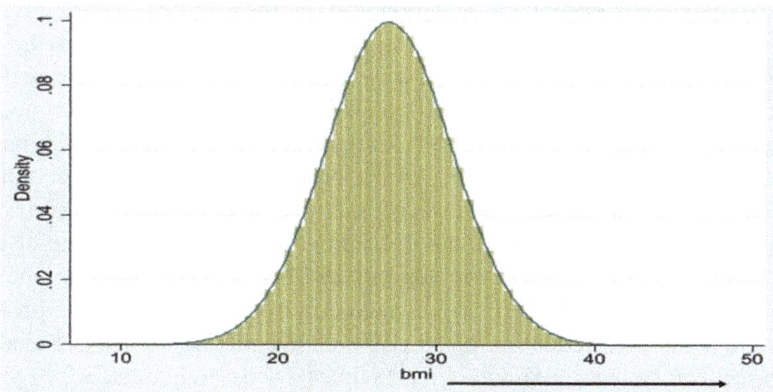

Fig. 3.7 Standard normal probability distribution; probability (z ≥ 0.75) = 0.22663

example, the mean body mass index is 27 and the standard deviation is 4. Based on these numbers, the value of interest can be standardized (See Eq. 3.4).

$$z = \frac{y - \bar{y}}{sd_y} \tag{3.4}$$

where z = value of the standard normal variable, y = value of interest, $\bar{y}$= mean value in the study population and sd_y = standard deviation in the study population.

Entering the data in Eq. 3.4, a body mass index of 30 corresponds with a standardized body mass index of 0.75 (i.e. (30–27)/4). So, the probability that a subject in the study population has a body mass index ≥30 is analogous to the probability that the standard normal variable z has a value ≥0.75. This probability can be calculated with statistical software. The probability that z is ≥0.75 is 0.23 (see Table 3.6 and Fig. 3.7). In other words, given the mean of 27 and a standard deviation of 4, there is a probability of 0.23 that a subject with a body mass index ≥30 will be found.

3.3 Statistical Testing and Effect Estimation

3.3.1 Statistical Testing

In Sect. 3.2 the probability distribution has been introduced and the calculation of probabilities based on these probability distributions has been explained. The examples used concerned the probability of finding a certain value in the study population. These kinds of questions do not really play an important role in medical research. Medical research deals more with the question whether what is observed in the study population can be generalized to the source population from which the study population was taken. To illustrate this, the example will be used in which the pain reduction was investigated in a group of 100 patients who used a new pain medication (see Table 3.1 and Table 3.2).

In the example, the mean pain reduction is 10 points and the standard deviation is 6.8. The question to what extent this result can be generalized to the source population can be answered in different ways. First, the probability can be calculated of finding a mean pain reduction of 10 points in the situation when the medication has no effect. Importantly, the interest is no longer the probability of a particular observation in the study population, but the probability of finding a certain mean value. Because the mean value is involved, the uncertainty of the observed result is not only due to the standard deviation of the individual observations, but also to the number of subjects in the study population (see Sect. 3.1). As has been mentioned before, this uncertainty is known as the standard error of the mean. The probability of finding a mean pain reduction of 10 points in the situation when the medication has no effect can be answered with the principles discussed in Sect. 3.2.2. Since the variable is continuous, the probability of an exact value of 10 is by definition 0. So, in this case, the probability must be calculated of finding a mean value ≥ 10 when the mean value is actually 0 (the medication has no effect). First, a z-value has to be calculated (see Eq. 3.5).

$$z = \frac{O - E}{sd/\sqrt{n}} \tag{3.5}$$

where z = standard normally distributed variable, O = observed mean; E = expected mean, sd = standard deviation in the study population and n = number of subjects in the study population.

When the relevant numbers are entered into Eq. 3.5, the z-value is 14.7.

$$z = \frac{10 - 0}{6.8/\sqrt{100}} = 14.7$$

When 14.7 is located in the standard normal probability distribution (see Fig. 3.8), it gives a very small probability (<0.001).

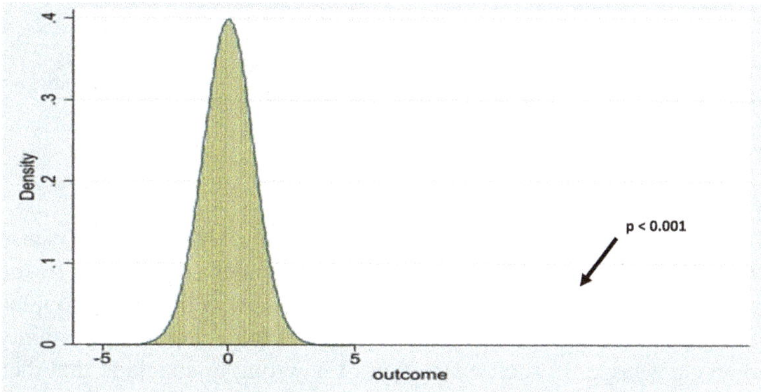

Fig. 3.8 Standard normal probability distribution; probability ($z \geq 14.7$) < 0.001

In fact, the procedure that has been performed is part of statistical testing. The z-value obtained from Eq. 3.5 is therefore called the test statistic. The value 0 (the medication has no effect) is known as the null hypothesis. So, the probability is calculated that a value $\geq$10 (or even further away from the null hypothesis) is observed when the null hypothesis is true. This probability is known as the (statistical) p-value. Basically, it is determined how well the observed mean value (i.e. 10) fits the null hypothesis (i.e. 0). It should be clear that the lower the p-value, the worse the observed result fits the null hypothesis, so the more unlikely the null hypothesis is. A general agreement within explanatory statistics is that, when the probability is $\leq$0.05, the observed result is statistically significant. In other words, when the probability of finding a mean value of 10 (or even further away from the null hypothesis) when the null hypothesis is true is very small, then the null hypothesis is assumed not to be true. This implies that the medication in the example has a statistically significant effect. In statistical terminology it is said that the null hypothesis is rejected.

In this approach, a probability distribution is made around the value of the null hypothesis in which the observed value can be located. This value must, of course, first be standardized. The calculation of a p-value and whether or not an observed result is statically significant is known as statistical testing. While there is not much wrong with calculating a p-value, one of the biggest problems with statistical testing is the fact that the concept of statistical significance is misinterpreted by almost everyone. In principle, statistical testing has to do with whether or not to reject a certain null hypothesis. Many researchers believe that when a null hypothesis cannot be rejected, i.e. when an observed result (for example, the effect of an intervention) is not statistically significant, there is no effect. This is a serious misconception (Twisk, 2024a).

When no statistically significant effect is obtained, then there is in general an effect (the effect is seldom 0), but that effect is not statistically significant in the study population. The fact that an observed result is not statistically significant can have several causes. First of all, it is possible that the effect is indeed small. In that case,

Table 3.7 Principles of testing theory

	Reality (unknown)	
	Null hypothesis true	Null hypothesis not true
Accept null hypothesis	$1 - \alpha$	β
Reject null hypothesis	α	$1 - \beta$

the conclusion that there is no effect is not totally wrong. However, it may also be the case that the effect is quite large but that the number of subjects in the study population is low and/or that the individual differences in the study population are large. In that case, the standard error of the mean is large and the uncertainty of the observed result is large. In such a situation, it is wrong to conclude that there is no effect. Finally, statistical testing, or whether or not an observed result is statistically significant, presupposes an all or nothing situation: there is an effect or there is no effect. An interpretation which is far too black white thinking. Using this dichotomy, for example, means that an effect estimate for which a p-value of 0.06 is obtained indicates that there is no effect, while an effect estimate for which a p-value of 0.04 is obtained suggests that there is an effect. The magnitude of both effects will hardly differ, but the conclusion is completely different. It is very important to realize that the concept of statistical significance should be treated and interpreted with caution (Twisk, 2024a).

In addition to statistical significance, also the concept of power plays an important role in statistical testing. Both statistical significance and power have to do with rejecting or not rejecting the null hypothesis. It has already been mentioned that, as a threshold for whether or not a result is statistically significant, a p-value of 0.05 is generally used. This basically means that in 5% of the situations the null hypothesis is rejected while it is actually true. Of course, it is not known whether the null hypothesis is true or not, but a 0.05 error is accepted. This error is called a first-order error and is also known as α-error. It is of course also possible that the null hypothesis is not rejected (i.e. the p-value is >0.05) while actually the null hypothesis is not true (i.e. there is an effect). The error made in this case is a second-order error or β-error. The statistical power of a statistical test is equal to $1 - \beta$ (see Table 3.7).

3.3.2 *One-Sided or Two-Sided Statistical Testing*

Within the scientific world, a debate has been going on for years about whether statistical testing should be carried out one-sided or two-sided. As mentioned before, statistical testing involves a certain null hypothesis. The p-value is the probability of finding the observed result (or even further away from the null hypothesis) when the null hypothesis is true. When the p-value is ≤ 0.05, the null hypothesis is rejected and the observed result is statistically significant. Whether or not a statistical test is one-sided has to do with the formulation of the null hypothesis. In many cases, the null hypothesis will be something like: there is no effect of the intervention, or, there is no association between two variables, and so on. The alternative hypothesis in these situations is: there is an effect of the intervention, or, there is an association between two variables. The formulation of the hypotheses implies that both a negative and a positive effect of the intervention or that both a negative and a positive association between two variables can be obtained. Because the alternative hypothesis can go both ways, the statistical test related to this hypothesis is two-sided.

However, there are researchers who suggest that one-sided testing can be performed in some situations. For a one-sided test, the null hypothesis is: there is no positive effect of the intervention or there is no positive association between two variables. The alternative hypothesis is then of course: there is a positive effect of the intervention or there is a positive association between two variables. In this situation, the alternative hypothesis can only go one way, and therefore it is suggested to test this type of null hypothesis one-sided. Although the discussion is there, it is basically a discussion about nothing. The advantage of a one-sided statistical test is that the p-value is twice as low as the p-value of a two-sided statistical test. For example, when the p-value of a two-sided statistical test is 0.08, the p-value of a one-sided statistical test based on the same data is 0.04. In that case, the two-sided p-value does not give a statistically significant result, but the one-sided p-value does, and the conclusion is therefore different although the effect estimate and the corresponding standard error do not differ. It should be clear that the discussion about one-sided or two-sided statistical testing is especially important when the researcher is very keen in finding a statistically significant result. Earlier in this chapter, however, the importance or non-importance of statistical significance of an observed result was already put in the right perspective, so the discussion about one-sided or two-sided statistical testing is basically irrelevant (Twisk, 2024a).

The statistical analyses discussed in this book are known as frequentist statistics. This approach assumes that there is no prior knowledge, and that the effect or relationship investigated can be both positive or negative. Because of that, within frequentist statistics always two-sided testing is used. Therefore, when p-values are mentioned in the forthcoming chapters and sections of this book, they are always two-sided. The counterpart of frequentist statistics is Bayesian statistics, which assumes prior knowledge. Bayesian statistics is mathematically difficult, so, therefore, a discussion about Bayesian statistics is beyond the scope of this book.

Figure 3.9 shows the principle of a one-sided statistical test and Fig. 3.10 shows the principle of a two-sided statistical test.

3.3.3 *Effect Estimation*

The question to what extent the observed result can be generalized to the source population can also be approached from another angle. The other approach is effect estimation, which is much more informative than statistical testing. Within effect

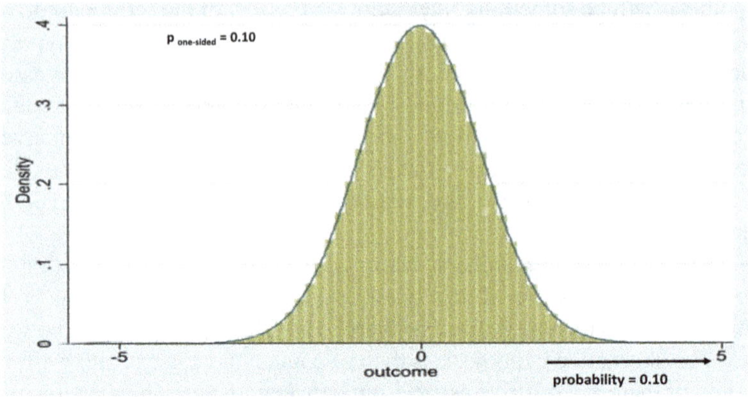

Fig. 3.9 Principle of a one-sided statistical test

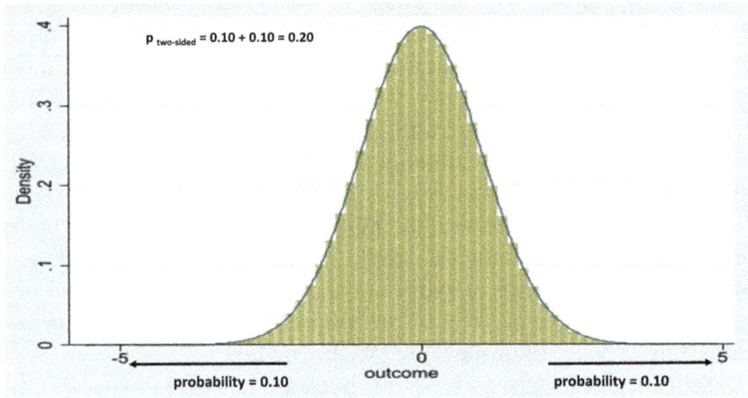

Fig. 3.10 Principle of a two-sided statistical test

estimation, the observed result is taken as a starting point and around the observed result a probability distribution is made. Using this probability distribution, a so-called confidence interval around the observed result is calculated. Mostly, a 95% confidence interval is used. Although the definition of this concept is difficult, the bottom line is that the result in the source population will be, with 95% certainty, somewhere between the limits of the 95% confidence interval. Thus, going back to the example, a 95% confidence interval can be calculated around the observed effect of 10. Of course, again the standard normal probability distribution is used. In this case, the value of the standard normal probability distribution is needed for which 95% of the observed results lie between them (see Table 3.8 and Fig. 3.11).

This number is 1.96, which is found in many statistical applications. In other words, the probability that the standard normal variable is between −1.96 and +1.96 is 0.95.

Table 3.8 Two-sided probabilities associated with different values of the standard normal probability distribution

z-value	p-value
0.00	1.00
0.67	0.50
0.84	0.40
1.28	0.20
1.64	0.10
1.96	0.05
2.33	0.02
2.58	0.01
3.29	0.001

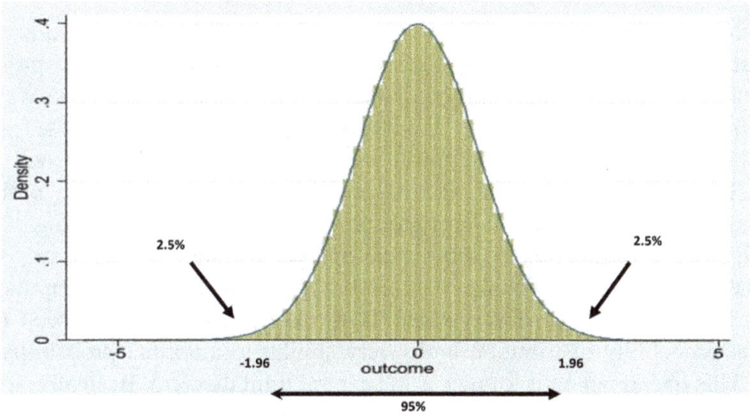

Fig. 3.11 Principle of the 95% confidence interval

Equation 3.6 shows the way in which the limits of a 95% confidence interval are calculated.

$$95\%CI = \bar{y} \pm 1.96 \times \left({}^{sd_y}/_{\sqrt{n}} \right) \tag{3.6}$$

where 95% CI = 95% confidence interval, $\bar{y}$ = mean value in the study population, sd_y = standard deviation in the study population and n = number of subjects in the study population.

When the data from the example are entered into Eq. 3.6, the 95% confidence interval ranges between 8.7 and 11.3.

$$95\% \ CI = 10 \pm 1.96 \times \left({}^{6.8}/_{\sqrt{100}} \right) = [8.7 - 11.3]$$

So, with 95% certainty the effect of the new medication (i.e. the pain reduction) in the source population (which is sometimes referred to as the real effect) is somewhere between 8.7 and 11.3 points.

In summary, statistical testing based on the data from a study population involves a probability distribution around the null hypothesis. With this probability distribution, the probability of finding the observed result can be calculated. Because there is a continuous probability distribution (a probability density), the probability is calculated that the observed result or a result further away from the null hypothesis is obtained. Effect estimation on the other hand, is based on a probability distribution around the observed result. The 95% confidence interval is then calculated based on this probability distribution.

3.4 The Central Limit Theorem

Probability distributions play an important role in both effect estimation and statistical testing. In Sect. 3.2.2 it was discussed that the (standard) normal probability distribution is used for a continuous variable. In principle, this only works well when the continuous variable is normally distributed on its own. When this is the case, then the probability distribution of the mean value in the study population will also be normal. However, looking at Figs. 3.2, 3.3 and 3.4, in which the binomial probability distribution was shown, an interesting phenomenon occurred. In Fig. 3.2, the probability distribution was shown for the number of times 6 when a die is rolled twice, i.e. when there are two observations. In Fig. 3.3, there are 10 observations and in Fig. 3.4, there are 100 observations. In the latter case, it can be seen that the binomial probability distribution looks very similar to a normal probability distribution. This phenomenon is known as the central limit theorem. Basically, when the number of observations is large, the mean in the study population has a normal probability distribution, regardless of the original distribution of the variable. The first question to be answered is: what is large? A question which is difficult to answer. Firstly, because there is no exact cut-off value (it is a sliding scale, i.e. as the number of observations becomes larger, the distribution of the mean in the study population becomes more and more normal) and secondly because the potential cut-off value depends on the original distribution of the variable (the more normal the original distribution, the lower the number of observations needed).

It is important to realize that although the probability distribution around the mean becomes more and more normal as the number of observations increases, the interpretation of the mean for a non-normally distributed variable is still complicated. Suppose there is a skewed to the right distributed continuous variable. In Sect. 2.4 it is indicated that when the distribution is skewed to the right, the mean is not a good indicator for the middle of the observations. The mean value is influenced too much by the high values (i.e. it is pulled to the right). The central limit theorem states that when the number of subjects in the study population is large, the mean has a normal distribution. This means that statistical testing can be performed using a normal probability distribution (see Sect. 3.2.2). However, this does not mean that the mean value is suddenly a good indicator for the middle of the observations. In order to obtain a clearly interpretable result when the variable is not normally distributed, a different procedure must be used (see Sect. 4.2.1 and 4.4.7).

3.5 Statistical Testing Based on the 95% Confidence Interval

Because statistical testing still seems to play an important role in medical research, the 95% confidence interval is also often used for statistical testing. When the value of the null hypothesis is outside the 95% confidence interval, it can be concluded that, when the null hypothesis is true, the probability of the observed result (or even further away from the null hypothesis) is in any case lower than 0.05 (i.e. the observed result is statistically significant). The other way around, of course, exactly the same applies; when the value of the null hypothesis is inside the 95% confidence interval, the observed result is not statistically significant (see Fig. 3.12).

3.6 The t-distribution

In the previous sections, two probability distributions were discussed: the binomial probability distribution was used for dichotomous variables and the (standard) normal probability distribution was used for continuous variables. Many other probability distributions will be discussed in the upcoming chapters of this book. This will be done when the particular probability distributions is used. An exception is made for the t-distribution, which is also known as the Student t-distribution. The t-distribution is used as an alternative for the standard normal distribution. One of the problems with the standard normal distribution is that it can only be used when the standard deviation in the source population is known. It has already been indicated that the source population consists not only of all other patients from which the study population is taken, but also of all future patients. In other words, the standard deviation in the source population is never known. Given the central limit theorem (see Sect. 3.4), the standard normal distribution can always be used when the number

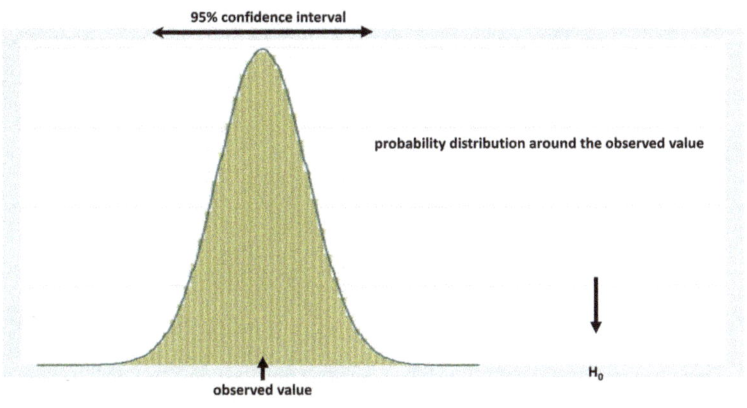

Fig. 3.12 Principle of statistical testing based on the 95% confidence interval

Table 3.9 t-values for a two-sided p-value of 0.05 for t-distributions with a different number of degrees of freedom

Degrees of freedom	t-value
5	2.571
10	2.228
20	2.086
50	2.009
100	1.984
∞	1.960

of observations is large. When the number of subjects in the study population is relatively small, there is a problem which can be solved using the t-distribution as an alternative for the standard normal distribution. The t-distribution is very similar to the standard normal distribution (symmetric, bell-shaped, has one top, the range of the x-axis is -∞ to +∞, and so on), but it is slightly wider. The difference in width between the t-distribution and the standard normal distribution depends on the number of subjects in the study population or, more general, it depends on the number of degrees of freedom. In principle, there are many different t-distributions, depending on the number of degrees of freedom. The concept of degrees of freedom is not really complicated. Suppose there is a mean value of 10 and there are five observations. To get a mean value of 10, any number can be entered for the first observation. For the second to the fourth observation, the same applies. However, when four values have been entered randomly, the last value is fixed. After all, the mean value has to be 10. So, in a situation with five observations, four numbers can be chosen randomly, which indicates that there are four degrees of freedom. In general, the number of degrees of freedom in a t-distribution is equal to the number of observations −1. Therefore, when confidence intervals and/or p-values are calculated for relatively small study populations, the t-distribution should be used instead of the standard normal distribution. In practice, this means that the number 1.96 (which is used in a standard normal distribution to calculate the 95% confidence interval) must be replaced by a number from the t-distribution. This number can be calculated by statistical software (see Table 3.9). Because the t-distribution is always wider than the standard normal distribution, the number in question will always be a bit higher than 1.96 (see Table 3.9).

Chapter 4
The Analysis of a Continuous Outcome Variable

Abstract For the analysis of a continuous outcome variable, different methods are available. When two observations within the same subject are compared to each other the paired t-test can be used. However, when two groups are compared to each other the independent t-test can be used, while analysis of variance is suitable for the comparison of more than two groups. However, mostly, linear regression is used for the analysis of a continuous outcome variable. The advantage of linear regression analysis is that the method can be used in all situations, including to analyse the relationship between a continuous outcome variable and a continuous independent variable. The starting point of a linear regression analysis is a scatter plot which includes all observations. The next step is to draw a straight line through the observations for which the distance between the observations and the line is as small as possible. This regression line is characterised by two parameters which always have the same interpretation. The b_0 is always the value of the outcome variable when the independent variable is 0 and the b_1 always indicates that when the independent variable differs with one unit, the outcome variable differs with b_1 units. In this chapter, examples are given for the analysis of a continuous outcome variable with a dichotomous, a categorical and a continuous independent variable. Furthermore, it is discussed what can be done when the continuous outcome variable is skewed, how to evaluate whether the relationship between a continuous outcome variable and a continuous independent variable is linear or not and how to adjust for confounding and how to investigate effect modification.

4.1 Comparing Two Observations Within the Same Subject

The first example used to illustrate the analysis of a continuous outcome variable is Example 4.1. Example 4.1 is an observational prospective cohort study, in which cholesterol is measured in 100 subjects. The question of the study is whether cholesterol changes over a certain period of time (i.e. 6 months). To answer this question cholesterol is measured twice with an interval of 6 months. Table 4.1 shows descriptive information of the variables used in this study.

J. W. R. Twisk, *Basic Principles of Applied Medical Statistics*,
https://doi.org/10.1007/978-3-031-86278-6_4

Table 4.1 Descriptive information of the variables used in Example 4.1

	Number of subjects	Minimum	Maximum	Mean	Standard deviation
Cholesterol at t0	100	2.96	7.06	4.72	0.81
Cholesterol at t6	100	3.49	6.96	5.09	0.85

Table 4.2 Descriptive information of changes in cholesterol over 6 months

	Number of subjects	Minimum	Maximum	Mean	Standard deviation
Change in cholesterol	100	−1.29	2.14	0.37	0.64

Table 4.1 shows that cholesterol increased from 4.72 to 5.09 in 6 months. So, the change in cholesterol is 0.37. The question now, of course, is to what extent this result (the change over time) also applies to other subjects who are not included in the study. As explained in Chap. 3, the purpose of the statistical analysis is to quantify the uncertainty of the observed result regarding the generalization to the source population.

In Sect. 3.1, it was discussed that two aspects of the study play a role in quantifying this uncertainty, i.e. the number of subjects in the study population and the standard deviation of the individual observations. It is important to realize that in this example it is not the standard deviation in cholesterol at both measurements which is important, but the standard deviation in the individual changes. In the example, when in all subjects after 6 months, more or less the same change is observed, then it is expected that this change will also apply to all other subjects in the source population. On the other hand, when a sharp increase in cholesterol is observed for one subject and a sharp decrease for another subject, then the uncertainty of the mean change between the two measurements will be greater. The number of subjects in the study population and the standard deviation of the individual observations are combined in the standard error of the mean (see Eq. 3.1). Using the standard error of the mean, the 95% confidence interval around the observed change can be calculated. To do this, first, the standard deviation of the individual changes has to be calculated. Table 4.2 shows the descriptive information of the change in cholesterol.

In Table 4.2 it can be seen that the mean change in cholesterol over 6 months is 0.37 (this was also calculated from the descriptive information shown in Table 4.1) and that the standard deviation of the individual changes is 0.64. Besides these numbers, also a value from a probability distribution is needed by which the standard error of the mean must be multiplied to obtain the limits of the 95% confidence interval. Because the change in cholesterol is a continuous outcome variable, the t-distribution has to be used (see Sect. 3.6). From the t-distribution, the value that corresponds with a 95% confidence interval has to be used (i.e. the alternative for the 1.96 from the standard normal distribution). This value depends on the number of degrees of freedom of the t-distribution and therefore on the number of subjects in the study population. In the example, there are 100 subjects with a change score and the t-distribution therefore has 99 degrees of freedom (see Sect. 3.6). The value of this t-distribution used to calculate a 95% confidence interval is 1.98 (see Table 3.9). The 95% confidence interval around the 6 months change in cholesterol can now be calculated with Eq. 4.1.

$$d\overline{y} \pm t_{\left(1-\alpha/2\right);\,(n-1)df} \times sd/\sqrt{n} \tag{4.1}$$

where $d\overline{y}$ = mean change in outcome variable, $t_{\left(1-\alpha/2\right)}$ = value of the t-distribution for which $(1-\alpha/2)\%$ of the distribution is below that value, sd = standard deviation of the outcome variable and n = number of subjects in the study population.

When the numbers of Table 4.2 are entered into Eq. 4.1, the 95% confidence interval ranges between 0.24 and 0.50.

$$0.37 \pm 1.98 \times 0.64/\sqrt{100} = [0.24 - 0.50]$$

In addition to quantifying the uncertainty using a 95% confidence interval around the observed mean change, it can of course also be statistically tested whether the observed mean change fits the value of the null hypothesis. The null hypothesis (almost) always states that nothing is going on, so in this case the value of the null hypothesis is a change in cholesterol of 0. The test statistic that has to be used to obtain the p-value always has a similar form: the observed value is compared to the expected value when the null hypothesis is true and that difference is divided by the uncertainty around the observed result, i.e. the standard error of the mean (see Eq. 4.2).

$$t = \frac{d\overline{y} - 0}{sd/\sqrt{n}} \tag{4.2}$$

where t = test statistic, $d\overline{y}$ = mean change in outcome variable, sd = standard deviation of the outcome variable and n = number of subjects in the study population.

The statistical method that can be used to perform the statistical test is the paired t-test. Paired because the individual changes are used as an outcome variable and t-test because a t-distribution is used. Output 4.1 shows the result of the paired t-test performed to analyse the 6 months change in cholesterol.

Output 4.1 Result of the paired t-test to analyse the 6 months change in cholesterol

				95% confidence interval				
	Mean	sd	sem	Lower	Upper	t-value	df	p-value
Change in cholesterol	0.37	0.64	0.06	0.24	0.50	5.78	99	<0.001

sd standard deviation, *sem* standard error of the mean, *df* degrees of freedom

In Output 4.1 it can be seen that around the mean change of 0.37 the 95% confidence interval ranges between 0.24 and 0.50 and that the p-value of the mean change is <0.001. In other words, the probability that a 6 months change of 0.37 (or even further away from the null hypothesis) is observed, when the change is actually 0, is very low. It should be noted, that the output of the paired t-test shows the change between the first and the second measurement and because cholesterol is higher in the second measurement, the mean change in cholesterol shown in the output is a negative value.

4.1.1 *Comparing an Observed Mean with a Standard Value*

A more or less similar situation occurs when evaluating whether the mean value of a particular outcome variable observed in a study population deviates from a certain standard value. Suppose, based on the data from Example 4.1, the research question is how much the mean cholesterol at the first measurement is different from 6.2. The value 6.2 is sometimes used in the literature as a cut-off value for high risk cholesterol. To answer this question, first the difference between the individual observations and the standard value is calculated (see Table 4.3).

Table 4.3 shows that the mean difference with the standard value is −1.49 and analogous to the paired t-test, a 95% confidence interval around this mean difference can be calculated with Eq. 4.1. When the numbers from Table 4.3 are entered into Eq. 4.1, the 95% confidence interval ranges between −1.65 and −1.33.

$$-1.49 \pm 1.98 \times 0.81/\sqrt{100} = [-1.65 - -1.33]$$

Using the test statistic from Eq. 4.2, also the p-value can be calculated. Output 4.2 shows the result of this one-sample t-test.

In Output 4.2 it can be seen that the mean difference between cholesterol of the subjects in the study population and the standard value of 6.2 is −1.49 and that the 95% confidence interval ranges between −1.65 and −1.33. The test statistic has a value of −18.39 and the corresponding p-value (based on a t-distribution with 99 degrees of freedom; the number of subjects in the study population − 1) is very low (<0.001).

Table 4.3 Part of the dataset from Example 4.1 comparing cholesterol with a standard value of 6.2

Id	Cholesterol	Standard value	Difference
1	3.92	6.2	−2.28
2	5.18	6.2	−1.01
3	3.48	6.2	−2.72
.			
.			
100	3.98	6.2	−2.22
Mean (sd)			−1.49 (0.81)

Output 4.2 Result of the one-sample t-test to analyse the difference in cholesterol with a standard value of 6.2

Test value = 6.2					95% confidence interval	
	t-value	df	p-value	Mean difference	Lower	Upper
Cholesterol at t0	−18.39	99	<0.001	−1.49	−1.65	−1.33

Table 4.4 Descriptive information of cholesterol for subjects with low social class and high social class

	Cholesterol		
	Number of subjects	Mean	Standard deviation
Low social class	53	4.865	0.755
High social class	47	4.545	0.840

4.2 Comparing Two Groups

Example 4.2 is used to illustrate the analysis to compare a continuous outcome variable between two groups. Example 4.2 is an observational cross-sectional cohort study that was also partly used in Chap. 2 (Example 2.1). In 100 subjects, the relationship between cholesterol and a number of independent variables such as age, sex, social class, smoking and alcohol consumption is investigated. One of the aims of the example is to analyse whether there is a difference in cholesterol between subjects with low social class and subjects with high social class. The easiest way to answer that question is to compare the mean value of cholesterol for the subjects with low social class with the mean value of cholesterol for the subjects with high social class. Table 4.4 shows the descriptive information for both groups.

Table 4.4 shows that the mean cholesterol of the 53 subjects with low social class is 4.865 and that the mean cholesterol of the 47 subjects with high social class is 4.545. Based on the descriptive information, it can be seen that there is a difference in mean cholesterol between the two groups. The subjects with high social class have a lower mean cholesterol than the subjects with low social class and that difference equals 4.545–4.865 = −0.319. The problem, of course, is that this difference applies to the 100 subjects in the study population, and it remains to be seen whether it also applies to all other subjects with low social class and high social class. As has been mentioned before, one of the aims of the statistical analysis is to quantify the uncertainty in the generalization of the observed result to the source population.

In Sect. 4.1 it has been indicated that two aspects of the study play an important role in the estimation of this uncertainty, i.e. the number of subjects in the study population and the standard deviation of the individual observations. Both are combined into the standard error of the mean. Using the standard error of the mean, a 95% confidence interval around the observed difference between the groups can be calculated. Again, a value from a probability distribution is needed by which the standard error of the mean has to be multiplied to get the lower and upper limit of this interval. In this case, of course, it is again a t-distribution and again this value depends on the number of degrees of freedom of the t-distribution, which is directly related to the number of subjects in the study population. In the example, 53 subjects with low social class are compared to 47 subjects with high social class and because for both groups the number of degrees of freedom is n − 1, the relevant t-distribution has 98 degrees of freedom. The value to be used to calculate the 95% confidence interval is, therefore, 1.98.

The example compares two groups that both have a different number of subjects and a different standard deviation. Because in the 95% confidence interval around the difference between the two groups only one standard error of the mean can be used, a sort of mean standard deviation must be calculated. This mean standard deviation is known as the population standard deviation and can be calculated with Eq. 4.3.

$$s_p = \sqrt{\frac{(n_1 - 1) \times s_1^2 + (n_2 - 1) \times s_2^2}{(n_1 - 1 + n_2 - 1)}} \tag{4.3}$$

where s_p = population standard deviation, s_1, s_2 = standard deviation of the outcome variable in both groups and n_1, n_2 = number of subjects in both groups.

Although Eq. 4.3 seems to be a bit complicated, it is not much more than the mean of the two variances of the two groups, weighted by the number of subjects in the two groups. When both groups have the same number of subjects, then the population standard deviation is the square root of the mean of the two variances. When the data of both groups are entered into Eq. 4.3, the population standard deviation is 0.796.

$$s_p = \sqrt{\frac{52 \times 0.755^2 + 46 \times 0.840^2}{(52 + 46)}} = 0.796$$

When two groups are compared to each other, the equation to calculate the 95% confidence interval (see Eq. 4.4) is slightly more complicated than Eq. 4.1, which was used to compare two measurements within one group.

$$(\overline{y}_1 - \overline{y}_2) \pm t_{(1-\alpha/2);(n_1+n_2-1)df} \times s_p \times \sqrt{(1/n_1 + 1/n_2)} \tag{4.4}$$

where $\overline{y}_1, \overline{y}_2$ = mean values of the outcome variable in both groups, $t_{(1-\alpha/2)}$ = value of the t-distribution for which $(1 - \alpha/2)\%$ of the distribution is below that value, s_p= population standard deviation and n_1, n_2 = number of subjects in both groups.

When the data from the example are entered into Eq. 4.4, the 95% confidence interval ranges between 0.003 and 0.636.

Output 4.3 Result of the independent t-test to analyse the difference in cholesterol between subjects with low social class and high social class

						95% confidence interval	
	t-value	df	p-value	Mean difference	se	Lower	Upper
Cholesterol	−2.003	98	0.048	−0.319	0.159	−0.636	−0.003

se standard error

$$-0.319 \pm 1.98 \times 0.796 \times \sqrt{(1/53 + 1/47)} = [-0.636 - -0.003]$$

In addition to quantifying the uncertainty using a 95% confidence interval around the observed mean difference, it can of course also be statistically tested whether the observed mean difference fits the value of the null hypothesis. The test statistic used to obtain the p-value is the same as has been mentioned before. The observed value is compared to the expected value when the null hypothesis is true (i.e. 0), which is then divided by the uncertainty of the observed result, i.e. the standard error of the mean (see Eq. 4.5).

$$t = \frac{\overline{y}_1 - \overline{y}_2 - 0}{s_p \times \sqrt{(1/n_1 + 1/n_2)}} \tag{4.5}$$

where t = test statistic, $\overline{y}_1, \overline{y}_2$ = mean values of the outcome variable in both groups, s_p = population standard deviation and n_1, n_2 = number of subjects in both groups.

When the data of the example are entered into Eq. 4.5, the test statistic is −2.003.

$$t = \frac{4.545 - 4.865 - 0}{0.796 \times \sqrt{(1/53 + 1/47)}} = -2.003$$

This t-value must be located in a t-distribution with 98 degrees of freedom to obtain the corresponding p-value. In Table 3.9 it can be seen that the corresponding p-value is just below 0.05. Output 4.3 shows the result of the t-test performed to analyse the difference in cholesterol between subjects with low social class and high social class. The t-test for two independent groups is also knows as the independent t-test.

The most interesting part of Output 4.3 is the mean difference between the two groups (−0.319) and the corresponding 95% confidence interval, which ranges between −0.636 and −0.003. Output 4.3 also shows the result of the t-test. In this example, the test statistic is −2.003 and the corresponding p-value, assuming a t-distribution with 98 degrees of freedom, is 0.048. So, when the null hypothesis is true, the probability of finding the difference between subjects with low social class and high social class observed in the study population (or even further away from the null hypothesis) is 0.048. This means that the observed difference is statistically significant. The p-value is ≤0.05. This conclusion can also be drawn using the 95% confidence interval, because the value of the null hypothesis (i.e. 0) is outside the 95% confidence interval. It is important to keep in mind again that the distinction

Output 4.4 Result of the F-test for equality of variances regarding cholesterol for subjects with low social class and high social class

	F-value	p-value
Cholesterol	0.781	0.379

Output 4.5 Result of the adjusted independent t-test to analyse the difference in cholesterol between subjects with low social class and high social class

						95% confidence interval	
	t-value	df	p-value	Mean difference	se	Lower	Upper
Cholesterol	−1.990	93.199	0.050	−0.319	0.160	−0.638	−0.0006

se standard error

between statistically significant or non-significant is based on an arbitrary cut-off value of 0.05 and should therefore be interpreted with caution. Furthermore, the p-value does not say anything about the magnitude of the difference in cholesterol between subjects with low social class and high social class.

In addition to the fact that the outcome variable (i.e. cholesterol) must have a more or less normal distribution (see Sect. 2.4), there is a second assumption for the independent t-test to be performed properly. This assumption is that the shape of the two normal distributions for the two groups must be more or less equal. In statistical terminology, this means that the variances in the two groups should be more or less equal. This assumption can be evaluated using the so-called F-test for equality of variances. The F (from Fisher) represents a test statistic that has an F probability distribution. The F probability distribution will not be discussed in detail, but in some statistical software, the F-test for equality of variances is performed automatically prior to the independent t-test. When the data does not meet this assumption, then a kind of alternative independent t-test can be performed, which is also known as Welch's adjustment. This adjustment mainly involves an adjustment of the number of degrees of freedom of the t-distribution. Output 4.4 shows the result of the F-test for the equality of variances regarding cholesterol for subjects with low social class and high social class.

As expected (based on the descriptive information shown in Table 4.4) the result of the F-test for the equality of variances gives a statistically non-significant p-value (i.e. 0.379). So, the null hypothesis (which implies that the two variances are equal) is not rejected. The result of the F-test for equality of variances, therefore, indicates that the assumption of equal variances holds. When the assumption of the equality of variances does not hold, the adjusted version of the independent t-test can be used (see Output 4.5).

In Output 4.5 it can be seen that the adjustment mainly involves an adjustment of the number of degrees of freedom (i.e. 93.199 instead of 98). As a result of the adjustment, the 95% confidence interval becomes somewhat wider and the p-value somewhat higher.

4.2.1 A Skewed Distributed Outcome Variable

It has already been mentioned that, in order to properly perform an independent t-test, the outcome variable must be more or less normally distributed. This is not surprising, because when two groups are compared to each other on a continuous outcome variable, the two mean values are compared to each other. When the distribution is skewed, the mean is (highly) influenced by the extreme values (see also Sect. 2.4) and is not a good indicator for the middle of the distribution. The most common skewed distribution is the skewed to the right distribution. Many blood parameters, for example, have a skewed to the right distribution. The question now, of course, is what to do when the outcome variable has such a skewed to the right distribution and the aim of the study is to compare two groups with each other. The first possibility is to apply a transformation to the original data in such a way that the transformed data has a more or less normal distribution. This transformed data can be used to calculate the difference between the two groups and the corresponding 95% confidence interval and, when necessary, to perform a statistical test. Then the result (i.e. the difference between the groups and the 95% confidence interval) must be transformed back to the original data. This procedure will be illustrated by Example 4.3; an observational cross-sectional cohort study aiming to analyse the difference in triglyceride between subjects with normal weight and overweight. Table 4.5 shows the descriptive information of triglyceride for subjects with normal weight and overweight.

Table 4.5 shows that for both groups, the mean is higher than the median. This is especially evident in the subjects with overweight; in these subjects the standard deviation is also relatively high compared to the mean. Based on the descriptive information it can be concluded that the distribution among subjects with overweight in particular is skewed to the right (for the evaluation whether or not data are normally distributed, see Sect. 2.4). In order to view the entire distribution, a histogram is made for both groups (see Fig. 4.1).

Both histograms show that the data is skewed to the right and that a regular independent t-test, therefore, cannot be performed. One could argue, of course, that an independent t-test can be performed, because the number of subjects in the study population is large enough ($n = 300$) and therefore the central limit theorem applies (see Sect. 3.4). However, in the discussion of the central limit theorem, it was already indicated that the mean from a skewed distribution, regardless of the number of subjects in the study population, has still no straightforward interpretation. In order to be able to say something about the magnitude of the difference between the two groups, the data must be transformed in such a way that the transformed data has a

Table 4.5 Descriptive information of triglyceride for subjects with normal weight and overweight

	Triglyceride			
	Number of subjects	Mean	Standard deviation	Median
Normal weight	150	0.76	0.39	0.70
Overweight	150	0.91	0.75	0.70

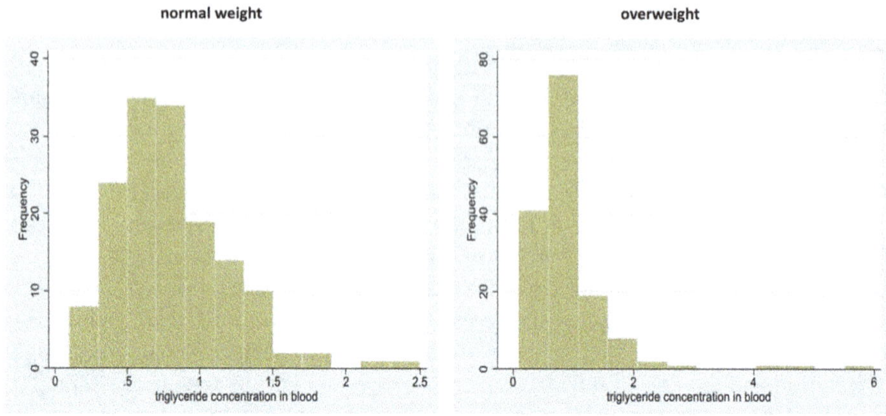

Fig. 4.1 Histogram of triglyceride for subjects with normal weight and overweight

more or less normal distribution. For a skewed to the right distribution, a log transformation is mostly used. The property of a log transformation is that the (right) tail of the distribution is pulled inwards and, therefore, disappears. Although all types of logarithms can be used for the transformation, in practice the natural logarithm is mostly used. The base of the natural logarithm is the natural number e, and the natural logarithm is usually denoted by ln. So, a log transformation (using the natural logarithm) is performed on all observations of the study population. After the transformation, the descriptive information and the histograms can be used to evaluate whether the log transformation was successful in making the distributions more or less normal. Figure 4.2 shows the histograms of the log transformed triglyceride for both groups.

In Fig. 4.2 it can be seen that the log transformation has been quite successful and that the new variable, i.e. the natural logarithm of triglyceride can be analysed as a more or less normally distributed continuous outcome variable. Because the interest is in the difference in triglyceride between subjects with normal weight and overweight, an independent t-test is performed with the log transformed triglyceride. Output 4.6 shows the result of this analysis.

In Output 4.6 it can be seen that the difference in the natural logarithm of triglyceride between subjects with normal weight and overweight is 0.127 and the corresponding 95% confidence interval ranges between −0.002 and 0.256. In order to be able to say something about the original data, the observed result must be transformed back. To do this, a classical calculation rule for logarithms is used, i.e. the difference between two logarithms with the same base is equal to the logarithm of the ratio of the two numbers (see Eq. 4.6).

$$a_{\log b} - a_{\log c} = a_{\log b/c} \tag{4.6}$$

where a = arbitrary base of the logarithm.

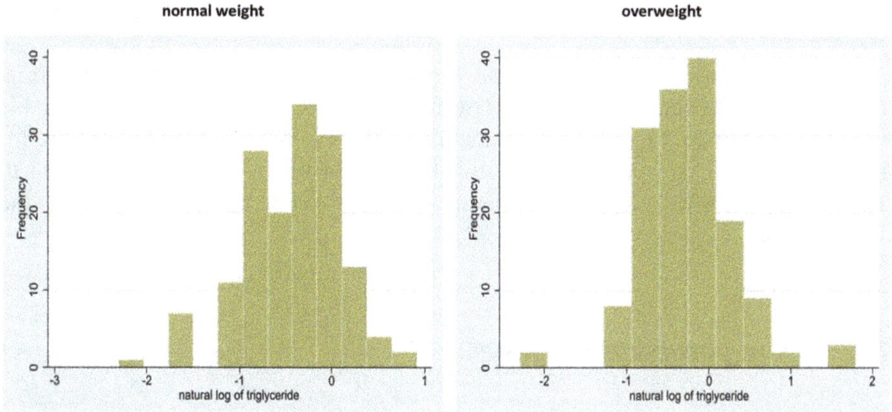

Fig. 4.2 Histogram of the natural logarithm of triglyceride for subjects with normal weight and overweight

Output 4.6 Result of the independent t-test to analyse the difference in the log transformed triglyceride between subjects with normal weight and overweight

						95% confidence interval	
	t-value	df	p-value	Mean difference	se	Lower	Upper
Log transformed triglyceride	1.941	298	0.053	0.127	0.066	−0.002	0.256

se standard error

This calculation rule for logarithms can be used to transform back the result of the analysis on the log transformed triglyceride. To do this, the inverse from the natural logarithm has to be taken, i.e. the e-power. The e-power is often notated with EXP.

$$ln_{\ overweight} - ln_{\ normal\ weight} = ln_{\ overweight/normal\ weight}$$

$$ln_{\ overweight/normal\ weight} = 0.127$$

$$_{overweight/normal\ weight} = EXP(0.127) = 1.14$$

So, the mean triglyceride in overweight subjects is 1.14 times greater than in subjects with normal weight. The mean in this case is not the normal mean (after all, the mean could not be used because of the skewed distribution), but the geometric mean. The geometric mean is defined as the transformed back mean of the log transformed values and can be seen as a sort of median. Transforming back the 95% confidence interval yields the 95% confidence interval around the ratio of geometric means. In the example, the 95% confidence interval is: [EXP(−0.002)—EXP (0.256)] = [0.998–1.292]. To obtain the corresponding p-value, the result of the t-test can be used directly (see Output 4.6). The corresponding p-value is therefore 0.053.

There are many possibilities to transform outcome variables with a non-normal distribution. For example, a square root transformation can be used for a variable with a skewed to the right distribution, while a square transformation can be used for a variable with a skewed to the left distribution. However, it is very important to realize that only after a log transformation the result can be transformed back to the original data.

4.2.2 *Non-parametric Testing*

An alternative approach to analyse a skewed continuous outcome variable is to use a non-parametric statistical test. For a non-parametric statistical test, there is no assumption about the distribution of the continuous outcome variable. The most important characteristic of a non-parametric statistical test is that the observed values are not analysed themselves, but they are converted into rank numbers and the rank numbers are then analysed. One of the biggest drawbacks of a non-parametric statistical test is the fact that it is just a statistical test. With a non-parametric statistical test it is not possible to calculate an effect estimate and a 95% confidence interval. The result of a non-parametric statistical test is a p-value.

To compare two groups with each other (for example, the situation in Example 4.3), the following procedure can be used. First of all, every observation, regardless the group it belongs to, is given a rank number. Then the sum of the rank numbers is calculated for both groups and finally the sum of the rank numbers of the two groups are compared to each other leading to a p-value. It should be realised that when comparing the sum of the rank numbers between the groups, the amount of observations in both groups have to be taken into account. This rank sum test (developed by Wilcoxon) is also known as the Mann-Whitney test and is widely used in medical research. Output 4.7 shows the result of the Mann-Whitney test to compare triglyceride between subjects with normal weight and overweight (see Example 4.3).

In Output 4.7 it can be see that a higher sum of rank numbers is observed for subjects with overweight than for subjects with normal weight and that the p-value related to this difference is 0.175. The p-value obtained from the Mann-Whitney test is known as an asymptotic p-value, because it is based on a normal approximation of the non-parametric statistical test. This normal approximation is also the reason why a z-value is given in the output. It seems rather strange to use a normal

Output 4.7 Result of the Mann-Whitney test to compare triglyceride between subjects with normal weight and overweight

	Number of subjects	Sum of ranks	z-value	p-value
Normal weight	150	21559.5	1.358	0.175
Overweight	150	23590.5		

Output 4.8 Result of the independent t-test to analyse the difference in triglyceride between subjects with normal weight and overweight

						95% confidence interval	
	t-value	df	p-value	Mean difference	se	Lower	Upper
Triglyceride	2.233	298	0.027	0.155	0.069	−0.018	0.291

se standard error

approximation for a non-parametric statistical test (which is used because the outcome variable is not normally distributed) but that is the way it is. It is possible to calculate the exact p-value, but the more subjects in the study population, the more complicated the calculation of the exact p-value is and the better the normal approximation is.

Although the non-parametric statistical tests are very often used, their use is not necessary when the number of subjects in the study population is relatively large. According to the central limit theorem (see Sect. 3.4), the mean of study population with a relatively large number of subjects (say more than 100), regardless of the original distribution, has a normal distribution. This means that in Example 4.3 the independent t-test on the original data could also be used to obtain a p-value. It is important to realize that this independent t-test does not provide a good estimate of the difference (and corresponding 95% confidence interval) of triglyceride between the groups, because the mean values remains too much influenced by the skewed distribution. Output 4.8 shows the result of the independent t-test, performed on the original data.

In Output 4.8 it can be seen that the p-value of this t-test is 0.027. So, basically, up to now, three statistical tests are performed to obtain a p-value to compare triglyceride between subjects with normal weight and overweight. The independent t-test on the original data gives a p-value of 0.027, the independent t-test on the log transformed data, a p-value of 0.053 and the non-parametric Mann-Whitney test, a p-value of 0.175. All three methods are statistically valid, but they all give a different p-value and it is unclear which of the three is the best method to determine the p-value. One thing which is generally observed is that non-parametric statistical tests are a bit more conservative than statistical tests assuming a normal distribution (which are also known as parametric statistical tests). In general, the log transformation is preferred, because a log transformation can be used to estimate a valid effect with a corresponding 95% confidence interval.

A non-parametric approach is also available for Example 4.1, i.e. for a study with two measurements in the same subject. The available statistical test for this situation is the Wilcoxon signed rank test. The idea behind this test is to indicate which change has a negative sign and which change has a positive sign. To perform this test, first, regardless of the sign, a rank number is assigned to the change. The smallest change gets rank number 1 and the biggest change gets the highest rank number (in Example 4.1, the highest rank number is 100). Next, the sum of the rank numbers with a positive sign (i.e. subjects with an increase in cholesterol) and the sum of the rank numbers with a negative sign (i.e. subjects with an decrease in cholesterol) are

Output 4.9 Result of the Wilcoxon signed rank test to analyse the 6 months change in cholesterol

	Number of subjects	Sum of ranks	z-value	p-value
Negative	29	1021.5	5.179	<0.001
Positive	71	4028.5		

calculated. The null hypothesis of the statistical test is that the sum of the rank numbers associated with a positive change is equal to the sum of the rank numbers associated with a negative change. The more the sum of rank numbers differ from each other, the more the observed changes tend to a go in a certain direction. Output 4.9 shows the result of the Wilcoxon signed rank test applied to the data from Example 4.1.

In Output 4.9 it can be seen that the sum of the rank numbers with a positive sign is much higher than the sum of the rank numbers with a negative sign. A positive sign in this case indicates an increase in cholesterol. Furthermore, it can be seen that a normal approximation of the non-parametric test is also used in this case. Again a z-value is calculated with an asymptotic p-value.

4.3 Comparing More than Two Groups

In some situations, it can be interesting to compare more than two groups to each other in one analysis. The method used to test differences between multiple groups is known as analysis of variance and is basically an extension of the independent t-test. Analysis of variance is widely used, for example in psychology, but has as greatest disadvantage that it is based on statistical testing. Analysis of variance will be explained using a simple numerical example. In this numerical example three groups are compared to each other (see Table 4.6).

To test whether the mean values of the three groups differ from each other, analysis of variance uses so-called sum of squares. A sum of squares is the sum of the squared differences between the observations and a mean value. First, the total sum of squares is calculated. The total sum of squares is the sum of the squared differences between the individual observations and the overall mean (see Eq. 4.7).

$$SS_t = \sum_{g=1}^{G} \sum_{i=1}^{n} (y_{ig} - \bar{y})^2 \tag{4.7}$$

where SS_t= total sum of squares, G = number of groups, n = number of subjects in each group, y_{ig} = value of the outcome variable for the subject i in group g and $\bar{y}$ = overall mean value of the outcome variable.

This total sum of squares is then split into the between group sum of squares (SS_b) and the within group sum of squares (SS_w). For the between group sum of squares, the mean values of the three groups are compared to the overall mean (see Eq. 4.8),

Table 4.6 Simple example dataset for comparing three groups

	Y_{group1}	Y_{group2}	Y_{group3}	Total
	5	3	5	
	5	3	4	
	4	2	4	
	6	3	5	
	6	3	3	
	4	4	3	
Mean	5	3	4	4

Table 4.7 Sum of squares calculated on the data of the example shown in Table 4.6

$SS_t = (5–4)^2 + (5–4)^2 + \cdots + (3–4)^2 = 22$
$SS_b = 6 \times (5–4)^2 + 6 \times (3–4)^2 + 6 \times (4–4)^2 = 12$
$SS_w = (5–5)^2 + (5–5)^2 + \cdots + (3–4)^2 + (3–4)^2 = 10$

while for the within group sum of squares, the individual observations are compared to the group mean (see Eq. 4.9).

$$SS_b = \sum_{g=1}^{G} n_g \left(\overline{y}_g - \overline{y}\right)^2 \tag{4.8}$$

where SS_b = between group sum of squares, G = number of groups, n_g = number of subjects in each group, $\overline{y}_g$ = mean value of the outcome variable of group g and $\overline{y}$ = overall mean value of the outcome variable.

$$SS_w = \sum_{g=1}^{G} \sum_{i=1}^{n} \left(y_{ig} - \overline{y}_g\right)^2 \tag{4.9}$$

where SS_w = within group sum of squares, G = number of groups, n = number of subjects in each group, y_{ig} = value of the outcome variable for subject i of group g and $\overline{y}_g$ = mean value of the outcome variable of group g.

In the simple numerical example shown in Table 4.6, the three sums of squares are easy to calculate (see Table 4.7).

Using analysis of variance, the calculated sums of squares can be used to test whether the mean values of the three groups differ statistically significant from each other. Output 4.10 shows the result of the analysis of variance.

In Output 4.10 first the three sums of squares are shown. The third column shows the corresponding degrees of freedom. For the total sum of squares, which is based on the overall mean value, the number of degrees of freedom is equal to the number of observations − 1. Because three groups are compared, a degree of freedom is lost for all three groups (analogous to the number of degrees of freedom by performing an independent t-test) and thus 15 degrees of freedom remain for the within group sum of squares. The between group sum of squares has two degrees of freedom (the number of groups − 1). When the between and within group sum of squares are

Output 4.10 Result of the analysis of variance to compare the three groups from the numerical example shown in Table 4.6

	Sum of squares	df	Mean square	F-value	p-value
Between groups	12.0	2	6.0	9.0	0.003
Within groups	10.0	15	0.667		
Total	22.0	17			

df degrees of freedom

Output 4.11 Result of the analysis of variance to analyse the difference in cholesterol between subjects with low social class and high social class

	Sum of squares	df	Mean square	F-value	p-value
Between groups	2.538	1	2.538	4.010	0.048
Within groups	62.029	98	0.633		
Total	64.567	99			

df degrees of freedom

divided by the number of degrees of freedom, the mean square is obtained. The ratio of the mean squares gives an F-value, which is the test statistic from which the p-value is derived. The greater the difference between the groups, the greater will be the between group sum of squares in relation to the within group sum of squares and, therefore, more reason to reject the null hypothesis, which implies that the mean values of the groups are equal. In the numerical example shown in Table 4.6, the p-value obtained from the analysis of variance is 0.003, i.e. a statistically significant difference between the mean values of the three groups. How big the difference is and between which groups there is a difference cannot be derived from the result of the analysis of variance.

Analysis of variance can also be used to compare two groups. Going back to the example of the comparison of cholesterol between subjects with low social class and high social class (Example 4.2), Output 4.11 shows the result of the analysis of variance to analyse this difference.

Output 4.11 shows that the p-value obtained from an analysis of variance (i.e. 0.048) is identical to the p-value obtained from the independent t-test (see Output 4.3).

In Example 4.2, the aim of the study is to investigate the relationship between cholesterol and a number of independent variables. One of these independent variables is alcohol consumption, which consists of three groups: non-drinkers, moderate drinkers and heavy drinkers. Table 4.8 shows descriptive information of cholesterol of three groups of alcohol consumption.

Table 4.8 shows that cholesterol differs considerably between the three groups. For the non-drinkers the mean value is 4.86, for the moderate drinkers the mean value is slightly lower, i.e. 4.29, while mean cholesterol is highest for the heavy drinkers (i.e. 5.18). Using analysis of variance the difference in cholesterol between the three groups of alcohol consumption can be analysed (see Output 4.12).

Table 4.8 Descriptive information of cholesterol of three groups of alcohol consumption

	Cholesterol		
	Mean	Number of subjects	Standard deviation
Non-drinkers	4.86	40	0.63
Moderate drinkers	4.29	38	0.77
Heavy drinkers	5.18	22	0.83

Output 4.12 Result of the analysis of variance to analyse the difference in cholesterol between three groups of alcohol consumption

	Sum of squares	df	Mean square	F-value	p-value
Between groups	12.593	2	6.296	11.751	<0.001
Within groups	51.974	97	0.536		
Total	64.567	99			

df degrees of freedom

Output 4.12 shows that the p-value of the analysis of variance is very low (< 0.001), So, there is a statistically significant difference in cholesterol between the three groups of alcohol consumption. Because the result of the analysis of variance only indicates that there is a statistically significant difference somewhere between the three groups, the next step in the analysis must answer the question which groups differ statistically significant from each other. To answer this question, a post-hoc procedure can be used, i.e. pairwise comparisons between the groups.

In principle, three independent t-tests can be performed. The problem with performing three independent t-tests to obtain p-values for each pairwise comparison is multiple testing. The multiple testing problem arise when a lot of statistical tests are performed on the same data and indicates that the probability of finding a statistically significant result is higher, the more statistical tests are performed. So, basically, when multiple statistical tests are performed, the cut-off value of 0.05 cannot be used anymore, but a lower value has to be used. There are many possibilities available for the correction for multiple testing. The most famous are the Bonferroni correction, the Scheffe correction or the Tukey correction. For example, using the Bonferroni correction, the cut-off value for statistical significance that has to be used is equal to 0.05 divided by the number of statistical tests performed. So, in this example, using the Bonferroni correction, a cut-off value for statistical significance of $0.05/3 = 0.017$ has to be used. It should be realized that within analysis of variance, the multiple testing problem is tackled in a slightly different way. It is tackled by making the 95% confidence interval around the observed difference a bit wider and by increasing the calculated p-value. Because of that, the cut-off value for statistical significance remains 0.05. Output 4.13 shows the result of several pairwise post-hoc comparisons of cholesterol (corrected for multiple testing) between three groups of alcohol consumption.

In Output 4.13, three blocks can be distinguished, each referring to a different correction method. In the first block the Tukey correction is used, in the second block

Output 4.13 Result of the post-hoc procedures to analyse the difference in cholesterol between three groups of alcohol consumption

					95% confidence interval	
Method	Comparison		Mean difference	p-value	Lower	Upper
Tuckey	Non-drinker	Moderate drinker	0.58	0.002	0.18	0.97
	Non-drinker	Heavy drinker	−0.32	0.23	−0.78	0.14
	Moderate drinker	Heavy drinker	−0.89	<0.001	−1.36	−0.43
Scheffe	Non-drinker	Moderate drinker	0.58	0.03	0.16	0.99
	Non-drinker	Heavy drinker	−0.32	0.27	−0.80	0.16
	Moderate drinker	Heavy drinker	−0.89	<0.001	−1.38	−0.41
Bonferroni	Non-drinker	Moderate drinker	0.58	0.02	−0.98	−0.17
	Non-drinker	Heavy drinker	−0.32	0.31	−0.79	0.16
	Moderate drinker	Heavy drinker	−0.89	<0.001	−1.37	0.42

Output 4.14 Results of three independent t-tests to analyse the difference in cholesterol between three groups of alcohol consumption

				95% confidence interval	
Comparison		Mean difference	p-value	Lower	Upper
Non-drinker	Moderate drinker	0.58	0.001	0.26	0.89
Non-drinker	Heavy drinker	−0.32	0.10	−0.69	0.06
Moderate drinker	Heavy drinker	−0.89	<0.001	−1.32	−0.47

the Scheffe correction and in the third block the Bonferroni correction. In each block, the results of three pairwise comparisons can be seen: non-drinkers versus moderate drinkers, non-drinkers versus heavy drinkers, and moderate drinkers versus heavy drinkers. For each pairwise comparison, the difference in cholesterol, the p-value and the 95% confidence interval are shown. Output 4.13 shows that the three correction methods differ slightly from each other (which is indicated by the p-values and the 95% confidence intervals), but that the conclusions (if they are based on whether or not the differences between the three groups are statistically significant) do not differ from each other. It should also be noted that although analysis of variance is mainly a testing method, when a post-hoc procedure is performed, also the differences in mean values between the groups are reported as well as the 95% confidence intervals around the mean differences.

For comparison, Output 4.14 shows the results of three independent t-tests.

The comparison between the, for multiple testing corrected, post-hoc procedures and the independent t-tests is obvious. The corrected post-hoc procedures provide wider 95% confidence intervals and higher p-values for the pairwise comparisons.

As with comparing two groups, when comparing more than two groups, the assumption is that the outcome variable is more or less normally distributed. When statements are made about mean values, then the mean should be a good indicator for the middle of the distribution and should not be too much influenced by extreme values. When the outcome variable is not normally distributed, the outcome variable can be transformed in such a way that the transformed variable is more or less normally distributed (as with the comparison between two groups). The transformed variable can then be analysed using analysis of variance. As with the comparison between two groups, the final result, i.e. the difference and the 95% confidence interval obtained from the post-hoc procedure must be transformed back (see Sect. 4.2.1).

Instead of transforming the non-normally distributed outcome variable (which is always preferable), also a non-parametric method can be used to compare more than two groups. As mentioned before, non-parametric methods do not assume any kind of distribution of the outcome variable, because they are performed on rank numbers rather than on the original data. As a non-parametric alternative to the analysis of variance, the Kruskal-Wallis test can be used. Output 4.15 shows the result of the Kruskal-Wallis test for the comparison of cholesterol between three groups of alcohol consumption.

Output 4.15 first shows the sum and the mean of the rank numbers of the three groups and then the result of the statistical test. The p-value is <0.001, which indicates that there is a statistically significant difference between the three groups. Comparing the mean rank numbers shows that the moderate drinkers have the lowest cholesterol, followed by the non-drinkers and the heavy drinkers. It can also be seen that the p-value is based on a chi-square value. Like the standard normal distribution and the t-distribution, the chi-square distribution is also a probability distribution. The chi-square probability distribution will be discussed in detail in Chap. 5.

Output 4.15 Result of the Kruskal-Wallis test to analyse the difference in cholesterol between three groups of alcohol consumption

	Number of subjects	Sum of ranks	Mean rank	Chi-square value	df	p-value
Non-drinker	40	2291.50	57.29	19.35	2	<0.001
Moderate drinker	38	1318.00	34.68			
Heavy drinker	22	1440.50	65.48			

4.4 Linear Regression Analysis

4.4.1 Introduction

The situations described in Sects. 4.2 and 4.3 (comparing two groups and comparing more than two groups) can also be analysed using linear regression analysis. Linear regression analysis is a general method for analysing a continuous outcome variable. Where an independent t-test is suitable for comparing two groups (i.e. a dichotomous independent variable) and analysis of variance is suitable for comparing more than two groups (i.e. a categorical independent variable), a linear regression analysis can be used to analyse all types of independent variables, i.e. dichotomous, categorical and continuous.

To explain the principles of linear regression analysis, it is best to start with the relationship between a continuous outcome variable (i.e. cholesterol) and a continuous independent variable (i.e. age). First, a scatter plot is made including all observations, with on the y-axis the outcome variable cholesterol and on the x-axis the independent variable age (see Fig. 4.3).

The purpose of a linear regression analysis is to analyse the relationship between the outcome variable cholesterol and the independent variable age as good as possible. This is done by making a straight line through the observations shown in Fig. 4.3. The question then is which straight line best describes the relationship between cholesterol and age. In the linear regression analysis, the best fitting line is defined as the line for which the (vertical) distance from the individual observations to the line is as small as possible (see Fig. 4.4). This method is known as the least squares method. It should be noted that within linear regression analysis, the

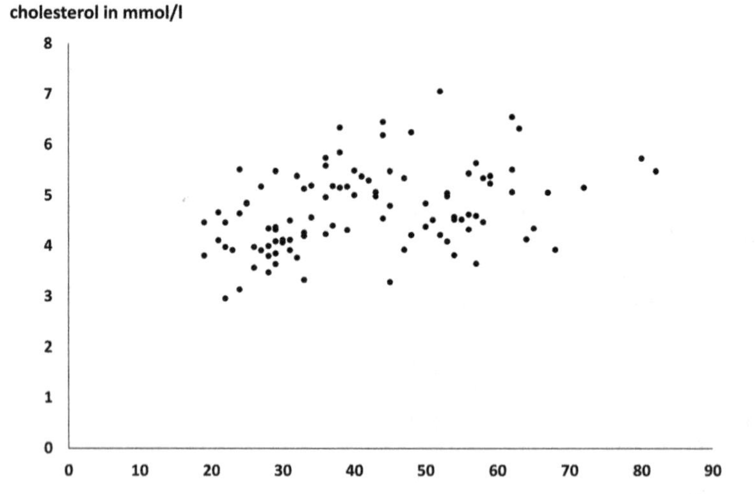

Fig. 4.3 Scatterplot to illustrate the relationship between cholesterol and age

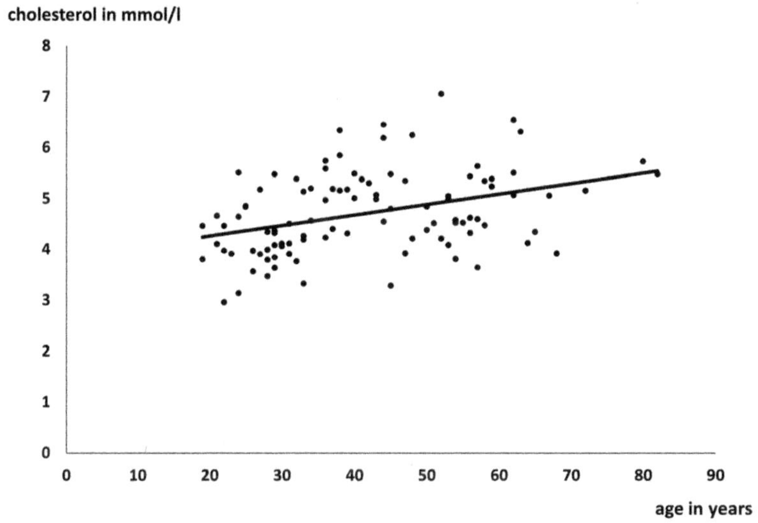

Fig. 4.4 Scatterplot to illustrate the relationship between cholesterol and age including the linear regression line

(vertical) distances from the individual observations to the estimated regression line are known as the residuals.

When this method is applied to the example with cholesterol and age, that relationship is best described with the following equation:

$$cholesterol = 3.859 + 0.021 \times age$$

The result of a linear regression analysis with one independent variable is described by two parameters, the intercept, which is also known as the constant or b_0, and the regression coefficient for the independent variable, also known as the slope or b_1. The b_0 (the intercept, the constant) can be interpreted as the value of the outcome variable (i.e. cholesterol) when the value of the independent variable (i.e. age) is 0. This can easily be seen by filling in the regression equation. When 0 is entered for age, the regression equation is reduced to the following:

$$cholesterol = 3.859 + 0.021 \times 0 = 3.859$$

So, at the age of 0 years, the estimated cholesterol is 3.859. A number which also can be obtained by extrapolating the estimated line to the y-axis (see Fig. 4.5). It should be noted that the value is interpretable but not very informative in this particular example, because after all, there are no subjects with age 0 in the study population.

The regression coefficient for age (b_1) has a much more interesting interpretation. For every 1-year difference in age, the estimated difference in cholesterol is 0.021. Again, this can easily be seen by entering two consecutive values for the independent

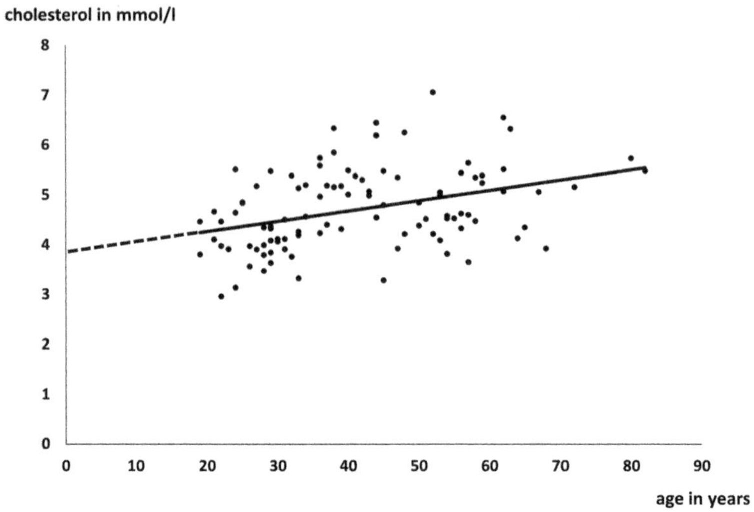

Fig. 4.5 Scatterplot to illustrate the relationship between cholesterol and age including the linear regression line extrapolated to the y-axis

variable age (e.g. 30 and 31) into the regression equation. The difference in cholesterol between the two ages becomes 0.021.

$$cholesterol_{30} = 3.859 + 0.021 \times 30 = 4.489$$

$$cholesterol_{31} = 3.859 + 0.021 \times 31 = 4.51$$

$$cholesterol_{31} - cholesterol_{30} = 4.51 - 4.489 = 0.021$$

Although in practice the regression coefficients are (obviously) not calculated by hand, it is possible to calculate the value of the regression coefficients with a relative simple equation (see Eqs. 4.10 and 4.11).

$$b_1 = \frac{\sum(x_i - \overline{x})(y_i - \overline{y})}{\sum(x_i - \overline{x})^2} \tag{4.10}$$

$$b_0 = \overline{y} - b_1\overline{x} \tag{4.11}$$

where b_1 = regression coefficient for independent variable x, x_i = value of the independent variable x for subject i, $\overline{x}$ = mean value of x, y_i = value of the outcome variable y for subject i, $\overline{y}$ = mean value of y and b_0 = intercept.

It should be noted that the regression coefficients always have the same interpretation irrespective of what kind of regression analysis is performed. The b_0 is always the value of the outcome variable when the independent variable is 0 and the regression coefficient for an independent variable (b_1) is always the difference in the outcome variable when the independent variable differs with one unit.

4.4.2 Linear Regression Analysis with a Dichotomous Independent Variable

As has been mentioned before, linear regression analysis can be used for all types of independent variables. So, also in the example where cholesterol was compared between subjects with low social class and high social class (see Sect. 4.2) linear regression analysis can be used. Before performing the linear regression analysis to analyse the relationship between cholesterol and social class, first a scatterplot is made. Figure 4.6 shows the scatterplot to illustrate the relationship between cholesterol and social class.

Because social class has only two values, the scatterplot in Fig. 4.6 seems a bit strange. Also in this situation the most appropriate line can be drawn through the observed data using the least squares method. In a situation where the independent variable can only take two values (in the example, low social class is coded 0 and high social class is coded 1), the point at which the distance from the observations to that point is as small as possible should be chosen for both groups. The best fitting line then runs through those two points. The point that satisfies this requirement is the mean value of the outcome variable for the particular group. So, the most appropriate line for the relationship between cholesterol and social class runs from the mean cholesterol of the subjects with low social class to the mean cholesterol of the subjects with high social class (see Fig. 4.7).

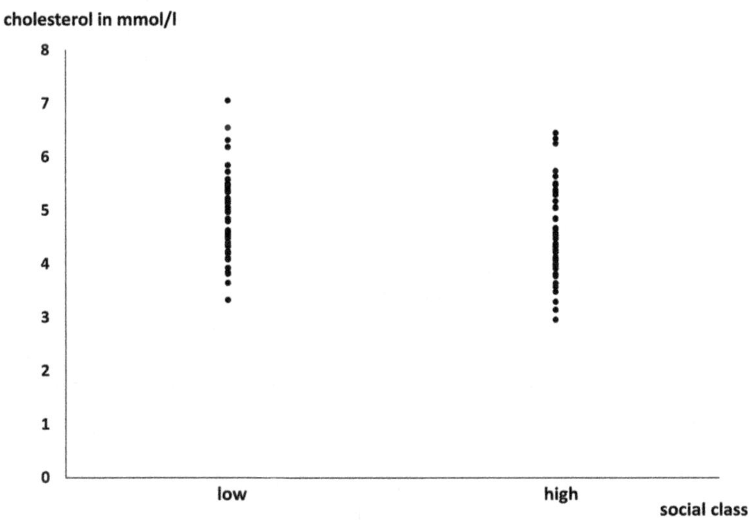

Fig. 4.6 Scatterplot to illustrate the relationship between cholesterol and social class

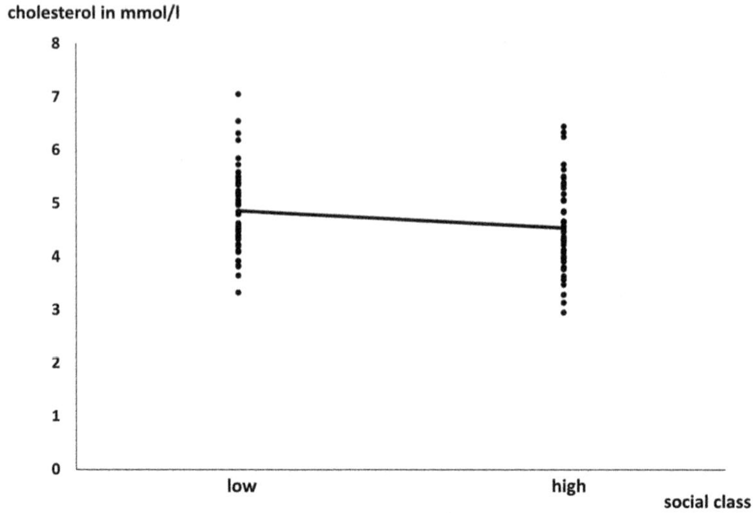

Fig. 4.7 Scatterplot to illustrate the relationship between cholesterol and social class including the linear regression line

Output 4.16 Result of the linear regression analysis to analyse the relationship between cholesterol and social class

					95% confidence interval	
	Coefficient	se	t-value	p-value	Lower	Upper
Social class	−0.32	0.16	−2.00	0.048	−0.64	−0.003
Constant	4.86	0.11	44.51	<0.001	4.65	5.08

se standard error

The estimated linear regression equation is then:

$$cholesterol = 4.86 - 0.32 \times social\ class$$

The interpretation of the regression coefficients is analogous to the linear regression analysis in which age was the independent variable. The b_0 (4.86) is the value of the outcome variable (i.e. cholesterol) when the independent variable (i.e. social class) is 0. In this situation, the b_0 is informative, because it is the mean cholesterol of the subjects with low social class. The b_1 (−0.32) is the difference in outcome variable (i.e. cholesterol) when the independent variable (i.e. social class) differs with one unit. When the independent variable differs with one unit indicates the difference between subjects with high social class and low social class.

So, the difference in cholesterol between subjects with high (coded 1) and low (coded 0) social class is −0.32. When social class = 1 is entered into the regression equation, the mean cholesterol for subjects with high social class is obtained (i.e. 4.86–0.32 = 4.54). Output 4.16 shows the result of the linear regression analysis to analyse the relationship between cholesterol and social class.

In Output 4.16 first the two regression coefficients are shown (−0.32 for the b_1 and 4.86 for the b_0). Next, the corresponding standard errors of both coefficients are given (0.16 and 0.11 respectively). These standard errors are the standard errors of the mean and they can be used to quantify the uncertainty in generalizing the observed result to the source population. Based on the regression coefficient and the standard error, the test statistic is calculated (i.e. the regression coefficient divided by its standard error), which is then used to obtain the p-value. Finally, the 95% confidence intervals around the regression coefficients are given.

The most important part of the output is the regression coefficient for social class, because that is the regression coefficient that indicates the difference in cholesterol between subjects with high social class and low social class and that is the answer to the research question. For this regression coefficient, the t-value is −2.00 (−0.32/ 0.16). In fact, this is exactly the same as the test statistic used in the independent t-test for comparing two groups (see Sect. 4.2).

In the independent t-test, the test statistic is calculated by subtracting the expected difference when the null hypothesis is true from the observed difference, and dividing the result by the standard error of the mean. Exactly the same applies to linear regression analysis. Here, the expected difference when the null hypothesis is true (i.e. 0) is subtracted from the observed regression coefficient (the difference between subjects with high social class and low social class) and the result is divided by the standard error of the regression coefficient (i.e. the standard error of the mean).

It is therefore not surprising that the t-value calculated with linear regression analysis is exactly the same as the t-value calculated with the independent t-test (see Output 4.3).

To determine the p-value, a t-distribution with n − 2 degrees of freedom is of course also used in the linear regression analysis. The p-value of the regression coefficient for social class has already been seen in Output 4.3 (i.e. 0.048). The last two columns of Output 4.16 show the limits of the 95% confidence interval around the regression coefficient for social class. This 95% confidence interval is calculated in the same way as for the independent t-test (see Eq. 4.5).

In the output also for the b_0 the standard error, t-value and p-value are given. It should be noted, that this information is not interesting, because the null hypothesis for the statistical test is that the intercept value is 0. Or in other words, the null hypothesis states that cholesterol for subjects with low social class is 0. A ridicule hypothesis.

4.4.3 Linear Regression Analysis with a Categorical Independent Variable

It has already been mentioned that linear regression analysis can be used for the analysis of a continuous outcome variable and all types of independent variables.

The question whether cholesterol is associated with alcohol consumption, which is divided into three groups (Example 4.2) can therefore also be answered using linear regression analysis. As usual in a linear regression analysis, first a scatterplot can be made to visualize the relationship between cholesterol and alcohol consumption (see Fig. 4.8).

Output 4.17 shows the result of the linear regression analysis to analyse the relationship between cholesterol and alcohol consumption.

Based on Output 4.17 the following regression equation can be made:

$$cholesterol = 4.65 + 0.07 \times alcohol\ consumption$$

The b_0 (4.65) shown in Output 4.17 can be interpreted as the value of the outcome variable when the independent variable is 0, i.e. as the mean cholesterol for the

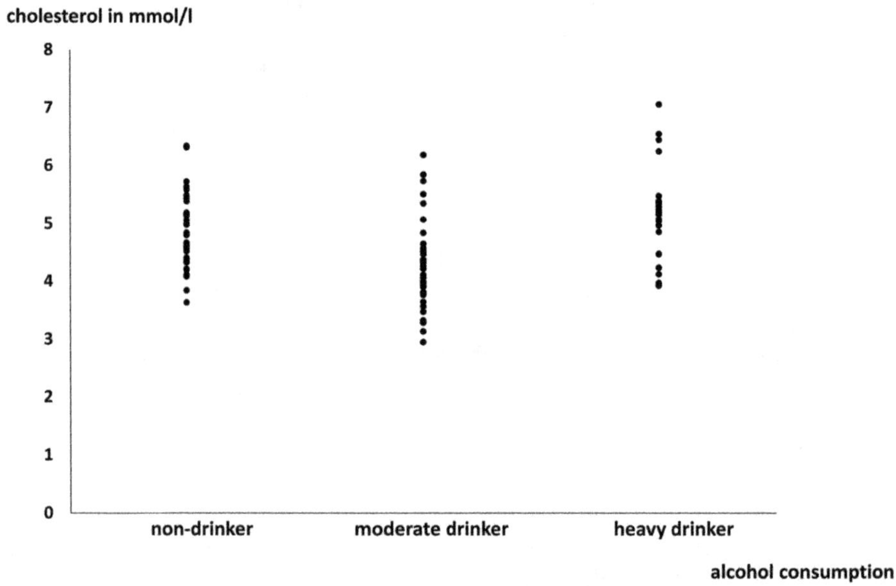

Fig. 4.8 Scatterplot to illustrate the relationship between cholesterol and alcohol consumption

Output 4.17 Result of the linear regression analysis to analyse the relationship between cholesterol and alcohol consumption

					95% confidence interval	
	Coefficient	se	t-value	p-value	Lower	Upper
Alcohol	0.07	0.11	0.70	0.49	−0.14	0.28
Constant	4.65	0.12	39.25	<0.001	4.42	4.89

se standard error

non-drinkers (because non-drinkers are coded 0). Next, the 0.07 for the regression coefficient for alcohol consumption indicates that for one unit difference of alcohol consumption, cholesterol differs by 0.07 units. In other words, 0.07 is the difference in mean cholesterol between moderate drinkers and non-drinkers (after all, the group of moderate drinkers is coded 1) and also the difference between heavy drinkers (which is coded 2) and moderate drinkers. When 0, 1 and 2 are entered into the regression equation, the estimated mean cholesterol for the three groups can be calculated. For non-drinkers, the estimated mean cholesterol is 4.65, for moderate drinkers 4.72 and for heavy drinkers 4.79.

When these estimated values are compared to the observed values in the three groups (see Table 4.8), it has to be concluded that the estimates based on the linear regression analysis are not even close to the observed mean values. The reason for this can be obtained from the scatterplot which is shown in Fig. 4.9.

With linear regression analysis the best straight line through the observations is estimated, but in the scatterplot it can be seen that the relationship between cholesterol and alcohol consumption cannot be described well with a straight line. The mean cholesterol of moderate drinkers is lower than the mean cholesterol of non-drinkers, while the mean cholesterol of heavy drinkers is slightly higher than the mean cholesterol of non-drinkers. The question now, of course, is how linear regression analysis can be used to adequately estimate the relationship between cholesterol and alcohol consumption. This requires the use of dummy variables (also known as indicator variables). To represent the categorical variable alcohol

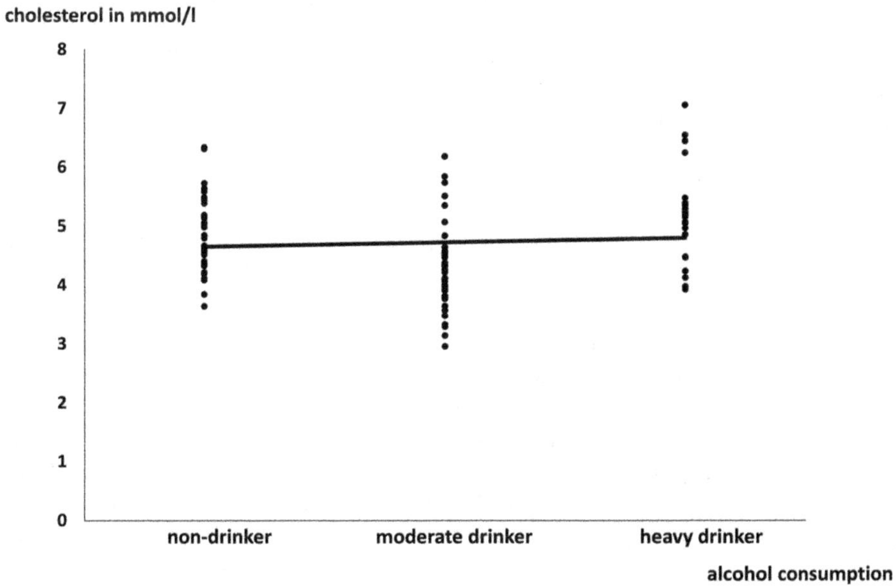

Fig. 4.9 Scatterplot to illustrate the relationship between cholesterol and alcohol consumption including the linear regression line

Table 4.9 Dummy coding for the variable alcohol consumption

	Dummy 1	Dummy 2
Non-drinker	0	0
Moderate drinker	1	0
Heavy drinker	0	1

consumption (which consists of three groups), two dummy variables must be made (see Table 4.9).

Table 4.9 shows that the first dummy variable is 0 for non-drinkers, 1 for moderate drinkers and 0 for heavy drinkers. The second dummy variable is 0 for both non-drinkers and moderate drinkers and 1 for heavy drinkers. The group for which all dummy variables are coded 0 is known as the reference group. To analyse the relationship between cholesterol and alcohol consumption in an appropriate way, both dummy variables has to be added to the regression equation. It should be noted that the two dummy variables should always be analysed together, because otherwise the interpretation of the regression coefficients for both dummy variables will change and will not be appropriate anymore. The regression equation with the two dummy variables is:

$$cholesterol = b_0 + b_1 \times dummy_1 + b_2 \times dummy_2$$

It is important to understand the interpretation of the different regression coefficients in this regression equation. The b_0 is the value of the outcome variable (i.e. cholesterol) when the independent variables are both 0. Because both dummy variables are coded 0 for non-drinkers, the b_0 is the mean cholesterol for non-drinkers. The mean cholesterol for moderate drinkers can be obtained by entering 1 for the first dummy variable and 0 for the second dummy variable. The mean cholesterol for moderate drinkers is therefore equal to $b_0 + b_1$. Now, b_1 can be interpreted as the difference in cholesterol between moderate drinkers and non-drinkers. For heavy drinkers, the same procedure can be followed: 0 is entered for the first dummy variable and 1 for the second dummy variable. The mean cholesterol for heavy drinkers is therefore equal to $b_0 + b_2$. In other words, b_2 can be interpreted as the difference in cholesterol between heavy drinkers and non-drinkers (see Table 4.10).

Output 4.18 shows the result of the linear regression analysis to analyse the relationship between cholesterol and alcohol consumption, where alcohol consumption is represented by two dummy variables.

In Output 4.18 it can be seen that cholesterol for non-drinkers is 4.86 (b_0), that the difference in cholesterol between moderate drinkers and non-drinkers is −0.58 (b_1) and that the difference in cholesterol between heavy drinkers and non-drinkers is 0.32 (b_2). Based on Output 4.18, the estimated mean cholesterol for the different groups can be calculated. For moderate drinkers, the mean cholesterol is 4.29 (4.86–0.58) and for heavy drinkers, the mean cholesterol is 5.18 (4.86 + 0.32). When the estimated values are now compared to the observed values for the three

Table 4.10 Interpretation of the regression coefficients for the relationship between cholesterol and two dummy variables (coded as shown in Table 4.9) for alcohol consumption

$$cholesterol_{non-drinkers} = b_0 + b_1 \times 0 + b_2 \times 0 = b_0$$
$$cholesterol_{moderate\ drinkers} = b_0 + b_1 \times 1 + b_2 \times 0 = b_0 + b_1$$
$$cholesterol_{heavy\ drinkers} = b_0 + b_1 \times 0 + b_2 \times 1 = b_0 + b_2$$
$$cholesterol_{moderate\ drinkers} - cholesterol_{non-drinkers} = b_0 + b_1 - b_0 = b_1$$
$$cholesterol_{heavy\ drinkers} - cholesterol_{non-drinkers} = b_0 + b_2 - b_0 = b_2$$

Output 4.18 Result of the linear regression analysis to analyse the relationship between cholesterol and alcohol consumption (represented by dummy variables)

					95% confidence interval	
	Coefficient	se	t-value	p-value	Lower	Upper
Dummy 1	−0.58	0.17	−3.47	0.001	−0.90	−0.25
Dummy 2	0.32	0.19	1.64	0.11	−0.07	0.70
Constant	4.86	0.12	42.02	<0.001	4.63	5.09

se standard error

groups (see Table 4.8), they are exactly the same. In other words, the linear regression analysis in which alcohol consumption is represented by dummy variables gives an accurate estimation of the relationship between cholesterol and alcohol consumption (see Fig. 4.10).

4.4.4 Linear Regression Analysis with a Continuous Independent Variable

It has already been mentioned that linear regression analysis can be used to analyse the relationship between a continuous outcome variable and a continuous independent variable. Going back to the relationship between cholesterol and age (see Sect. 4.4.1), Output 4.19 shows the result of the linear regression analysis to analyse this relationship.

In Output 4.19 it can be seen that the regression coefficient for age is 0.02. This indicates that for every unit difference in age, cholesterol differs by 0.02 units. The 95% confidence interval around the regression coefficient ranges between 0.01 and 0.03. The b_0 (3.86) indicates the mean cholesterol for subjects aged 0 years, i.e. a non-informative number. The result of a linear regression analysis is a straight line, which in this case means that it makes no difference which ages are compared to each other. Each difference of 1 year in age (e.g. between 21 and 20 years, 41 and 40 years, 65 and 64 years, etc.) is associated with an equally large difference in cholesterol, i.e. 0.02. Of course, it is questionable whether the assumption of a linear relationship is justified. The same phenomenon has already emerged when analysing the relationship between cholesterol and alcohol consumption. In that example,

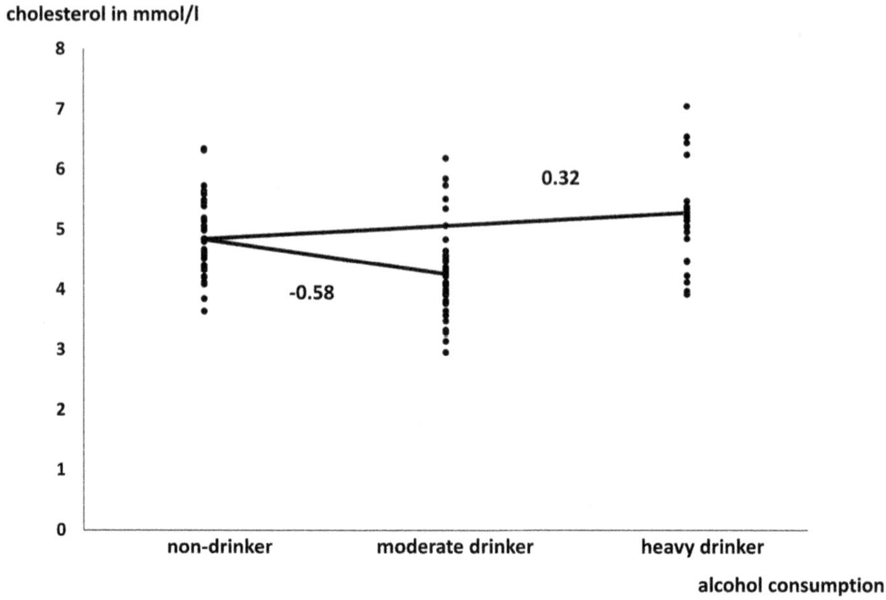

Fig. 4.10 Scatterplot to illustrate the relationship between cholesterol and alcohol consumption including the two linear regression lines based on the regression analysis with dummy variables

Output 4.19 Result of the linear regression analysis to analyse the relationship between cholesterol and age

					95% confidence interval	
	Coefficient	se	t-value	p-value	Lower	Upper
Age	0.02	0.005	3.96	<0.001	0.01	0.03
Constant	3.86	0.23	16.68	<0.001	3.41	4.31

se standard error

dummy variables had to be used to analyse the relationship correctly (see Sect. 4.4.3). For a continuous independent variable, dummy variables cannot be used directly, but there are several other ways to evaluate whether the observed relationship is linear (see Sect. 4.4.4.1).

4.4.4.1 Evaluation of the Linear Relationship with a Continuous Independent Variable

The first possibility to evaluate whether the relationship with a continuous independent variable is linear is to analyse the relationship between the two variables with a different mathematical function. For example, a quadratic relationship (a hyperbolic or parabolic relationship), a cubic relationship (an S-shaped relationship), a logarithmic relationship and so on. Which mathematical function one chooses, of course, depends to a large extent on the pattern in the scatterplot and the biologically expected relationship. Looking at the scatterplot in Fig. 4.3, at first glance there does not seem to be much wrong with the linear relationship between cholesterol and age. Perhaps a quadratic relationship is slightly better, in which a somewhat weaker relationship is estimated at the older ages. Whether this is indeed necessary can be evaluated with a linear regression analysis in which age squared is added as an independent variable in addition to age. Output 4.20 shows the result of this analysis.

The most important part of Output 4.20 is the regression coefficient for age squared. When this coefficient is important, then the quadratic relationship is a better description of the relationship than the linear relationship. When the coefficient is not important, then a linear relationship is just as good as a quadratic relationship and then a straight line can be used to describe the relationship. The importance of the regression coefficient in these situations is often based on the p-value. That the importance is evaluated on the p-value is mainly because the magnitude of the regression coefficient for age squared is difficult to interpret and therefore difficult to use. The result of the linear regression analysis including age squared more or less confirms what was already seen in the scatter plot, i.e. the linear relationship is a good way to describe the relationship between cholesterol and age. This is because the regression coefficient for age squared is not statistically significant ($p = 0.13$), so the null hypothesis, which implies that this regression coefficient is 0, is not rejected. Although in this case a decision is made based on whether a regression coefficient is statistically significant or not, it should be realized that statistical significance still needs to be interpreted with caution.

The biggest disadvantage of the above procedure is that when a quadratic relationship is found to be better than a linear relationship (i.e. when the regression coefficient for age squared is statistically significant) the interpretation of the regression coefficients becomes difficult. Because the variable age is present three times in the regression equation (one time for the linear part and two times for the quadratic part), the interpretation of each coefficient is dependent on the other coefficient. So, there is no straightforward interpretation. Therefore, in practice an alternative procedure is often used to evaluate whether a certain relationship is linear or not. The general idea of this procedure is that the continuous independent variable is divided into a number of groups (e.g. quartiles) and then the relationship between the outcome variable and the newly made categorical variable is analysed using dummy variables. Based on the increasing (or decreasing) trend in the regression

Output 4.20 Result of the linear regression analysis to analyse the relationship between cholesterol and age including age squared

					95% confidence interval	
	Coefficient	se	t-value	p-value	Lower	Upper
Age	0.06	0.03	2.22	0.029	0.007	0.12
Age squared	−0.0005	0.0003	−1.54	0.13	−0.001	0.0001
Constant	2.97	0.62	4.77	<0.001	1.73	4.20

se standard error

Table 4.11 Dummy coding for the variable age

	Dummy 1	Dummy 2	Dummy 3
Quartile 1	0	0	0
Quartile 2	1	0	0
Quartile 3	0	1	0
Quartile 4	0	0	1

Output 4.21 Result of the linear regression analysis to analyse the relationship between cholesterol and age as categorical variable

					95% confidence interval	
	Coefficient	se	t-value	p-value	Lower	Upper
Dummy 1	0.53	0.22	2.47	0.015	0.10	0.96
Dummy 2	0.82	0.21	3.96	<0.001	0.41	1.22
Dummy 3	0.74	0.21	3.56	<0.001	0.33	1.15
Constant	4.20	0.14	29.16	<0.001	3.92	4.49

se standard error

coefficients for the dummy variables, it can be evaluated whether there is a linear relationship or not.

In the example, the relationship between cholesterol and age is analysed. To evaluate whether this relationship is linear, first the continuous independent variable age is categorized into four equal groups, based on quartiles. Then, based on this new categorical variable, three dummy variables are made (see Table 4.11), and analysed in a linear regression analysis. Output 4.21 shows the result of this regression analysis.

The interpretation of the regression coefficients in Output 4.21 is as follows: the regression coefficient for the first dummy variable (0.53) indicates the difference in cholesterol between the second and the first age quartile. The regression coefficient for the second dummy variable (0.82) indicates the difference in cholesterol between the third and first age quartile, and the regression coefficient for the third dummy variable (0.74) indicates the difference in cholesterol between the fourth and the first age quartile. From the fact that the regression coefficient for the third dummy variable is lower than the regression coefficient for the second dummy variable, it can be concluded that the relationship between cholesterol and age is not linear. Because there is no linear relationship, the result of the analysis with the dummy variables has to be reported. It should be noted that besides the regression coefficients for the dummy variables, also the mean age values for the different quartiles must be reported, because otherwise, it is still not clear what the interpretation of the regression coefficients is.

It is important to realise that when there is an increasing or decreasing trend in the regression coefficients for the dummy variables, the relationship is only linear when the steps in the trend are equal to the steps in the mean values of the four quartiles. Table 4.12 shows two examples to illustrate this.

Table 4.12 Two examples to illustrate the comparison between the trend in regression coefficients and the mean values for the age quartiles

Example 1	Regression coefficient	Mean age
		30
Dummy 1	1.1	25
Dummy 2	2.0	26
Dummy 3	2.9	35
Example 2	Regression coefficient	Mean age
		30
Dummy 1	0.5	25
Dummy 2	0.6	26
Dummy 3	1.5	35

Based on the regression coefficients of Table 4.12 it can be concluded that the relationship in the first example is linear (each step in the trend of the regression coefficients is more or less the same) and that the relationship in the second example is not linear (each step in the trend of the regression coefficients is not the same). However, when the trend in regression coefficients is compared to the trend in mean values of the four quartiles, the conclusion is totally different. The relationship in the first example is not linear, while the relationship in the second example is linear.

One should realise that also dividing the continuous independent variable into groups is not the holy grail for dealing with a non-linear relationship with a continuous independent variable. Also this method has some disadvantages. One of them is that subjects in the same group are considered to be the same as far as the outcome variable is concerned, which is of course never true. Another problem is that the cut-off values for the groups are arbitrary. Mostly quartiles are used, but it is possible that using other cut-off values, lead to different conclusions.

Of course, in general, one can also choose to express the relation between the two continuous variables with a different mathematical function. When there is no interest in the direct interpretation of the regression coefficients, using a different mathematical function is probably the best option. For example, when the aim of the analysis is to predict the outcome variable, a different mathematical function for the relationship with a continuous independent variables makes a lot of sense (see Chap. 7). It should be noted that the methods used to evaluate whether the relationship between cholesterol and age is linear lead to a different conclusion. When age squared is added to the analysis, it is concluded that a quadratic relationship is not better than a linear relationship and that, therefore, a linear relationship can best be used. When the relationship is analysed with age as a categorical variable represented by dummy variables, on the other hand, it is concluded that the relationship between cholesterol and age is not linear. One of the reasons why the different methods can lead to different conclusions is that when age squared is added to the analysis, only the quadratic relationship is analysed as an alternative for the linear relationship. Using dummy variables, basically all non-linear relationships are evaluated.

Another method to evaluate whether a relationship between a continuous outcome variable and a continuous independent variable is linear or not, is the use of splines (Schuster et al., 2022). The general idea of this method is that the independent variable is divided into separate parts in which a different relationship between the outcome variable and the independent variable is estimated. The most simple spline regression analysis that can be applied is a linear spline regression analysis with two parts; an analysis which is also known as a linear spline regression analysis with one knot. Figure 4.11 illustrates this linear spline regression analysis for the relationship between cholesterol and age in which the independent variable age is divided into two parts by the median (i.e. 39).

Figure 4.11 shows nicely that two regression lines are estimated. One regression line for the ages from 19 (the lowest value in the dataset) till 39 (the median value) and one regression line for the ages from 39 till 82 (the highest value in the dataset). It can also be seen that the regression coefficient for the first regression line is highly positive and that the regression coefficient for the second regression line is almost zero. Table 4.13 shows part of the dataset that is used in the linear spline regression analysis to analyse the relationship between cholesterol and age and Output 4.22 shows the results of the linear spline regression analysis with one knot to analyse the relationship between cholesterol and age.

So, in the linear spline regression analysis, the regression coefficient for age1 (0.057) indicates the relationship between cholesterol and age for the ages ≤39 years, while the regression coefficient for age2 (0.001) indicates the relationship

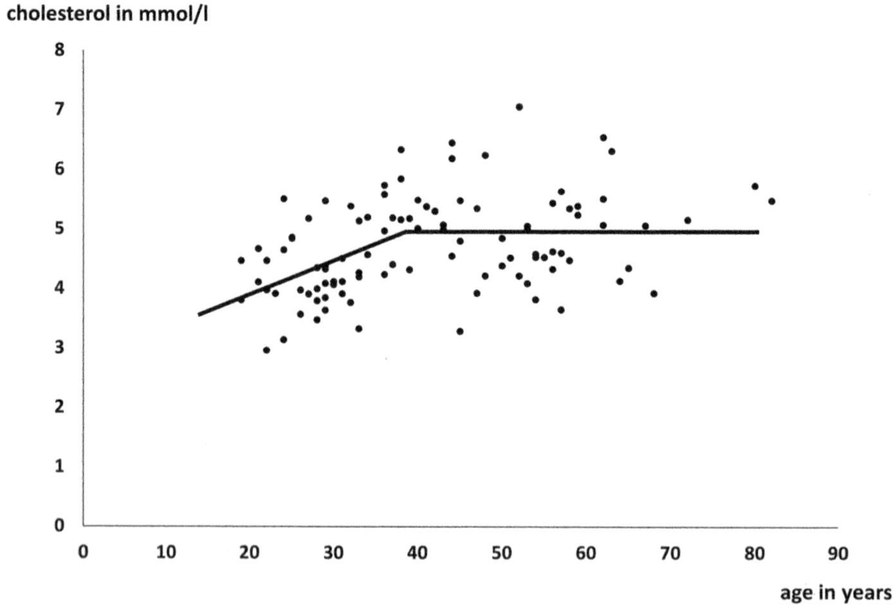

Fig. 4.11 Scatterplot to illustrate the relationship between cholesterol and age including linear splines

Table 4.13 Part of the dataset that is used in the linear spline regression analysis to analyse the relationship between cholesterol and age

Id	Cholesterol	Age	Age1	Age2
1	3.92	23	23	0
2	5.18	39	39	0
3	3.48	28	28	0
.				
8	3.82	54	39	15
9	4.22	52	39	13
.				
100	3.98	26	26	0

Output 4.22 Result of the linear spline regression analysis with one knot to analyse the relationship between cholesterol and age

					95% confidence interval	
	Coefficient	se	t-value	p-value	Lower	Upper
Age1	0.057	0.015	3.93	<0.001	0.028	0.086
Age2	0.001	0.009	0.12	0.91	−0.016	0.019
Constant	2.74	0.47	5.83	<0.001	1.81	3.68

se standard error

between cholesterol and age for the ages >39 years. To evaluate whether the relationship between cholesterol and age is linear, the two regression coefficients for age derived from the linear spline regression analysis have to be compared to each other. When the two regression coefficients are more or less equal it can be concluded that the relationship between cholesterol and age is linear.

It is also possible to analyse age and age2 (see Table 4.13) together in a linear spline regression analysis. In this regression analysis the regression coefficient for age indicates the relationship between cholesterol and age for the ages ≤39 years while the regression coefficient for age2 indicates the difference in the relationship between cholesterol and age for the ages ≤39 years and the relationship between cholesterol and age for the ages >39 years. Output 4.23 shows the result of this analysis.

In Output 4.23 it can be seen that the difference in the relationship between cholesterol and age for the ages ≤39 years and the relationship between cholesterol and age for the ages >39 years is −0.056. When this value is subtracted from the regression coefficient for age it gives the regression coefficient for age for the ages >39 years. This regression coefficient (0.001) was already directly estimated in the first linear spline regression analysis (see Output 4.22). Because the regression coefficient for age2 (−0.056) indicates the difference between the regression coefficients for the two periods, to evaluate whether the relationship between cholesterol and age is linear, the p-value of the regression coefficient for age2 can be used. When the p-value of this regression coefficients is not statistically significant, it can be concluded that the relationship between cholesterol and age can be assumed to be linear. It is often mentioned that the advantage of using the second linear spline regression analysis is that this statistical test is performed directly. In the example the

Output 4.23 Result of the linear spline regression analysis with one knot to analyse the relationship between cholesterol and age

					95% confidence interval	
	Coefficient	se	t-value	p-value	Lower	Upper
Age	0.057	0.015	3.93	<0.001	0.028	0.086
Age2	−0.056	0.021	−2.69	0.008	−0.098	−0.015
Constant	2.74	0.47	5.83	<0.001	1.81	3.68

se standard error

p-value for the difference between the two regression coefficient is 0.008, which indicates that the regression coefficients are statistically significant different from each other and that, therefore, the relationship between cholesterol and age cannot be assumed to be linear. However, also with the first linear spline analysis it can be seen that this is the case when evaluating the 95% confidence intervals around the regression coefficients for both age ranges. Because the regression coefficient for the first age range is outside the 95% confidence interval of the regression coefficient for the second age range and because the regression coefficient for the second age range is outside the 95% confidence interval of the regression coefficient for the first age range, it can also be concluded that there is a statistically significant difference between the two regression coefficients. The advantage of the use of the first linear spline regression analysis is that directly a regression coefficient (and a 95% confidence interval) for the two age ranges is estimated.

The linear spline regression analysis with one knot is the most simple analysis using splines. It is, of course, also possible to use a linear spline regression analysis with more than one knot. It is, however, quite complicated to define where the knots should be placed. It could be based on the scatterplot, but the scatterplot is mostly not very clear, especially not when the number of subjects in the study population is high. In many situations, percentiles are used for defining the knots, but that is, of course, a rather arbitrary choice.

Besides linear spline regression analysis, it also possible to use cubic spline regression analysis (Schuster et al., 2022). Instead of estimating a linear regression line for each age range, a cubic relationship (i.e. an S-shaped relationship) is used for each age range. It was already mentioned that the interpretation of the results of a regression analysis with a different mathematical function for the independent variable is difficult, it is obvious that the regression coefficients obtained from a cubic spline regression analysis are not interpretable at all. Nevertheless, it is a very popular method to deal with non-linear relationships with a continuous independent variable. Because of the difficulty in the interpretation of the regression coefficients, the method is mostly used in situations when the interpretation of the regression coefficients is not important. This is, for example, the case in prediction modelling (see Chap. 7).

4.4.5 Standardized Regression Coefficient–Correlation Coefficient

The outputs of linear regression analyses shown so far are a limited selection of the outputs generated by statistical software. One coefficient often reported is the standardized regression coefficient. The standardized regression coefficient is also known as the Pearson correlation coefficient and can be calculated by multiplying the regular regression coefficient with the standard deviation of the independent variable and divide this by the standard deviation of the outcome variable (see Eq. 4.12) .

$$b_{sta} = \frac{b_{reg} \times sd(x)}{sd(y)} \tag{4.12}$$

Where b_{sta} = standardized regression coefficient, b_{reg}= regular regression coefficient, $sd(x)$= standard deviation of the independent variable and $sd(y)$= standard deviation of the outcome variable.

To calculate the standardized regression coefficient for age in the relationship with cholesterol, the standard deviations of both variables must be used (see Table 4.14).

When both the standard deviations and the regular regression coefficient for age (from the analysis assuming a linear relationship between cholesterol and age; see Output 4.19) are entered into Eq. 4.12, the standardized regression coefficient is 0.36 (i.e. 0.02 × 14.62/ 0.81 = 0.36). When the standardized regression coefficient is calculated with statistical software, due to rounding, a slightly higher value is obtained (i.e. 0.372).

The standardized regression coefficient can be seen as a regression coefficient in which the x-axis and the y-axis of the scatterplot are stretched or shrunken in such a way that they have the same unit (i.e. number of standard deviations). It has already been mentioned that the standardized regression coefficient is also known as the Pearson correlation coefficient and by that name it is widely used.

The regular regression coefficient provides different information than the standardized regression coefficient. This is nicely illustrated by Fig. 4.12. Figure 4.12a, b show the results of two linear regression analyses, where the same regular regression coefficient is obtained (0.10), but because the observations illustrated in Fig. 4.12a are closer to the regression line than the observations illustrated in Fig. 4.12b, the standardized regression coefficient is higher in the first analysis (0.866 versus 0.655). Figure 4.12c shows the result of a linear regression analysis in which the

Table 4.14 Descriptive information of cholesterol and age

	Number of subjects	Mean	Standard deviation	Minimum	Maximum
Cholesterol	100	4.72	0.81	2.96	7.06
Age	100	41.67	14.62	19	82

standardized regression coefficient between the outcome variable and the independent variable is the same as in the linear regression analysis illustrated in Fig. 4.12a (both standardized regression coefficients are 0.866), but where the regular regression coefficient is twice as high (0.20 versus 0.10).

4.4.6 Explained Variance

In the output of a linear regression analysis provided by statistical software, mostly also the explained variance is provided. The explained variance is known as the R-square. In the example where the relationship between cholesterol and age is analysed (assuming a linear relationship between cholesterol and age; see Output 4.19), the R-square is 0.138. The value of the R-square indicates that 13.8% of the variance in cholesterol is explained by age. It should be noted that the R-square from a linear regression analysis with only one independent variable is the same as the squared Pearson correlation coefficient between the outcome variable and the independent variable. It was already mentioned that the Pearson correlation coefficient between cholesterol and age was 0.372 and 0.372 squared is 0.138.

The explained variance is often used in multiple regression analyses, as an indication of the quality of a multiple regression model (see Sect. 7.3.6). Besides the R-square, also the adjusted R-square is mostly provided. The adjusted R-square is a modified version of R-square, which is adjusted for the number of independent variables in the model. The adjusted R-square is always lower than the R-square itself.

Because linear regression analysis and analysis of variance use the same principles, the output of a linear regression analysis mostly provides the output of an analysis of variance as well. It should be noted that the analysis of variance part of the output of a linear regression analysis is, of course, not much used in practice, because the purpose of performing a linear regression analysis is to obtain effect estimates and 95% confidence intervals.

4.4.7 Linear Regression Analysis with a Non-normally Distributed Outcome Variable

One of the assumptions of linear regression analysis is that the outcome variable must be more or less normally distributed. A linear regression analysis makes statements about mean values and the mean value of a non-normal distribution is not very informative. As has been mentioned before, the most common non-normal distribution is the skewed to the right distribution. Earlier it was indicated that in the case of a skewed to the right distribution, a log transformation can be performed to obtain a more or less normal distribution of the outcome variable.

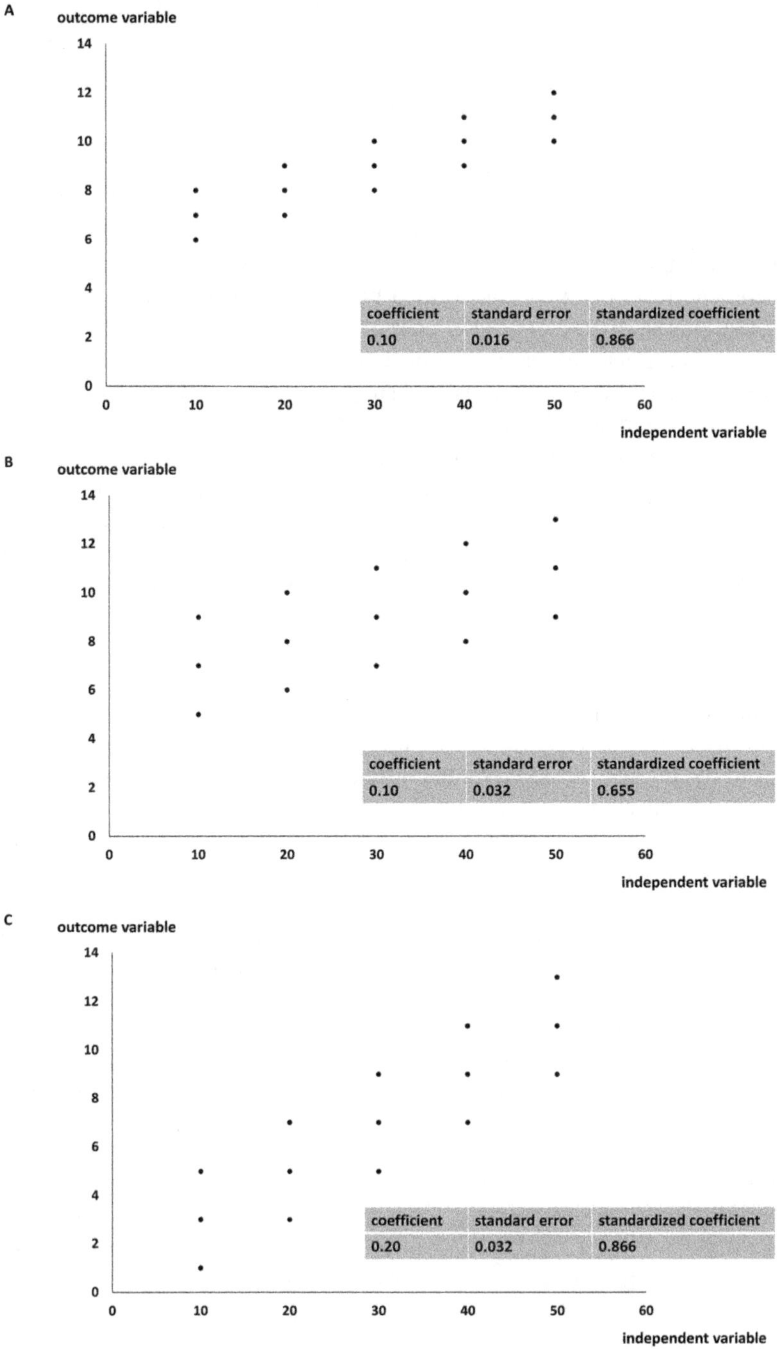

Fig. 4.12 Illustration of the differences between the regular regression coefficient and the standardized regression coefficient (i.e. the Pearson correlation coefficient)

In Sect. 4.2.1, the analysis of a skewed outcome variable has already been discussed in detail using Example 4.3. The aim of the study is to analyse the relationship between triglyceride and overweight. Of course, this relationship can also be analysed with a linear regression analysis. Output 4.24 shows the result of the linear regression analysis with the log transformed triglyceride as outcome variable and overweight as independent variable.

The regression coefficient for overweight shown in Output 4.24 (0.13) is the difference in outcome variable between subjects with normal weight and overweight. Since the outcome variable is the natural logarithm of triglyceride, this regression coefficient can be transformed back into an interpretable effect measure using the e-power of the regression coefficient, i.e. EXP(0.13) = 1.14. The interpretation of this effect measure is of course the same as the interpretation of the effect estimated with the independent t-test, i.e. subjects with overweight have a 1.14 times higher triglyceride than subjects with normal weight.

Regarding the assumption of the more or less normally distributed outcome variable in a linear regression analysis, it should be noted that it is not the normality of the outcome variable which is the key issue, but it is the normality of the residuals. The residuals are the differences between the observations and the estimated values of the regression line. In many situations, a non-normal distribution of the outcome variable results in a non-normal distribution of the residuals as well, but sometimes it is different. To explain this a bit further, suppose the relationship between a continuous outcome variable and a dichotomous independent variable is investigated and suppose that the distribution of the outcome variable is highly skewed. When both groups are more or less equally skewed, both mean values are equally influenced by this skewness. When the difference between these two mean values is estimated, this difference is a valid estimate. In this situation, the residuals will be more or less normally distributed, even though the distribution of the outcome variable is highly skewed.

Of course, this is not always the case. To illustrate this, going back to Example 4.3 in which the relationship between triglyceride and overweight is investigated. Output 4.25 shows the result of a linear regression analysis on the original data (i.e. triglyceride without log transformation), while Fig. 4.13 shows the corresponding distribution of the residuals.

In Fig. 4.13 it can be seen that the residuals are not normally distributed and that, therefore, the performed linear regression analysis is not valid. Therefore, the

Output 4.24 Result of the linear regression analysis to analyse the relationship between log transformed triglyceride and overweight

					95% confidence interval	
	Coefficient	se	t-value	p-value	Lower	Upper
Overweight	0.13	0.07	1.94	0.053	−0.001	0.26
Constant	−0.41	0.05	−8.91	<0.001	−0.50	−0.32

se standard error

Output 4.25 Result of the linear regression analysis to analyse the relationship between triglyceride and overweight

	Coefficient	se	t-value	p-value	95% confidence interval Lower	Upper
Overweight	0.15	0.07	2.23	0.03	0.02	0.29
Constant	0.76	0.05	15.45	<0.001	0.66	0.85

se standard error

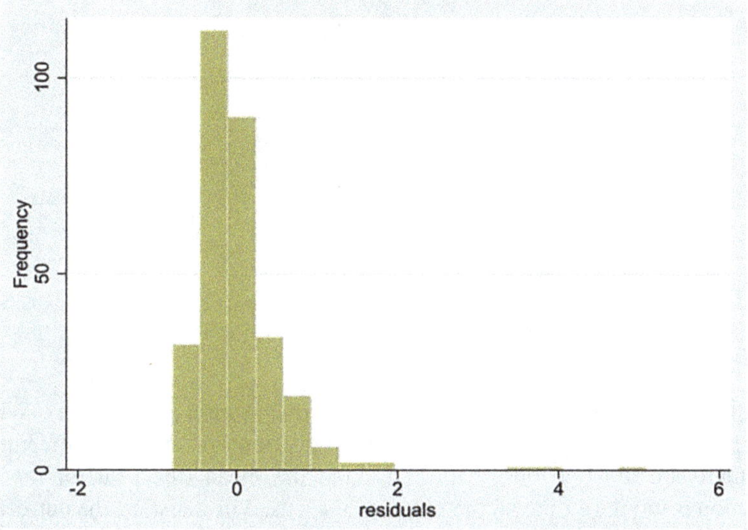

Fig. 4.13 Distribution of the residuals obtained from the linear regression analysis between triglyceride and overweight

triglyceride values are log transformed and a linear regression analysis is performed on the log transformed data (see Output 4.24). Figure 4.14 shows the distribution of the residuals resulting from this analysis. It obvious that the distribution of the residuals derived from the linear regression analysis with log transformed triglyceride as outcome variable is much more normal than the one derived from the linear regression analysis with triglyceride as outcome variable. So, the results derived from the analysis with the log transformed triglyceride as outcome variable must be reported.

It should be noted that there are many other possibilities to evaluate whether the residuals are normally distributed. First of all, there are the so-called skewness and kurtosis. When a distribution is perfectly normal, both skewness and kurtosis are 0. The values for skewness and kurtosis are of course never 0, but it is assumed that there is a more or less normal distribution when the values for skewness and kurtosis are between −1 and +1. When the skewness is >1, there is a skewed to the right distribution, and when the kurtosis is >1, there is a distribution in which most values

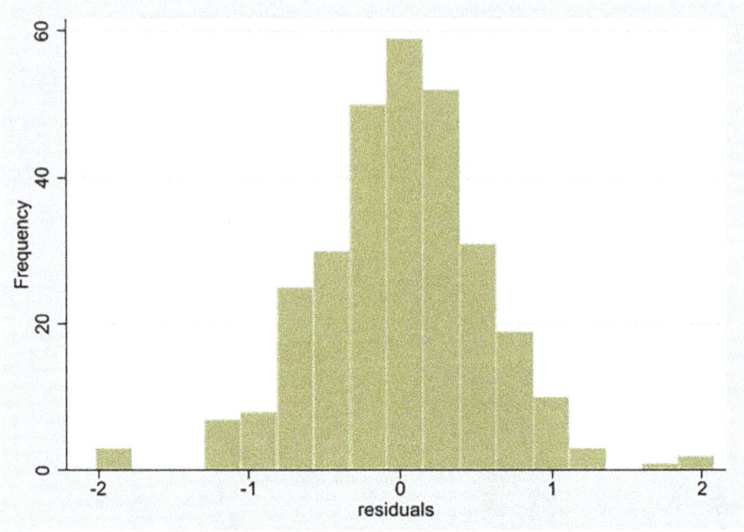

Fig. 4.14 Distribution of the residuals obtained from the linear regression analysis between log transformed triglyceride and overweight

are around the mean (the peak of the normal distribution is too high). When the skewness is <-1, there is a skewed to the left distribution, and when the kurtosis is <-1, there are too few observations around the mean (the peak of the normal distribution is too flat). Like all the cut-off values used in statistics, the cut-off values for skewness and kurtosis (-1 and $+1$) are arbitrary and should therefore be used with caution. In addition to skewness and kurtosis, a statistical test is often used to evaluate whether a certain distribution is more or less normal. The two mostly used statistical tests to test whether a distribution is more or less normal are the Kolmogorov-Smirnov test and the Shapiro-Wilks test. As with all statistical tests, the problem is that the p-value depends on the number of subjects in the study population. When the number of subjects in the study population is small, then the tests do not have enough power to make even large deviations from normality statistically significant, and when the number of subjects in the study population is large, the tests will always give a significant p-value, indicating that the distribution is not normal. Because the result of these tests depend so much on the number of subjects in the study population, the use of these tests is (strongly) discouraged.

In earlier sections of this chapter it has already been indicated that non-parametric methods can be used to analyse non-normally distributed outcome variables. And although there are many different regression analyses available to analyse outcome variables with different distributions (see Chap. 9), for linear regression analysis, there is no direct non-parametric alternative available. The only possibility is to use the non-parametric correlation coefficient.

4.4.8 Non-parametric Correlation Coefficient

In Sect. 4.4.5 it was mentioned that the Pearson correlation coefficient can be used for normally distributed outcome variables. For non-normally distributed outcome variables, the Spearman correlation coefficient can be used. The difference between the two is that the Spearman correlation coefficient is not calculated with the original data but it is calculated with the rank numbers. When the Spearman correlation coefficient is, for example, calculated between cholesterol and age, the coefficient is 0.395, which is slightly higher than the Pearson correlation coefficient, which is 0.372. That the Spearman correlation coefficient is exactly the same as the Pearson correlation coefficient calculated with rank numbers can be illustrated by first determining the rank numbers for both cholesterol and age and then calculating the Pearson correlation coefficient between the two new (rank numbered) variables. The Pearson correlation coefficient calculated with the rank numbers is indeed 0.395.

4.5 Confounding and Effect Modification

When interpreting the result of a statistical analysis, confounding and effect modification can play an important role. Effect modification means that the observed relationship is different for different values of the possible effect modifier. For example, the relationship may be different for males and females, different for young people and old people, and so on. Confounding has to do with the fact that the observed relationship is totally or partly caused by something else. For example, looking at the relationship between cholesterol and age. Suppose that subjects with low social class in the study population are older than subjects with high social class. From an earlier analysis it is known that subjects with low social class have higher cholesterol than subjects with high social class (see Output 4.16). In this situation, the observed relationship between cholesterol and age can be partly or totally caused by social class, which means that the result of the analysis only including age would be an overestimation of the real relationship between cholesterol and age. When that occurs, social class is a confounder in the relationship between cholesterol and age. Of course, confounding can also lead to an underestimation of the relationship. Suppose that the situation is the other way round and that subjects with low social class in the study population are younger than subjects with high social class. In this situation, the observed relationship between cholesterol and age (without taking social class into account) may well be an underestimation of the real relationship between cholesterol and age. The question now is how to use linear regression analysis to take into account confounding and/or to evaluate effect modification.

Going back to the linear regression analysis between cholesterol and age in which a linear relationship between cholesterol and age was assumed. Now, it is evaluated to what extent social class is a confounder in this relationship. Therefore, besides the

Output 4.26 Result of two linear regression analyses to analyse the relationship between cholesterol and age

					95% confidence interval	
Unadjusted	Coefficient	se	t-value	p-value	Lower	Upper
Age	0.02	0.005	3.96	<0.001	0.01	0.03
Constant	3.86	0.23	16.68	<0.001	3.41	4.31
					95% confidence interval	
Adjusted	Coefficient	se	t-value	p-value	Lower	Upper
Age	0.02	0.006	3.34	<0.001	0.01	0.03
Social class	−0.004	0.18	−0.02	0.98	−0.36	0.35
Constant	3.86	0.31	12.17	<0.001	3.23	4.49

se standard error

linear regression analysis with cholesterol and age (i.e. the unadjusted or crude analysis), a second linear regression analysis is performed in which social class is included as an independent variable in the linear regression analysis in addition to age (i.e. the adjusted analysis). Output 4.26 shows the result of both analyses.

In the adjusted analysis, the regression coefficient for age can be interpreted as the relationship between cholesterol and age independent of social class. This means that a comparison is made between subjects who differ in age, but are of the same social class. How can it be assessed whether the relationship between cholesterol and age is confounded by social class? The definition of confounding is that the observed relationship is totally or partly caused by something else. Thus, when this definition is used in the present example, a comparison has to be made between the result of the linear regression analysis without social class (i.e. the unadjusted analysis) and the result of the linear regression analysis with social class (i.e. the adjusted analysis). In this case, the result refers to the magnitude of the regression coefficient for age, because that is the relationship of interest. When the results of both analyses are compared to each other, it can be seen that the regression coefficient for age in the adjusted analysis is the same as in the unadjusted analysis. So, there is no confounding by social class. When the regression coefficient in the adjusted analysis is different from the regression coefficient in the unadjusted analysis it is important to evaluate whether confounding is relevant or not. Mostly the (arbitrary) cut-off value of 10% difference in the magnitude of the regression coefficient between the adjusted and the unadjusted analysis is used.

As stated before, effect modification involves different relationships for different values of the possible effect modifier. Effect modification can also be investigated using linear regression analysis. To do this, an interaction term must be made. This is done by multiplying the independent variable of interest with the possible effect modifier. Next, a linear regression analysis is performed which includes the independent variable of interest, the possible effect modifier, and the interaction term. To explain the principle of effect modification, the linear regression analysis with cholesterol and social class will be used. The question is whether smoking is an effect modifier in this relationship. In other words: whether the relationship between cholesterol and social class is different for smokers and non-smokers. To evaluate whether smoking is an effect modifier in the relationship between cholesterol and social class, first an interaction term is made by multiplying social class with smoking. Second, a linear regression analysis is performed with social class, smoking and the interaction between social class and smoking as independent variables. Output 4.27 shows the result of this analysis.

To understand the interpretation of the different regression coefficients shown in Output 4.27, it is useful to write out the regression equation:

$$cholesterol = b_0 + b_1 \times social\_class + b_2 \times smoking + b_3 \times social\_class \times smoking$$

$$cholesterol = 4.78 - 0.36 \times social\_class + 0.24 \times smoking + 0.59 \times social\_class \times smoking$$

It can be seen that the regression coefficient for social class is 0.36 and it is important to understand the interpretation of this regression coefficient. The regression coefficient can still be interpreted as the difference in cholesterol between subjects with high social class and low social class, but it does not hold for the whole population anymore. Because of the interaction term in the analysis, which includes social class, the regression coefficient for social class only holds for non-smokers (which are coded 0 in the example). This can be seen when the number for the non-smokers is entered into the regression equation.

$$cholesterol = 4.78 - 0.36 \times social\_class + 0.24 \times 0 + 0.59 \times social\_class \times 0$$

The difference in cholesterol between subjects with high social class and low social class can be calculated by first calculating cholesterol for subjects with high social class (i.e. social class = 1) and then by calculating cholesterol for subjects with low social class (i.e. social class = 0):

$$cholesterol_{high\ social\ class} = 4.78 - 0.36 \times 1 + 0.24 \times 0 + 0.59 \times 1 \times 0 = 4.78 - 0.36$$

Output 4.27 Result of the linear regression analysis to analyse the relationship between cholesterol and social class including smoking and the interaction between social class and smoking

					95% confidence interval	
	Coefficient	se	t-value	p-value	Lower	Upper
Social class	−0.36	0.18	−1.98	0.051	−0.71	0.001
Smoking	0.24	0.22	1.07	0.29	−0.20	0.68
Social class*smoking	0.59	0.39	1.52	0.13	−0.18	1.35
Constant	4.78	0.13	36.07	<0.001	4.52	5.04

se standard error

$$cholesterol_{low\ social\ class} = 4.78 - 0.36 \times 0 + 0.24 \times 0 + 0.59 \times 0 \times 0 = 4.78$$

So, the difference in cholesterol between non-smoking subjects with high social class and non-smoking subjects with low social class is 0.36.

The next question is, of course, what is the difference in cholesterol between high social class and low social class for smokers. Again, this can be calculated by entering the number for smokers (i.e. smoking = 1) into the regression equation:

$$cholesterol_{high\ social\ class} = 4.78 - 0.36 \times 1 + 0.24 \times 1 + 0.59 \times 1 \times 1 = 4.78 - 0.36 + 0.24 + 0.59$$

$$cholesterol_{low\ social\ class} = 4.78 - 0.36 \times 0 + 0.24 \times 1 + 0.59 \times 0 \times 1 = 4.78 + 0.24$$

The difference in cholesterol between smokers with high social class and low social class is equal to the sum of the regression coefficient for social class (−0.36) and the regression coefficient for the interaction term (0.59). So, for smokers, the difference in cholesterol between subjects with high social class and low social class is 0.23. The magnitude of the difference between smoking and non-smoking regarding the relationship between cholesterol and social class is, therefore, indicated by the regression coefficient for the interaction term (0.59). So, to answer the question whether there is effect modification by smoking, the magnitude and importance of the regression coefficient for the interaction term must be evaluated.

One way to do that (and by far the most commonly used way) is using the p-value of the interaction term. When the regression coefficient for the interaction term is not statistically significant, there is no statistically significant effect modification. In Output 4.27 it can be seen that the p-value of the interaction term is 0.13, which indicates no statistically significant effect modification due to smoking. So, although the use of statistical significance is questionable, in the evaluation of possible effect modification, statistical significance plays an important role. One of the problems with using statistical significance for evaluating whether or not there is effect modification is that in the analysis including an interaction term, basically the study population is divided into different groups and when the number of subjects in one of the groups is relatively small, the p-value of the interaction term is relatively high due to the relatively small number of subjects in one of the groups. To illustrate this, in the example there is a fairly large difference in the relationship between cholesterol and social class for smokers and non-smokers (0.59) but the corresponding p-value is not statistically significant. To overcome this problem, in many cases a somewhat higher cut-off value (i.e. 0.10) is used for the p-value to evaluate whether there is significant effect modification or not.

Output 4.27 directly shows the difference in cholesterol between subjects with high social class and low social class for non-smokers (−0.36), while the difference between subjects with high social class and low social class for smokers requires two regression coefficients to be added (−0.36 + 0.59). Although that is not a big problem, the standard error of the combined regression coefficient cannot be obtained directly from the output. It is therefore not possible to directly calculate

Output 4.28 Result of the linear regression analysis to analyse the relationship between cholesterol and social class including smoking and the interaction between social class and smoking recoded

					95% confidence interval	
	Coefficient	se	t-value	p-value	Lower	Upper
Social class	0.23	0.34	0.67	0.50	−0.45	0.91
Smoking_recoded	−0.24	0.22	−1.07	0.29	−0.68	0.20
Social_class*smoking_recoded	−0.59	0.39	−1.52	0.13	−1.35	0.18
Constant	5.01	0.18	28.30	<0.001	4.66	5.37

se standard error

the 95% confidence interval for the relationship between cholesterol and social class for smokers. To do this, the variable smoking has to be recoded (i.e. 0 for smokers and 1 for non-smokers). Output 4.28 shows the result of the linear regression analysis with the recoded variable for smoking and the corresponding interaction term.

In Output 4.28 it can be seen that the regression coefficient for social class is 0.23. Due to the different coding for smoking, this regression coefficient now indicates the difference in cholesterol between subjects with high social class and low social class for smokers. This number was already calculated with the result of the first analysis using the interaction term between social class and smoking. However, now it can also be seen that the 95% confidence interval around this difference ranges between −0.45 and 0.91 and that the corresponding p-value is 0.50.

Basically, two things can be done now. The first possibility is that, based on the large difference in the relationship between cholesterol and social class for smokers and non-smokers, it is concluded that there is relevant effect modification. The consequence of this decision is that the magnitude of the relationship between cholesterol and social class for both smokers and non-smokers is reported including the corresponding 95% confidence intervals and p-values. The second possibility is that, based on the statistically non-significant interaction term, it is concluded that there is no relevant effect modification due to smoking. The consequence of this decision is that only the overall relationship between cholesterol and social class is reported. It should be realised that when separate regression coefficients are reported for smokers and non-smokers, it is common practice, also to report the overall relationship (i.e. the relationship in the total population).

Because the interpretation of the regression coefficients in a linear regression analysis with an interaction term is rather complicated, Table 4.15 summarizes the different interpretations.

The interpretation of a regression analysis including an interaction term is a bit more difficult when effect modification is evaluated with a possible continuous effect modifier. Suppose the question is whether age is an effect modifier in the relationship between cholesterol and social class. To evaluate this, an interaction term between social class and age is made, i.e. a multiplication between social class

Table 4.15 Interpretation of the regression coefficients in a linear regression analysis with an interaction term

$y = b_0 + b_1 \times x + b_2 \times em + b_2 \times x \times em$
$y_{0,\,0} = b_0 + b_1 \times 0 + b_2 \times 0 + b_3 \times 0 \times 0 = b_0$
$y_{1,\,0} = b_0 + b_1 \times 1 + b_2 \times 0 + b_3 \times 1 \times 0 = b_0 + b_1$
$y_{0,\,1} = b_0 + b_1 \times 0 + b_2 \times 1 + b_3 \times 1 \times 0 = b_0 + b_2$
$y_{1,\,1} = b_0 + b_1 \times 1 + b_2 \times 1 + b_3 \times 1 \times 1 = b_0 + b_1 + b_2 + b_3$
b_1 = regression coefficient for x when em = 0
$b_1 + b_3$ = regression coefficient for x when em = 1

y outcome variable, *x* independent variable, *em* effect modifier

Output 4.29 Result of the linear regression analysis to analyse the relationship between cholesterol and social class including age and the interaction between social class and age

					95% confidence interval	
	Coefficient	se	t-value	p-value	Lower	Upper
Social class	−0.51	0.53	−0.97	0.34	−1.56	0.54
Age	0.015	0.008	1.98	0.051	−0.000	0.031
Social class*age	0.013	0.013	1.02	0.31	−0.012	0.038
Constant	4.11	0.40	10.35	<0.001	3.31	4.89

se standard error

and age. The importance of this interaction term is then evaluated in a linear regression analysis including social class, age and the interaction between social class and age. Output 4.29 shows the result of this linear regression analysis.

In Output 4.29 it can be seen that the interaction between social class and age is not statistically significant; the p-value of the interaction term is 0.31. Furthermore, it can be seen that the regression coefficient for the interaction term is 0.013. The interpretation of this number is that the magnitude of the relationship between cholesterol and social class (i.e. the difference in cholesterol between subjects with high social class and low social class) is 0.013 higher per age year. It is important to remember that the regression coefficient for social class in Output 4.29 (−0.51) has a different interpretation than in the previous analyses. This regression coefficient now indicates the difference in cholesterol between subjects with high social class and low social class for subjects aged 0. After all, when age is 0, the interaction term is 0. Age is 0 is not present in the dataset, so this number is non-informative. Moreover, the analysis performed assumes that the relationship between cholesterol and social class differs linearly per age year (each year the difference is 0.013 higher) and it is questionable whether this linear difference in the regression coefficient is true.

In this example there is no statistically significant interaction between social class and age (the p-value is 0.31). But, suppose that the interaction term is statistically significant. The question then is what to do with this statistically significant effect modification? When statistically significant effect modification is observed with a dichotomous effect modifier, separate regression coefficients are reported for the two groups of the effect modifier. When statistically significant effect modification is observed with a continuous effect modifier, this procedure is not possible. An alternative, often used solution is to create two groups of the continuous effect modifier (mostly split by the median) and report separate coefficients for the two groups. Another alternative is only to describe the statistically significant effect modification, i.e. by mentioning that the overall relationship is stronger or less strong for higher values of the continuous effect modifier.

4.5.1 *Effect Modification in Analysis of Variance*

In Sect. 4.3 analysis of variance (ANOVA) was introduced as a method to compare the mean value of more than two groups with each other. Within an analysis of variance, also possible effect modification can be investigated by adding an interaction term to the analysis. However, the interpretation of the different effects within an analysis of variance with an interaction is different from the interpretation of the different effects within a linear regression analysis with an interaction. To illustrate this difference, Example 4.4 is used. Example 4.4 is a very small intervention study in which 12 patients with hypertension are treated with either a new intervention or with usual care. The outcome variable of interest is the reduction in systolic blood pressure. Furthermore, overweight is measured as a possible effect modifier. First, the data is analysed with both an analysis of variance and a linear regression analysis in order to estimate the effect of the intervention (see Outputs 4.30 and 4.31).

In the two outputs, it can first be seen that the p-value for the intervention is exactly the same for both methods. So, it shows nicely that analysis of variance and linear regression analysis are basically the same. Furthermore, it can be seen that within a linear regression analysis, the effect of the intervention with the corresponding 95% confidence interval is estimated, while within an analysis of variance only the p-value is given.

Output 4.30 Result of the analysis of variance to analyse the difference in reduction in systolic blood pressure between the intervention and usual care group

	Sum of squares	df	Mean square	F-value	p-value
Between groups	48	1	48	5.2	0.045
Within groups	92	10	9.2		
Total	140	11			

df degrees of freedom

Output 4.31 Result of the linear regression analysis to analyse the relationship between the reduction in systolic blood pressure and the intervention

					95% confidence interval	
	Coefficient	se	t-value	p-value	Lower	Upper
Intervention	4.00	1.75	2.28	0.045	0.10	7.80
Constant	3.00	1.24	2.42	0.036	0.24	5.76

se standard error

Output 4.32 Result of the analysis of variance to analyse the difference in reduction in systolic blood pressure between the intervention and usual care group including the interaction with overweight

	Sum of squares	df	Mean square	F-value	p-value
Intervention	48	1	48	12	0.009
Overweight	48	1	48	12	0.009
Intervention*overweight	12	1	12	3	0.12
Error	32	8	4		
Total	140	11			

df degrees of freedom

Output 4.33 Result of the linear regression analysis to analyse the relationship between the reduction in systolic blood pressure and the intervention including the interaction with overweight

					95% confidence interval	
	Coefficient	se	t-value	p-value	Lower	Upper
Intervention	2.00	1.63	1.22	0.26	−1.77	5.77
Overweight	2.00	1.63	1.22	0.26	−1.77	5.77
Intervention*overweight	4.00	2.31	1.73	0.12	−1.33	9.33
Constant	2.00	1.24	1.73	0.12	−0.66	4.66

se standard error

In the second analysis, the interaction with overweight is added to both the analysis of variance (see Output 4.32) and the linear regression analysis (see Output 4.33).

Comparing the two outputs with each other, it can be seen that the p-value of the interaction term is exactly the same. With both methods, the p-value for the interaction term is 0.12, which indicates a non-statistically significant interaction between the intervention and overweight. It can also be seen that the p-value for the intervention and for overweight are totally different between the two methods. It has already been mentioned that within a linear regression analysis the regression coefficient for the intervention in Output 4.33 (2.00) indicates the difference between the intervention group and the usual care group for subjects with normal weight (i.e. overweight = 0). Within an analysis of variance including an interaction the interpretation of the effect of the intervention is different. It can be seen that the sum of squares for the intervention in the analysis with the interaction is exactly the same as the sum of squares in the analysis without the interaction. So, the interpretation of the p-value for the intervention is also exactly the same. It does not indicate the difference between the intervention group and the usual care group for subjects with normal weight, but it indicates the difference between the intervention group and the usual care group for the whole population. The effect is therefore sometimes called the main effect of the intervention. The reason why the p-value for the intervention derived from the analysis of variance with an interaction is less than the p-value derived from the analysis of variance without an interaction has to do with the increased efficiency of the analysis. Anyway, it is important to realize that an analysis of variance with an interaction should be interpreted differently from a linear regression analysis with an interaction. Not regarding the p-value for the interaction term, but for the variables itself. Within analysis of variance it indicates the main effect of the independent variable (i.e. the effect for the whole population). Within a linear regression analysis, it does not indicate the main effect, but it indicates the effect of the independent variable when the effect modifier is 0.

Chapter 5
The Analysis of a Dichotomous Outcome Variable

Abstract For the analysis of a dichotomous outcome variable cross-tables can be used for the comparison of two groups and the comparison of more than two groups. Based on the cross-table different effect estimates can be derived. Relative risk and risk difference can only be used when the study is prospective, while the odds ratio can be used in all study designs. For statistical testing of these effect estimates, the Fisher exact test or chi-square test can be used. For all these situations, also a regression method is available, i.e. logistic regression analysis. Logistic regression analysis is comparable to linear regression analysis in a way that the regression coefficients have the same interpretation, only the outcome variable is different. In a logistic regression analysis, the outcome variable is the natural log of the odds of having the dichotomous outcome variable. Because of that the regression coefficient for an independent variable can be transformed into an odds ratio. In this chapter, furthermore, the evaluation of linearity of the relationship with a continuous independent variable, the adjustment for confounding and the investigation of effect modification are discussed. The way this is done in logistic regression analysis is exactly the same as in linear regression analysis.

5.1 Comparing Two Groups

5.1.1 Introduction

To compare a dichotomous outcome variable between two groups, a simple way to present the result is a so-called 2 × 2 table. Table 5.1 shows the 2 × 2 table derived from Example 5.1. Example 5.1 is a randomized controlled trial in which 200 patients with low back pain are randomized into an intervention group and a control group. The intervention group received an activity program, while the control group received usual care. The outcome variable, perceived recovery, is dichotomous: the patient is recovered or not recovered. In Table 5.1, the number of patients recovered and not recovered are compared between the intervention group and the usual care group.

J. W. R. Twisk, *Basic Principles of Applied Medical Statistics*,
https://doi.org/10.1007/978-3-031-86278-6_5

Table 5.1 2 × 2 table with the number of patients recovered and not recovered in both groups

	Recovered	Not recovered	Total
Intervention	40	60	100
Usual care	20	80	100
Total	60	140	200

In Table 5.1 it can be seen that the probability of recovery is 0.40 (40/100) in the intervention group and 0.20 (20/100) in the usual care group. The two probabilities can be used to estimate the effect of the intervention. The first option is to calculate the difference between the two probabilities. This difference is called the risk difference, which is 0.20 (0.40–0.20) in the present example. The second possibility is to calculate the ratio of the two probabilities. This ratio is called the relative risk and is 2 (0.40/0.20). It should be noted that, even though the outcome variable in the example is positive, i.e. recovery, the term risk is used. Anyway, the conclusion of both effect estimates is that the intervention group performs better than the usual care group.

As has been mentioned before, in the next step, it is important to evaluate to what extend the observed result can be generalized to the source population. A risk difference of 0.20 is obtained in the study population, but does that also apply to all other patients who are going to receive the intervention? This information is essential in order to be able to make the final decision whether or not to implement the intervention (i.e. the activity program) to new patients. In this respect, it is important to quantify the uncertainty of the observed result.

5.1.2 95% Confidence Interval Around Risk Difference and Relative Risk

In Chap. 3, it has been mentioned that the uncertainty of an effect estimate depends on the number of subjects in the study population and on the standard deviation of the outcome variable. The probability to have a dichotomous outcome variable is basically a proportion, and the standard deviation of a proportion can be calculated with Eq. 5.1.

$$sd(p) = \sqrt{p(1-p)} \tag{5.1}$$

where $sd(p)$ = standard deviation of a proportion and p = proportion.

The standard error of a proportion can then be calculated (as with continuous outcome variables) by dividing the standard deviation by the square root of the number of subjects (see Eq. 5.2).

$$se(p) = \sqrt{\frac{p(1-p)}{n}} \tag{5.2}$$

where $se(p)$ = standard error of a proportion, p = proportion and n = number of subjects.

In the example, however, the effect estimate is a difference in proportions. The standard error of a difference in proportions can be calculated with Eq. 5.3.

$$se(p_1 - p_2) = \sqrt{\frac{p_1(1-p_1)}{n_1} + \frac{p_2(1-p_2)}{n_2}} \tag{5.3}$$

where $se(p_1 - p_2)$= standard error of a difference in proportions, p_1, p_2 = proportions in both groups and n_1, n_2 = number of subjects in both groups.

When the numbers from Table 5.1 are entered into Eq. 5.3, the standard error for the risk difference is 0.063.

$$se(p_1 - p_2) = \sqrt{\frac{0.40(1-0.40)}{100} + \frac{0.20(1-0.20)}{100}} = 0.063$$

The 95% confidence interval around the risk difference can then be calculated using a normal approximation (see Eq. 5.4).

$$p_1 - p_2 \pm z_{(1-\alpha/2)} \times se(p_1 - p_2) \tag{5.4}$$

where $p_1 - p_2$= difference in proportions, $z_{(1-\alpha/2)}$ = value of the standard normal distribution for which $(1-\alpha/2)\%$ of the distribution is below that value and $se(p_1 - p_2)$ = standard error of a difference in proportions.

When the results of the example are entered into Eq. 5.4, the 95% confidence interval ranges between 0.08 and 0.32.

$$0.20 \pm 1.96 \times 0.063 = [0.08 - 0.32]$$

Based on the 95% confidence interval, a statement can also be made about the statistical significance of the risk difference. To do this, it is necessary to evaluate whether the value of the null hypothesis is inside or outside the 95% confidence interval. The value of the null hypothesis in this case is 0 (i.e. there is no difference in recovery proportions between the two groups) and that number is outside the 95% confidence interval. So, there is a statistically significant difference in recovery proportions between the intervention and the usual care group.

It has been mentioned before that the calculation of the 95% confidence interval is based on a normal approximation. Because of that, 1.96 times the standard error is used as a measure of uncertainty. This normal approximation performs well when the number of subjects in the study population is large and when the observed

Table 5.2 Example of a 2 × 2 table

	Outcome variable +	Outcome variable −	Total
Independent variable +	a	b	a + b
Independent variable −	c	d	c + d
Total	a + c	b + d	a + b + c + d

proportions are closer to 0.50. Most statistical textbooks state that the normal approximation should only be used when the number of subjects multiplied by the observed proportion is ≥5 and when the number of subjects multiplied by the complement of the observed proportion is also ≥5. It should be noted that arbitrary cut-off values like this must be treated with caution and must certainly not be interpreted absolutely. Of course, it is not the case that the normal approximation goes wrong in a research situation where the numbers are just below the cut-off value, while it goes well in a research situation where the numbers are just above the cut-off value. There is more or less a continuum: the normal approximation performs better when the number of subjects in the study population become larger and the observed proportions are closer to 0.50.

Besides the risk difference, also the relative risk is an effect estimate which is often used. In Example 5.1, the relative risk to recover for the activity program compared to usual care is 2. For the calculation of the 95% confidence interval around the relative risk, it is important to realize that (when the null hypothesis is true) the relative risk has a skewed to the right distribution. After all, the value of the null hypothesis is 1, the minimum value is 0, and the maximum value is ∞. In order to calculate a 95% confidence interval, first a log transformation has to be performed. Second, the standard error of the log transformed value of the relative risk must be calculated (see Eq. 5.5).

$$se[ln(RR)] = \sqrt{\left[\frac{1}{a} - \frac{1}{(a+b)} + \frac{1}{c} - \frac{1}{(c+d)}\right]} \tag{5.5}$$

where $se[ln(RR)]$ = standard error of the natural logarithm of the relative risk and a, b, c and d = number of subjects in the cells of the 2 × 2 table (see Table 5.2).

When the numbers of Table 5.1 are entered into Eq. 5.5, the standard error of the natural logarithm of the relative risk is 0.23.

$$se[ln(RR)] = \sqrt{\left[\frac{1}{40} - \frac{1}{(40+60)} + \frac{1}{20} - \frac{1}{(20+80)}\right]} = 0.23$$

Subsequently, a 95% confidence interval can be calculated around the natural logarithm of relative risk with Eq. 5.6.

$$ln(RR) \pm z_{(1-\alpha/2)} \times se[ln(RR)] \tag{5.6}$$

where $ln(RR)$= natural logarithm of the relative risk, $z_{(1-\alpha/2)}$ = value of the standard normal distribution for which $(1 - \alpha/2)\%$ of the distribution is below that value and $se[ln(RR)]$= standard error of the natural logarithm of the relative risk.

When the different values are entered into Eq. 5.6, the 95% confidence interval around the natural logarithm of the relative risk ranges between 0.24 and 1.14.

$$ln(2) \pm 1.96 \times 0.23 = [0.24 - 1.14]$$

Because this confidence interval is around the natural logarithm of the relative risk, it needs to be transformed back to calculate a 95% confidence interval around the relative risk. This can be done by taking the e-power of both the upper and lower limit of the 95% confidence interval. When this is done, the 95% confidence interval around the relative risk ranges between 1.27 and 3.14. Based on this interval, it can also be concluded that the relative risk is statistically significant, because the value of the null hypothesis (in this case 1) is outside the 95% confidence interval. Because the relative risk is measured on a logarithmic scale, It should be noted that this confidence interval is not symmetric around the observed relative risk. The upper limit is further away from the observed relative risk than the lower limit (for a relative risk less than 1, it is, of course, just the other way around).

5.1.3 Statistical Testing of Risk Difference and Relative Risk

Based on the 95% confidence interval around the risk difference, it was concluded that the risk difference was statistically significant. To obtain the p-value for the risk difference, different approaches can be used. First of all, a test statistic can be generated (see Eq. 5.7).

$$z = \frac{(p_1 - p_2) - 0}{se(p_1 - p_2)_{H0}} \tag{5.7}$$

where z = test statistic, $(p_1 - p_2)$ = observed difference in proportions and $se(p_1 - p_2)_{H0}$= standard error of the difference in proportions when the null hypothesis is true.

It is important to realize that the standard error of the difference in proportions is not the same as the one shown in Eq. 5.3, which was used to calculate the 95% confidence interval. To calculate the confidence interval, the standard error of the observed difference in proportions is used, while the standard error of the difference in proportions when the null hypothesis is true is used for statistical testing. Because the proportions are directly related to the standard error (see, for example, Eqs. 5.2 and 5.3), the two standard errors are not the same. Equations 5.8a and 5.8b can be used to calculate the standard error of the difference between two proportions when the null hypothesis is true.

$$se(p_1 - p_2)_{H0} = \sqrt{\frac{\widehat{p}(1-\widehat{p})}{n_1} + \frac{\widehat{p}(1-\widehat{p})}{n_2}} \tag{5.8a}$$

$$\widehat{p} = \frac{(r_1 + r_2)}{(n_1 + n_2)} \tag{5.8b}$$

where $\widehat{p}$ = expected proportion when the null hypothesis is true, r_1, r_2=number of subjects with the outcome variable of interest in both groups and n_1, n_2= number of subjects in both groups.

When the results shown in Table 5.1 are entered into Eq. 5.7 the standard error is 0.065.

$$\widehat{p} = \frac{(40 + 20)}{(100 + 100)} = 0.3$$

$$se(p_1 - p_2)_{H0} = \sqrt{\frac{0.3 \times 0.7}{100} + \frac{0.3 \times 0.7}{100}} = 0.065$$

So, the standard error of the difference in proportions when the null hypothesis is true (0.065) is indeed slightly different from the standard error of the difference in observed proportions (0.063). With the standard error of the difference in proportions when the null hypothesis is true, the test statistic can be calculated and the corresponding p-value can be obtained.

$$z = \frac{(0.4 - 0.2) - 0}{0{,}065} = 3.08$$

The corresponding p-value of this z-value, which can be derived from the normal probability distribution (see Table 3.8), is 0.003. Because the statistical test and the 95% confidence interval use a different standard error, it is important to realize that in the context of statistical significance, the statistical test may lead to a different conclusion than the statistical test based on the 95% confidence interval. However, this will only happen in situations where the p-value is very close to the 0.05 cut-off value.

The second option to obtain the p-value for the risk difference is the chi-square test. Basically, the chi-square test does not provide a p-value only for the risk difference, the p-value is related to the whole 2 × 2 table. To perform a chi-square test, first, it is necessary to calculate how many subjects are expected in the different cells of the 2 × 2 table when the null hypothesis is true. In other words, how many subjects are expected to be in the different cells of the 2 × 2 table when there is no effect of the intervention or when there is no relationship between the dichotomous outcome variable and the independent group variable. To calculate this number, a

Table 5.3 Example of a simple 2 × 2 table

	Outcome variable +	Outcome variable −	Total
Independent variable +			10
Independent variable −			10
Total	10	10	20

Table 5.4 Example of a simple 2 × 2 table as a study result

	Outcome variable +	Outcome variable −	Total
Independent variable +	8	2	10
Independent variable −	2	8	10
Total	10	10	20

rule from probability theory can be used: when two probabilities are independent of each other, they can be multiplied. When, for example, a die is rolled twice, the probability of twice a 6 is equal to 1/6 (for the first roll) multiplied by 1/6 (for the second roll), which is 1/36. That is because both rolls of the die are independent of each other. So, using this rule, the probability that a subject is in a certain cell of a 2 × 2 table can be calculated. To do this, the probability that a subject is in a certain row must be multiplied by the probability that a subject is in a certain column. For illustrative purposes, Table 5.3 shows a simple 2 × 2 table.

The probability to be in the upper left cell in the 2 × 2 table when the null hypothesis is true is equal to the probability of being in the first row (10/20) multiplied by the probability of being in the first column (10/20). So, when the null hypothesis is true, that probability is 0.25. When this probability is multiplied by the number of subjects in the study population (20), the result is the expected number of subjects in the particular cell. In this simple example, when the null hypothesis is true, the upper left cell is expected to contain five subjects. Exactly the same calculation can be performed for the other cells. So, when the null hypothesis is true, five subjects are expected to be in all cells of the 2 × 2 table. Suppose now that Table 5.4 is observed as a result in a particular study.

To calculate the probability of finding this 2 × 2 table (or values even further away from the null hypothesis) when the null hypothesis is true, the observed number of subjects must be compared to the expected number of subject in each cell of the 2 × 2 table. The test statistic (i.e. chi-square) can be calculated as shown in Eq. 5.9.

$$\chi^2 = \sum \left[\frac{(O - E)^2}{E} \right] \tag{5.9}$$

where χ^2= chi-square test statistic, O = observed number of subjects, and E = expected number of subjects when the null hypothesis is true.

For each cell, the difference between the observed number of subjects and the expected number of subjects is squared and then divided by the expected number of subjects. Added together, the number is the chi-square test statistic. The chi-square

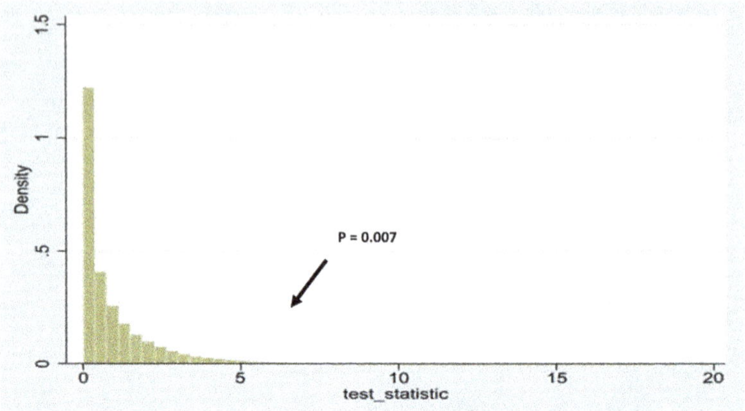

Fig. 5.1 Chi-square distribution with one degree of freedom; probability ($\chi^2 \geq 7.2$) = 0.007

Table 5.5 p-values of a chi-square distribution for different chi-square (χ^2) values and a different number of degrees of freedom

	Number of degrees of freedom			
p-value	1	2	3	10
	χ^2	χ^2	χ^2	χ^2
0.50	0.45	1.39	2.37	9.34
0.20	1.32	2.77	4.11	12.55
0.10	2.71	4.61	6.25	15.99
0.05	3.84	5.99	7.81	18.31
0.01	6.63	9.21	11.34	23.21
0.005	7.88	10.60	12.84	25.19
0.001	10.83	13.82	16.27	29.59

test statistic has a chi-square distribution with one degree of freedom. The chi-square distribution (like the t-distribution and the standard normal distribution) is a probability distribution, and like the t-distribution, the shape of the chi-square distribution depends on the number of degrees of freedom.

That there is one degree of freedom in this situation can easily be seen by taking an arbitrary 2 × 2 table with given total numbers of the rows and columns. In such a 2 × 2 table, one number can be chosen freely and the other three numbers are then fixed, which means that there is one degree of freedom.

In the simple example of Table 5.4, the chi-square test statistic is equal to: $(8–5)^2 / 5 + (2–5)^2 /5 + (2–5)^2 /5 + (8–5)^2 /5 = 7.2$. This value has a chi-square distribution with one degree of freedom and the corresponding p-value is 0.007 (see Fig. 5.1).

Table 5.5 shows the p-values for a chi-square distributions with different chi-square (χ^2) values and a different number of degrees of freedom.

It should be noted that using the chi-square test for calculating the p-value belonging to this 2 × 2 table is an approximation. The approximation improves as the expected numbers in the different cells are higher. Again, there is an arbitrary cut-off for this approximation, which is known as the rule of 5, i.e. the chi-square test is assumed to be correct when the expected numbers in 80% of the cells are ≥5 and when the expected numbers are >1 in all cells. In the example in Table 5.1, the chi-square test should work well, because in all cells the expected number is 5. It should be realized that the rule of 5 uses an arbitrary cut-off, where there is basically a continuum: when the expected numbers in the cells become larger, the p-value obtained from the chi-square test will be a better approximation of the exact p-value. So, again, the cut-off value should be treated with caution.

The exact p-value related to a 2 × 2 table can be calculated with the Fisher exact test. The calculation of the p-value of the Fisher exact test is explained using the simple example shown in Table 5.4. The first step in calculating the exact p-value is to make all the combinations that are possible with the row and column totals from Table 5.4. Table 5.6 shows all possible combinations.

In the next step, the probability of a particular combination (when the null hypothesis is true) can be calculated with Eqs. 5.10a and 5.10b. This can be done for all possible combinations.

$$p = \frac{(a+b)!(a+c)!(b+d)!(c+d)!}{n!a!b!c!d!} \tag{5.10a}$$

$$a! = 1 \times 2 \times 3 \times \ldots\ldots\ldots\ldots \times a \tag{5.10b}$$

where p = probability of a combination, a, b, c and d = numbers in the cells of the 2 × 2 table (see Table 5.2), n = number of subjects and $a!$ = a factorial.

For the first combination, for example, the probability is 0.0000054.

$$p = \frac{(10+0)!(10+0)!(0+10)!(10+0)!}{20!10!0!10!0!} = 0.0000054$$

In other words, when the null hypothesis is true (i.e. there is no relationship between the two variables), the probability of the most extreme combination away from the null hypothesis is 0.0000054. Table 5.7 gives an overview of the probability for all possible combinations. Of course, the sum of the probabilities for all possible combinations is 1.

The next step in the calculation of the exact p-value is to find the probability for the 2 × 2 table observed in the study and the probability of the combinations that are further away from the null hypothesis. The 2 × 2 table observed in the example is combination 3 and Table 5.7 shows that the probability of that combination (when the null hypothesis is true) is 0.01096. Further away from the null hypothesis are combination 2 and combination 1 and those probabilities must therefore be added to the probability of 0.01096. The total probability is then 0.01096 + 0.00054 + 0.0000054 = 0.0115. However, this is a one-tailed probability. For the two-tailed probability, the probabilities on the other side of the null hypothesis must also be taken into account. Because all row and column totals are equal, the probability distribution is symmetric (when the row and column totals are not equal the probability distribution is not symmetric) and because of the symmetry, the same

Table 5.6 All possible 2 × 2 tables, given the row and column totals shown in Table 5.4

1	
10	0
0	10

2	
9	1
1	9

3	
8	2
2	8

4	
7	3
3	7

5	
6	4
4	6

6	
5	5
5	5

7	
4	6
6	4

8	
3	7
7	3

9	
2	8
8	2

10	
1	9
9	1

11	
0	10
10	0

probability is added for the two-tailed probability. The two-tailed exact probability is therefore 0.0230. In other words, the probability of finding the observed 2 × 2 table (or even further away from the null hypothesis) when the null hypothesis is true is 0.0230. Output 5.1 shows the result of the Fisher exact test and the chi-square test for the result which were shown in Table 5.4.

In Output 5.1 it can be seen that the p-value based on the Fisher exact test is 0.023 and that the chi-square test gives a p-value of 0.007. So, despite the fact that according to the arbitrary rule of 5 the chi-square test can be used, the chi-square test provides a p-value which is (much) too low. It should be noted that the chi-square test always gives a lower p-value than the Fisher exact test, and perhaps

Table 5.7 Overview of the probabilities of possible combinations (see Table 5.6)

Combination	Probability
1	0.0000054
2	0.00054
3	0.01096
4	0.07794
5	0.23869
6	0.34372
7	0.23869
8	0.07794
9	0.01096
10	0.00054
11	0.0000054

Output 5.1 Result of the Fisher exact test and the chi-square test for the 2 × 2 table shown in Table 5.4

	Value	df	Asymptotic p-value	Exact p-value (1-sided)	Exact p-value (2-sided)
Fisher exact test				0.012	0.023
Chi-square test	7.200	1	0.007		

that is one of the reasons why the chi-square test is very popular. In fact, it is very strange that the approximation (i.e. the chi-square test) is so often used when analysing 2 × 2 tables, while it is also possible to obtain the exact p-value with the Fisher exact test.

The chi-square test was developed in a period when hardly any statistical software was available. Calculating the exact p-value with the Fisher exact test without statistical software was so extensive that the chi-square test was developed as a relatively simple way to approximate the p-value as closely as possible. Nowadays it is no longer necessary to approximate the p-value related to a certain 2 × 2 table using the chi-square test, because the exact p-value can be calculated very easily with statistical software. Despite this, most people use the chi-square test by default, and only use the Fisher exact test when the expected numbers in the 2 × 2 table are too small, i.e. do not meet the rule of 5. Again, a strange statistical misunderstanding.

There is another possibility to adjust the too low p-value of the chi-square test and that is the so-called continuity correction. The continuity correction is also known as Yates correction and because it is always better to use the Fisher exact test, nowadays, the continuity correction is not much used in practice.

Also in Example 5.1 it is of course possible to perform the Fisher exact test and the chi-square test for the comparison of recovery proportions in the intervention group and the usual care group. Output 5.2 shows this result.

Output 5.2 Result of the Fisher exact test and the chi-square test to analyse the difference in recovery proportions

	Value	df	Asymptotic p-value	Exact p-value (1-sided)	Exact p-value (2-sided)
Fisher exact test				0.002	0.003
Chi-square test	9.524	1	0.002		

Output 5.2 shows that there is only a small difference between the p-values of the Fisher exact test and the chi-square test. This has to do with the relatively large number of subjects in the study population.

In the previous section of this chapter, two approximation methods have been used to calculate the p-value of a risk difference. First, using the z-value and second, using the chi-square test. Basically, the calculated chi-square value is exactly the same as the z-value squared. This has to do with the fact that a chi-square distribution with one degree of freedom (the chi-square distribution used for a 2 × 2 table) is identical to the standard normal distribution squared. Although the two approaches appear to take a very different starting point, they are in fact identical.

In Sect. 5.1.2 it was concluded that, based on the 95% confidence interval, there was a statistically significant relative risk. To calculate the p-value associated with the relative risk, also the Fisher exact test (or the chi-square test) can be used. It is important to realize that the p-value for the risk difference and the p-value for the relative risk are the same. This is due to the fact that the p-value is calculated for the 2 × 2 table. So two different effect sizes, one p-value.

Because both the relative risk and the risk difference are calculated from the same 2 × 2 table, the question can be asked which of the two effect estimates can best be used. In practice, the relative risk is most commonly used, although the risk difference is better interpretable. When interpreting the relative risk, it is important to know the value of the absolute risk to get a certain dichotomous outcome variable. For example, when the effect of a certain risk factor on the development of a disease is analysed and the probability of getting the disease is very low, then a high relative risk for a particular risk factor will still mean that the absolute risk to get the disease for that particular risk factor is rather low. For the risk difference, this problem does not exist, because the absolute risk is part of the risk difference.

5.1.4 Comparing One Proportion to a Standard Value

Sometimes, researchers may be interested in the extent to which the observed proportion is different from a certain standard value. Output 5.1 showed, for instance, that the recovery proportion in the intervention group is 0.40. Now suppose that there is interest in the question whether this proportion is different from 0.50. The answer is simple: yes, the recovery proportion in the intervention group is less than 0.50. To evaluate whether this result can be generalized to the source population, the uncertainty of the observed result must be quantified. First of all, this can be done by calculating a 95% confidence interval around the observed proportion of 0.40 (see Eq. 5.11).

$$p \pm z_{(1-\alpha/2)} \times se(p) \tag{5.11}$$

where p = proportion, $z_{(1-\alpha/2)}$ = value of the standard normal distribution for which $(1-\alpha/2)\%$ of the distribution is below that value and $se(p)$ = standard error of the proportion.

The standard error of a proportion can be calculated using Eq. 5.2 and when this standard error is entered into Eq. 5.11, the 95% confidence interval ranges between 0.304 and 0.496.

$$0.4 \pm 1.96 \times \sqrt{\frac{0.4(1-0.4)}{100}} = [0.304 - 0.496]$$

The value of the null hypothesis (i.e. 0.50) is just outside the 95% confidence interval, so the observed proportion of 0.40 is statistically significantly different from 0.50. Also in this situation the normal approximation is used and again the approximation works better when the number of subjects in the study population is large and the observed proportion is closer to 0.50 (see Sect. 5.1.2). Of course, also the probability of finding a proportion of 0.40 (or even further away from the null hypothesis) when the null hypothesis (i.e. a proportion of 0.50) is true can be calculated. To do this, a similar test statistic must be calculated as has been done in Eq. 5.7 (see Eq. 5.12).

$$z = \frac{p - 0.50}{se(p)_{H_0}} \tag{5.12}$$

where z = value of the standard normal distribution, p = observed proportion and $se(p)_{H_0}$ = standard error of the proportion when the null hypothesis is true.

Also in this situation, the standard error used for statistical testing is different from the standard error used for calculating the 95% confidence interval. For statistical testing, the standard error of the value of the null hypothesis is used, while for the 95% confidence interval, the standard error of the observed value is used. When the numbers from the example are entered into Eq. 5.12, the test statistic (z-value) is 2, which leads to a p-value just below 0.05 (see Table 3.8 for the p-values belonging to different z-values).

$$z = \frac{0.40 - 0.50}{\sqrt{\frac{0.50(1 - 0.50)}{100}}} = 2$$

5.2 Comparing Two Observations Within the Same Subject

In Sect. 4.1 it was mentioned that for a continuous outcome variable, the differences between two observations within the same subject can be analysed with a paired t-test. For dichotomous outcome variables, a similar method is available. This method, which is known as the McNemar test, is much less known than the paired t-test. This probably has to do with the fact that paired observations with a dichotomous outcome variable are not as common as paired observations with a continuous outcome variable. One of the research designs in which these types of observations occur is a crossover intervention study which is also known as a crossover trial. In a crossover trial, the subjects are used as their own control and instead of randomizing the subjects, mostly the order of the intervention and control condition is randomized. In most crossover trials half of the subjects receive the intervention first and then the control condition, while the other half receive the control condition first and then the intervention. It should be clear that crossover trials are only suitable for interventions that produce a short-term effect, because otherwise the starting point for both conditions will differ and the conditions can no longer be compared within the same subject. Crossover trials are regularly used in studies investigating the effect of pain killers, blood thinners and so on.

The McNemar test will be illustrated using Example 5.2, a crossover trial in which two painkillers (drug A and drug B) are compared to each other. Fifty patients participated in the study; 25 patients received drug A first and then drug B, the other 25 patients received drug B first and then drug A. The dichotomous outcome variable is improvement. Table 5.8 shows the result of this study.

In Table 5.8 it can be seen that of the 50 patients who received drug A, 30 improved and that of the same 50 patients who received drug B, only 20 improved. In short, the difference in proportion improvement between drug A and B is 0.20. However, because in a crossover trial the same subjects receive both interventions, the groups that are compared are not independent of each other. The 2 × 2 table shown in Table 5.8 is, therefore, not a good representation of the result of the crossover trial. The result of the crossover trial should be presented in a different way (see Table 5.9).

Table 5.8 Result of a crossover trial to compare two painkillers

	Improved	Not improved	Total
Drug A	30	20	50
Drug B	20	30	50
Total	50	50	100

Table 5.9 Result of a crossover trial to compare two painkillers

		Drug B		
		Improved	Not improved	Total
Drug A	Improved	8	22	30
	Not improved	12	8	20
	Total	20	30	

Table 5.10 General 2 × 2 table for paired observations in a dichotomous outcome variable

		Drug B		
		Outcome variable +	Outcome variable –	Total
Drug A	Outcome variable +	a	b	
	Outcome variable –	c	d	
	Total			n

Table 5.9 shows that there are 50 subjects who used both drug A and drug B. When the proportion of subjects who improved using drug A is compared to the proportion of subjects who improved using drug B, this will of course again result in a difference of 0.20. The difference with an analysis based on independent observations is related to the calculation of the 95% confidence interval and the corresponding p-value.

Table 5.10 shows the general 2 × 2 table for paired observations in a dichotomous outcome variable.

The difference between the two proportions with outcome variable +, and the corresponding standard error can be calculated using Eqs. 5.13a and 5.13b.

$$p_1 - p_2 = \frac{(a+b)}{n} - \frac{(a+c)}{n} = \frac{(b-c)}{n} \tag{5.13a}$$

$$se(p_1 - p_2) = \frac{1}{n}\sqrt{b + c - \frac{(b-c)^2}{n}} \tag{5.13b}$$

where $p_1 - p_2 =$ difference in proportions, a, b, c and $d =$ number of subjects in the different cells of the 2 × 2 table as shown in Table 5.10, n = total number of subjects and $se(p_1 - p_2) =$ standard error of the difference in proportions.

When the numbers shown in Table 5.9 are entered into Eqs. 5.13a and 5.13b, the standard error is 0.133.

$$p_1 - p_2 = \frac{(8+22)}{50} - \frac{(8+12)}{50} = \frac{(22-12)}{50} = 0.2$$

$$se(p_1 - p_2) = \frac{1}{50}\sqrt{22 + 12 - \frac{(22-12)^2}{50}} = 0.133$$

Using the standard error, the 95% confidence interval around the observed difference in proportions can be calculated with Eq. 5.14.

$$p_1 - p_2 \pm z_{(1-\alpha/2)} \times se(p_1 - p_2) \tag{5.14}$$

where $p_1 - p_2 =$ difference in proportions, $z_{(1-\alpha/2)}$ = value of the standard normal distribution for which $(1 - \alpha/2)\%$ of the distribution is below that value and $se(p_1 - p_2) =$ standard error of the difference in proportions.

When the calculated standard error is entered into Eq. 5.14, the 95% confidence interval ranges between −0.02 and 0.42.

$$p_1 - p_2 \pm 1.96 \times 0.133 = [-0.02 - 0.42]$$

It can be seen that the value 0 (i.e. the value of the null hypothesis) is inside the 95% confidence interval and that, therefore, the observed difference in proportions of 0.20 is not statistically significant. The corresponding p-value can be calculated using the McNemar test (i.e. a chi-square test for paired observations).

The test statistic of the McNemar test can be calculated with Eq. 5.15a and 5.1b.

$$z = \frac{|b - c|}{\sqrt{b + c}} \tag{5.15a}$$

$$\chi^2 = \frac{(b - c)^2}{b + c} \tag{5.15b}$$

where $z =$ value of the standard normal distribution, b and $c =$ number of subjects in the different cells of the 2 × 2 table as shown in Table 5.10 and $\chi^2 =$ chi-square test statistic.

When the numbers of Table 5.8 (i.e. the result of the study) are entered into Eq. 5.15b, the chi-square value is 2.94 and based on a chi-square distribution with one degree of freedom, this gives to a p-value between 0.05 and 0.10 (see Table 5.5).

$$\chi^2 = \frac{(12 - 22)^2}{12 + 22} = \frac{100}{34} = 2.94$$

The equation to calculate the test statistic only contains the number of subjects who improve with one drug but not with the other. This is due to the fact that subjects who improve with both drugs or do not improve with both drugs do not provide information about the difference between the two drugs. Output 5.3 shows the result of the McNemar test (Example 5.2).

Output 5.3 shows the chi-square value of 2.94 and the corresponding p-value of 0.09 (which is indeed between 0.05 and 0.10). The output also shows the exact p-value of 0.12. This exact p-value is calculated including a continuity correction (see Sect. 5.1.3).

Output 5.3 Result of the McNemar test to compare two painkillers

	Chi-square	Degrees of freedom	p-value
McNemar test	2.94	1	0.09
Exact			0.12

Table 5.11 2 × 3 table with the number of patients recovered and not recovered in the three groups

	Recovered	Not recovered	Total
Intervention 1	40	60	100
Intervention 2	50	50	100
Usual care	20	80	100
Total	110	190	300

Intervention 1 = activity; intervention 2 = activity plus behavioural therapy

5.3 Comparing More than Two Groups

Suppose that in the study of Example 5.1, in which the effect of an activity program is investigated in patients with low back pain, a second intervention group is included. In addition to the activity program, this second intervention group also received behavioural therapy. The second intervention group also consists of 100 patients (Example 5.1a). The result of the study can be shown in a 2 × 3 table (see Table 5.11).

In Table 5.11 it can be seen that in the second intervention group, the recovery proportion is 0.50. The recovery proportions for the control group and the first intervention group are, of course, the same as in the example comparing two groups. The research situation described here is to a large extent comparable to the comparison of three groups for a continuous outcome variable. In that case, an analysis of variance was performed in which an overall p-value was provided for the association between the continuous outcome variable and the categorical independent variable (see Sect. 4.3). More or less the same can be done for the comparison of three groups for a dichotomous outcome variable. The overall association between the dichotomous outcome variable (i.e. recovery) and the independent variable (i.e. the three groups) can be statistically tested using the Fisher exact test or the chi-square test. The general idea of both methods is exactly the same as in the situation when two groups are compared to each other. For instance, for the chi-square test, for each cell in the 2 × 3 table, the expected number of patients must be calculated when the null hypothesis is true. Table 5.12 shows the expected numbers in the cells of the 2 × 3 table shown in Table 5.11.

In Table 5.12 it can be seen that, when the null hypothesis is true, in all three groups 63.3 patients are expected to be not recovered and 36.7 patients are expected to be recovered. Using Eq. 5.9, the chi-square value can be calculated. This value is 20.096 and has a chi-square distribution with two degrees of freedom. The number of degrees of freedom for any cross table can be calculated by multiplying the number of rows − 1 by the number of columns − 1. So, for a 2 × 3 table there are two degrees of freedom. The p-value associated with a chi-square value of 20.096

Table 5.12 2 × 3 table with the expected number of patients recovered and not recovered in the three groups when the null hypothesis is true

	Recovered	Not recovered	Total
Intervention 1	36.7	63.3	100
Intervention 2	36.7	63.3	100
Usual care	36.7	63.3	100
Total	110	190	300

Intervention 1 = activity; intervention 2 = activity plus behavioural therapy

Output 5.4 Result of the Fisher exact test and the chi-square test for the 2 × 3 table shown in Table 5.11

	Value	df	Asymptotic p-value	Exact p-value (2-sided)
Fisher exact test				<0.001
Chi-square test	20.096	2	<0.001	

(with two degrees of freedom) is <0.001. In this situation also the Fisher Exact test can be performed and the two-sided p-value of the Fischer Exact test is also <0.001 (see Output 5.4).

When a 2 × 3 table is analysed, sometimes a p-value is given for the linear-by-linear association. This statistical test is also known as the test for trend. The test for trend only has an interpretable p-value when the independent variable (i.e. the variable with more than two groups) is an ordinal categorical variable. The test for trend always has one degree of freedom, independent of the number of groups of the ordinal categorical independent variable. One degree of freedom because basically it is statistically tested whether the proportion in the groups of the ordinal categorical independent variable increase or decrease with the same amount.

In order to estimate effects with their corresponding 95% confidence intervals, the 2 × 3 table must be divided into three 2 × 2 tables. Risk differences or relative risks can then be calculated in the various 2 × 2 tables (see Sect. 5.1.1). Because there are no regular post-hoc procedures available, which are, for example, available after an analysis of variance the confidence intervals calculated for the 2 × 2 tables are not automatically corrected for multiple testing (see Sect. 4.3).

5.4 Odds Ratio

In the previous sections, the risk difference and the relative risk were used as effect estimates derived from a 2 × 2 table. However, these two effect estimates can only be used in a prospective study (see Sect. 1.1). In case-control studies and in retrospective and cross-sectional cohort studies it is not possible to calculate the absolute probability to have a dichotomous outcome variable and therefore the risk difference and the relative risk do not have a straightforward interpretation. For studies that are either cross-sectional or retrospective, the odds ratio can be used as an alternative effect estimate. The odds to have a dichotomous outcome variable is defined as the probability to have a dichotomous outcome variable divided by 1—that probability and is, therefore, interpretable as a relative probability (see Eq. 5.16).

$$odds(y=1) = \frac{p(y=1)}{1-p(y=1)} \tag{5.16}$$

where $p(y = 1)$ = probability to have the dichotomous outcome variable y.

How to calculate the odds ratio can best be explained using Example 5.3, a case control study among 100 patients (cases) with a myocardial infarction, and 100 control subjects. The aim of the study is to investigate whether certain risk factors (smoking, alcohol consumption and body mass index) are associated with the occurrence of a myocardial infarction. The first risk factor that is investigated is smoking. Table 5.13 shows the 2 × 2 table with the result of this study.

From Table 5.13 it can be calculated that the odds for smokers to have a myocardial infarction is equal to (39/53) / (14/53) = 2.79. For non-smokers the odds to have a myocardial infarction is equal to (61/147) / (86/147) = 0.71. So the odds ratio for smokers compared to non-smokers to have a myocardial infarction is 2.79/0.71 = 3.93. The same number can also be obtained by cross multiplication, i.e. (39 × 86) / (61 × 14) = 3.93, which is an easy way to calculate the odds ratio.

For effect estimates it is important also to report a 95% confidence interval. In order to calculate a 95% confidence interval around the odds ratio (like the relative risk), the odds ratio must first be log transformed. When the null hypothesis is true, then the odds ratio (like the relative risk) has a skewed to the right distribution, i.e. the value of the null hypothesis is 1, the minimum value is 0, and the maximum value is ∞. The standard error of the natural logarithm of the odds ratio is very easy to calculate (see Eq. 5.17).

$$se[ln(OR)] = \sqrt{\frac{1}{a} + \frac{1}{b} + \frac{1}{c} + \frac{1}{d}} \tag{5.17}$$

where $se[ln(OR)]$ = standard error of the natural logarithm of the odds ratio and a, b, c and d = number of subjects in the cells of the 2 × 2 table.

When the numbers of Table 5.13 are entered into Eq. 5.17, the standard error of the natural logarithm of the odds ratio is 0.35.

Table 5.13 2 × 2 table to show the relationship between having a myocardial infarction and smoking

	Myocardial infarction	No myocardial infarction	Total
Smoking	39	14	53
Non smoking	61	86	147
Total	100	100	200

$$se[ln(OR)] = \sqrt{\frac{1}{39} + \frac{1}{14} + \frac{1}{61} + \frac{1}{86}} = 0.35$$

Then, a 95% confidence interval around the natural logarithm of the odds ratio can be calculated with Eq. 5.18.

$$ln(OR) \pm z_{(1-\alpha/2)} \times se[ln(OR)] \tag{5.18}$$

where $ln\ (OR)$ = natural logarithm of the odds ratio, $z_{(1-\alpha/2)}$ = value of the standard normal distribution for which $(1 - \alpha/2)$% of the distribution is below that value and $se[ln(OR)]$ = the standard error of the natural logarithm of the odds ratio.

Entering the standard error into Eq. 5.18, the 95% confidence interval around the natural logarithm of the odds ratio ranges between 0.67 and 2.04.

$$ln(3.93) \pm 1.96 \times 0.35 = [0.67 - 2.04]$$

Again, this 95% confidence interval needs to be transformed back to get a 95% confidence interval around the odds ratio. Doing that, the 95% confidence interval ranges between 1.95 and 7.69. As for the relative risk, the confidence interval around the odds ratio is not symmetric. Again, the upper limit is further away from the observed odds ratio than the lower limit (for an odds ratio less than 1 this is of course the other way around) and just as for the relative risk, this is due to the logarithmic scale on which the odds ratio is measured.

To obtain the p-value for the observed odds ratio, again, the Fisher exact test or the chi-square test can be performed. Output 5.5 shows the result of both analyses.

In Output 5.5 it can be seen that the relationship between having a myocardial infarction and smoking is statistically significant. Both the Fisher exact test and the chi-square test give a p-value <0.001.

5.4.1 Odds Ratio Versus Relative Risk

Although it is often argued that the odds ratio should only be used in studies that are not prospective, the odds ratio is also often used in prospective studies. Also in

Output 5.5 Result of the Fisher exact test and the chi-square test to analyse the relationship between having a myocardial infarction and smoking

	Value	df	Asymptotic p-value	Exact p-value (1-sided)	Exact p-value (2-sided)
Fisher exact test				<0.001	<0.001
Chi-square test	16.044	2	<0.001		

randomized controlled trials (RCTs) such as Example 5.1, in which an activity program is compared to usual care, the odds ratio is often reported. When the odds ratio is calculated from the result reported in Table 5.1, the odds ratio is 2.67 ((80 × 40) / (60 × 20)).

Although the odds ratio is often interpreted as a relative risk, it can be seen that in this example the odds ratio is much higher than the relative risk (2.67 versus 2). When the odds ratio is calculated with data from the same 2 × 2 table as the relative risk, then the odds ratio is always higher than the relative risk. The magnitude of the difference depends on the prevalence of the outcome variable. In Example 5.1, of the 200 patients in the RCT, 60 patients recovered, leading to a prevalence of the outcome variable of 30%.

It is sometimes argued that the odds ratio is a good estimator of the relative risk when the prevalence of the outcome variable is less than 5%, but like all other cut-off values, this cut-off value is arbitrary. The fact is that the odds ratio is always higher than the relative risk (when calculated with data from the same 2 × 2 table) and that the difference increases as the prevalence of the outcome variable increases. It is important to realize that the p-value associated with the odds ratio of 2.67 is equal to the p-value associated with the relative risk of 2. After all, both are calculated from the same 2 × 2 table and both p-values are therefore calculated with the same Fisher exact test or chi-square test. The fact that the odds ratio is often used in prospective studies has everything to do with the fact that the odds ratio is the effect estimate that can be calculated from the result of a logistic regression analysis (see Sect. 5.5).

5.5 Logistic Regression Analysis

5.5.1 Introduction

Comparable to the analysis of a continuous outcome variable, there is also a regression method available for the analysis of a dichotomous outcome variable, i.e. logistic regression analysis. With logistic regression analysis it is possible to analyse the relationship between a dichotomous outcome variable and all kinds of independent variables. The idea behind logistic regression analysis is to transform the dichotomous outcome variable in such a way that a kind of linear regression analysis can be performed. This idea can be best explained in a number of steps. The first step is to use a linear regression analysis for the dichotomous outcome variable (see Eq. 5.19).

$$y_{dichotomous} = b_0 + b_1 x \tag{5.19}$$

where b_0= intercept, b_1 = regression coefficient for the independent variable and x = independent variable.

This relationship is impossible to analyse with a linear regression analysis, because the outcome variable is not continuous and not normally distributed. The second step is not to analyse the dichotomous outcome variable itself, but to analyse the probability to have the dichotomous outcome variable (see Eq. 5.20). This is a logical step because with a dichotomous outcome variable, the interest is in the probability to have the dichotomous outcome variable.

$$p(y_{dichotomous}) = b_0 + b_1x \tag{5.20}$$

Although the probability is a kind of continuous variable (ranging between 0 and 1), it is not normally distributed. As has been mentioned in Sect. 3.2, the probability has a binomial distribution. The next step is, therefore, not to analyse the probability, but to analyse the relative probability, i.e. the odds (see Eq. 5.21).

$$\frac{p(y_{dichotomous})}{1 - p(y_{dichotomous})} = b_0 + b_1x \tag{5.21}$$

This options seems to be a lot better, because the odds is a continuous variable ranging between 0 and ∞. The only problem, however, is that the odds is still not normally distributed. The odds is highly skewed to the right: a probability of 0.50 (the middle of the distribution) gives an odds of 1, a probability of 0 gives an odds of 0 and a probability of 1 gives an odds of∞. To deal with a skewed to right distribution, a log transformation can be applied (see Sect. 4.2.1), so the next step is to use the natural logarithm of the odds as outcome variable in the regression analysis (see Eq. 5.22).

$$ln\left(\frac{p(y_{dichotomous})}{1 - p(y_{dichotomous})}\right) = b_0 + b_1x \tag{5.22}$$

This new outcome variable of the regression analysis is continuous and normally distributed, so it seems to be an excellent option to be used as an outcome variable in a logistic regression analysis. The logistic regression analysis can also be written in another way (see Eq. 5.23). In this way, the probability of the dichotomous outcome variable can be calculated for each subject in the dataset, given the value of the independent variables (see further Sects. 5.5.3 and 7.4).

$$p(y_{dichotomous}) = \frac{1}{1 + e^{-(b_0 + b_1x)}} \tag{5.23}$$

5.5.2 Logistic Regression Analysis with a Dichotomous Independent Variable

Going back to Example 5.3, i.e. the case-control study in which the relationship between having a myocardial infarction and smoking is investigated. In Sect. 5.4 this relationship was shown using a 2 × 2 table and based on these numbers, the odds ratio with the corresponding 95% confidence interval was calculated. Furthermore, the p-value was obtained using either the Fisher exact test or the chi-square test. It was shown that the odds ratio for smoking compared to not smoking to have a myocardial infarction is 3.93, the corresponding 95% confidence interval ranges between 1.96 and 7.86, and the p-value is <0.001. The same result can be obtained using a logistic regression analysis, with myocardial infarction as a dichotomous outcome variable and smoking as a dichotomous independent variable. Output 5.6 shows the result of this analysis.

In Output 5.6 it can be seen that the regression coefficient for smoking is 1.37. Comparable to the interpretation of the regression coefficient in a linear regression analysis, the regression coefficient is the difference in the outcome variable per unit difference in the independent variable, in this case the difference between smokers and non-smokers (see Sect. 4.4.2). So, the difference in outcome variable between smokers and non-smokers is 1.37. Since the outcome variable of a logistic regression analysis is the natural logarithm of the odds to have the dichotomous outcome variable, the regression coefficient for the variable smoking can be seen as the difference between smokers and non-smokers in the natural logarithm of the probability to have a myocardial infarction divided by 1 − that probability, i.e. the difference in the natural logarithm of the odds to have a myocardial infarction (see Eqs. 5.24a and 5.24b).

$$b_1 = \ln\left(\frac{P(y=1)}{1-P(y=1)}\right)_{smoking} - \ln\left(\frac{P(y=1)}{1-P(y=1)}\right)_{non-smoking} \quad (5.24a)$$

$$b_1 = \ln\left(odds(y=1)\right)_{smoking} - \ln\left(odds(y=1)\right)_{non-smoking} \quad (5.24b)$$

In Sect. 4.2.1 it was explained that the difference of two logarithms with the same base is equal to the logarithm of the ratio of the two numbers. This can also be applied to the difference of the two natural logarithms from Eqs. 5.24a and 5.24b (see Eq. 5.25).

Output 5.6 Result of the logistic regression analysis to analyse the relationship between having a myocardial infarction and smoking

	Coefficient	se	Wald	df	p-value
Smoking	1.37	0.35	14.96	1	<0.001
Constant	−0.34	0.17	4.21	1	0.04

se standard error, *df* degrees of freedom

$$b_1 = \ln\left(\frac{odds(y=1)_{smoking}}{odds(y=1)_{non-smoking}}\right) \tag{5.25}$$

So, the regression coefficient is equal to the natural logarithm of the odds ratio. By taking the e-power of the regression coefficient, the odds ratio can be obtained (see Eq. 5.26).

$$EXP(b_1) = \frac{odds(y=1)_{smoking}}{odds(y=1)_{non-smoking}} \tag{5.26}$$

To calculate the 95% confidence interval around the odds ratio, the 95% confidence interval around the regression coefficient must first be calculated (see Eq. 5.27).

$$b_1 \pm z_{(1-\alpha/2)} \times se(b_1) \tag{5.27}$$

where b_1= regression coefficient, $z_{(1-\alpha/2)}$ = value of the standard normal distribution for which $(1-\alpha/2)$% of the distribution is below that value, i.e. 1.96 and $se(b_1)$ = standard error of the regression coefficient.

When the numbers shown in Output 5.6 are entered into Eq. 5.27, the 95% confidence interval ranges between 0.67 and 2.06.

$$1.39 \pm 1.96 \times 0.35 = [0.67 - 2.06]$$

The limits of the 95% confidence interval around the regression coefficient need to be transformed to get the 95% confidence interval around the odds ratio. This can, of course, be done by taking the e-power of both limits. In the example, around the odds ratio of 3.93, this results in a 95% confidence interval of EXP[0.67] = 1.96 to EXP [2.06] = 7.86. Output 5.7 shows the result of the logistic regression analysis which includes the odds ratio and the 95% confidence interval around the odds ratio.

The p-value for a regression coefficient in a logistic regression analysis is obtained from the Wald statistic. The Wald statistic can be calculated by taking the regression coefficient divided by its standard error, squared (see Eq. 5.28)

$$Wald = \left(b/_{se(b)}\right)^2 \tag{5.28}$$

where *Wald* = Wald statistic, *b* = regression coefficient and *se(b)* = standard error of the regression coefficient.

In Output 5.7 it can be seen that the Wald statistic is 14.96. The corresponding p-value can be obtained from a chi-square distribution with one degree of freedom and is <0.001.

The value of the Wald statistic can be compared to the chi-square value shown in Output 5.5 (i.e. 16.044). Although both analyses answer exactly the same question,

Output 5.7 Result of the logistic regression analysis to analyse the relationship between having a myocardial infarction and smoking

							95% confidence interval	
	Coefficient	se	Wald	df	p-value	Odds ratio	Lower	Upper
Smoking	1.37	0.35	14.96	1	<0.001	3.93	1.96	7.86
Constant	−0.34	0.17	4.21	1	0.04			

se standard error, *df* degrees of freedom

the chi-square value and the Wald statistic are not exactly the same. This has to do with the fact that both the chi-square value and the Wald statistic are approximations, and differ slightly from each other.

5.5.3 Maximum Likelihood

Within linear regression analysis, the values of the regression coefficients are estimated using the least squares method (see Sect. 4.4.1). Within logistic regression analysis, however, the values of the regression coefficients are estimated using maximum likelihood. The values of the regression coefficients are estimated in such a way that the likelihood of the logistic regression analysis (in this context mostly referred to as the logistic regression model) is as high as possible. The likelihood of the logistic regression model can be calculated using the probability of the dichotomous outcome variable for each subject in the study population based on the regression coefficients and then multiplying all these probabilities. Equation 5.23 can be used to calculate the different probabilities. When the values of the regression coefficients from Output 5.7 are entered into Eq. 5.23, the probability to have a myocardial infarction for both a smoker and a non-smoker can be calculated.

$$p(y=1)_{non-smoker} = \frac{1}{1+e^{-(-0.34+1.37\times 0)}} = 0.42$$

$$p(y=1)_{smoker} = \frac{1}{1+e^{-(-0.34+1.37\times 1)}} = 0.74$$

So, in the example, the probability to have a myocardial infarction is 0.74 for a smoker and 0.42 for a non-smoker. Of course, these probabilities should not be interpreted absolutely, but only relative to the 0.50 probability that exists a priori. This a priori probability is 0.50, because the same number of subjects with a myocardial infarction as without a myocardial infarction are included in the study (i.e. the same number of cases and controls). With the calculated probabilities, for each subject in the dataset, the probability to have the outcome variable can be calculated. In this case, there are four possibilities: (1) a smoker who has a myocardial infarction; (2) a smoker who does not have a myocardial infarction; (3) a

Table 5.14 Probabilities to have a myocardial infarction for smokers and non-smokers

Smoking	Myocardial infarction	Probability	Number of subjects
Yes	Yes	0.74	39
Yes	No	0.26	14
No	Yes	0.42	61
No	No	0.58	86

non-smoker who has a myocardial infarction and (4) a non-smoker who does not have a myocardial infarction.

The 2 × 2 table showing the relationship between having a myocardial infarction and smoking (Table 5.13) shows that there are 39 smokers who have a myocardial infarction. All these smokers have (based on the probabilities calculated with the logistic regression analysis) a probability of 0.74 to have a myocardial infarction. Furthermore, there are 14 smokers who do not have a myocardial infarction, and the probability to have no myocardial infarction for these subjects is 0.26. For the 61 non-smokers who have a myocardial infarction, the probability to have a myocardial infarction is 0.42 and for the 86 non-smokers who do not have a myocardial infarction, the probability to have no myocardial infarction is 0.58. Table 5.14 shows the probabilities of the four different possibilities based on the results of the logistic regression analysis.

The likelihood of the logistic regression model is therefore: $(0.74)^{39} \times (0.26)^{14} \times (0.42)^{61} \times (0.58)^{86} = 2.4 \times 10^{-57}$. Because the likelihood is a very small number, it is transformed into a value that is easier to handle and that also has a nice property, i.e. the −2 log likelihood (−2 × the natural logarithm of the likelihood). The nice property of the −2 log likelihood has to do with the fact that it can be used to compare different models with each other. The −2 log likelihood of the logistic regression model with smoking is equal to $-2 \times \ln[((0.74)^{39} \times (0.26)^{14} \times (0.42)^{61} \times (0.58)^{86})] = 260.7$. Because the general idea of using maximum likelihood is to estimate regression coefficients in such a way that the likelihood of the model is as high as possible, the −2 log likelihood should be as low as possible. The absolute value of the −2 log likelihood, like the absolute value of the likelihood, is not interpretable, but, as mentioned before, the −2 log likelihood can be used to compare models with each other. This is done with the likelihood ratio test.

In the present example, the −2 log likelihood of the logistic regression model with smoking can be compared to the −2 log likelihood of the logistic regression model without smoking. In the logistic regression model without smoking (i.e. the model without independent variables), the probability to have a myocardial infarction is 0.50 (because the number of cases is equal to the number of controls). Because there are 200 subjects, the −2 log likelihood of the logistic regression model without smoking is equal to: $-2 \times \ln[(0.50)^{200}] = 277.2$. For the likelihood ratio test, the difference between the −2 log likelihood of the logistic regression model without smoking and the −2 log likelihood of the logistic regression model with smoking has to be calculated. This difference is equal to 277.2–260.7 = 16.5 and appears to have a chi-square distribution. The number of degrees of freedom of this chi-square distribution is equal to the difference in the number of parameters estimated by the two logistic regression models. In the example, the difference of the −2 log likelihoods has a chi-square distribution with one degree of freedom. This is because only the variable smoking is added to the logistic regression model, so the difference in number of estimated parameters between the logistic regression models with and without smoking is one. The corresponding p-value is <0.001 (see Table 5.5).

It should be noted that the difference between the two −2 log likelihoods in the present example is again an answer to the question whether there is a statistically significant relationship between having a myocardial infarction and smoking. So, the value (16.6) basically answers the same question as the chi-square value (16.04) and the value of the Wald statistic (14.96). It should be noted that in practice the p-value derived from the Wald statistic is usually reported.

5.5.4 Logistic Regression Analysis with a Categorical Independent Variable

In the previous section, the principles of logistic regression analysis were discussed using an example with a dichotomous independent variable. In this section, logistic regression analysis with a categorical independent variable will be discussed, again using the case-control study in which the relationship between having a myocardial infarction and a number of possible risk factors is investigated. One of these risk factors is alcohol consumption, which is divided into three groups (non-drinkers, moderate drinkers and heavy drinkers). The relationship between having a myocardial infarction and alcohol consumption can, of course, be shown in a 2 × 3 table, and the p-value can be calculated using the Fisher exact test or the chi-square test (see Table 5.15 and Output 5.8).

Based on the numbers shown in Table 5.15 it can be seen that moderate drinking seems to be protective to have a myocardial infarction, compared to non-drinking and heavy drinking. In Output 5.8 it can be seen that there is a statistically significant relationship between having a myocardial infarction and alcohol consumption; both the Fisher exact test and the chi-square test show a p-value <0.001. As has been mentioned before, it is not possible to obtain an effect estimate directly from the 2 × 3 table. To obtain effect estimates, several 2 × 2 tables has to be created. However, it is, of course, also possible to perform a logistic regression analysis to obtain effect estimates.

In Sect. 4.4.3, in which linear regression analysis with a categorical independent variable was discussed, it was already shown that a categorical independent variable must be analysed using dummy variables. This is, because otherwise a linear relationship between the outcome variable and the different groups of the categorical

Table 5.15 2 × 3 table to analyse the relationship between having a myocardial infarction and alcohol consumption

	Myocardial infarction	No myocardial infarction	Total
Non-drinker	26	16	42
Moderate drinker	34	63	97
Heavy drinker	40	21	61
Total	100	100	200

Output 5.8 Result of the Fisher exact test and the chi-square test to analyse the relationship between having a myocardial infarction and alcohol consumption

	Value	df	Asymptotic p-value	Exact p-value (2-sided)
Fisher exact test				<0.001
Chi-square test	16.97	2	<0.001	

Table 5.16 Dummy coding for the variable alcohol consumption

	Dummy 1	Dummy 2
Non-drinker	0	0
Moderate drinker	1	0
Heavy drinker	0	1

independent variable is analysed, which basically makes no sense. Therefore, the categorical independent variable alcohol consumption (with three groups) is represented by two dummy variables in the logistic regression analysis. The two dummy variables are coded in such a way that the regression coefficient for the first dummy variable indicates the difference in the outcome variable (the natural logarithm of the odds to have a myocardial infarction) between moderate drinkers and non-drinkers, while the regression coefficient for the second dummy variable indicates the difference in the outcome variable between heavy drinkers and non-drinkers (see Table 4.10 for a detailed explanation). Table 5.16 shows the dummy coding for the variable alcohol consumption.

Output 5.9 shows the result of the logistic regression analysis to analyse the relationship between having a myocardial infarction and alcohol consumption.

As has been mentioned before, the odds ratio for the first dummy variable (0.33) is the odds ratio for moderate drinkers compared to non-drinkers to have a myocardial infarction, while the odds ratio for the second dummy variable (1.17) is the odds ratio for heavy drinkers compared to non-drinkers to have a myocardial infarction. In Output 5.9 it can further be seen that the odds ratio for moderate drinkers compared to non-drinkers is statistically significant ($p = 0.004$), while the odds ratio for heavy drinkers compared to non-drinkers is not statistically significant ($p = 0.70$).

With the performed logistic regression analysis, the odds ratios for moderate drinkers compared to non-drinkers and for heavy drinkers compared to non-drinkers were obtained. To obtain the odds ratio for moderate drinkers compared to heavy drinkers, the value of the outcome variable for moderate drinkers must be compared to the value of the outcome variable for heavy drinkers. Both values can be

Output 5.9 Result of the logistic regression analysis to analyse the relationship between having a myocardial infarction and alcohol consumption

							95% confidence interval	
	Coefficient	se	Wald	df	p-value	Odds ratio	Lower	Upper
Dummy 1	−1.10	0.38	8.31	1	0.004	0.33	0.16	0.70
Dummy 2	0.16	0.42	0.15	1	0.70	1.17	0.52	2.65
Constant	0.49	0.32	2.34	1	0.13			

se standard error, *df* degrees of freedom

Table 5.17 Alternative dummy coding for the variable alcohol consumption

	Dummy 1	Dummy 2
Non-drinker	1	0
Moderate drinker	0	1
Heavy drinker	0	0

calculated with the regression coefficients shown in Output 5.9. For moderate drinkers, the value of the outcome variable is equal to $b_0 + b_1$ (0.49–1.10) and for heavy drinkers the value of the outcome variable is equal to $b_0 + b_2$ (0.49 + 0.16). The difference between the two groups is therefore equal to the difference between the regression coefficients for both dummy variables (−1.10–0.16 = −1.26). This value can be transformed into an odds ratio by taking the e-power. The odds ratio is therefore 0.28, which means that the odds to have a myocardial infarction for moderate drinkers is 0.28 times as high as for heavy drinkers. The inverse of this odds ratio (1/0.28 = 3.53) indicates that the odds to have a myocardial infarction for heavy drinkers is 3.53 times as high as for moderate drinkers. The only problem with this analysis is that a 95% confidence interval and the corresponding p-value cannot be derived directly from the results shown in Output 5.9. To obtain the 95% confidence interval and the p-value for the comparison between moderate drinkers and heavy drinkers, the dummy variables have to be coded differently. Table 5.17 shows one of the possibilities for an alternative dummy coding and Output 5.10 shows the result of the logistic regression analysis with this alternative dummy coding.

In Table 5.17 it can be seen that the heavy drinkers are now used as reference group, because both dummy variables are coded 0 for heavy drinkers. Because of that the b_0 (0.64) is now the value of the outcome variable for heavy drinkers. The regression coefficient for the first dummy variable is the difference in outcome variable between non-drinkers and heavy drinkers, and the regression coefficient for the second dummy variable is the difference in outcome variable between moderate drinkers and heavy drinkers. It can be seen that this regression coefficient is indeed −1.26 and that the odds ratio is 0.28. The reason for doing this analysis is to obtain the 95% confidence interval around this odds ratio and the corresponding p-value. In Output 5.10 it can be seen that the 95% confidence interval ranges between 0.15 and 0.56 and that the p-value is <0.001.

Output 5.10 Result of the logistic regression analysis to analyse the relationship between having a myocardial infarction and alcohol consumption with the alternative dummy coding

							95% confidence interval	
	Coefficient	se	Wald	df	p-value	Odds ratio	Lower	Upper
Dummy 1	−0.16	0.42	0.15	1	0.70	0.85	0.38	1.93
Dummy 2	−1.26	0.34	13.49	1	<0.001	0.28	0.15	0.56
Constant	0.64	0.27	5.72	1	0.017			

se standard error, *df* degrees of freedom

In some statistical software, the output of a logistic regression analysis with a categorical independent variable also includes the so-called overall Wald test. The overall Wald test gives a Wald statistic and a corresponding p-value, which is comparable to the p-value obtained from the chi-square test on the 2 × 3 table. The test statistic of the overall Wald test in the present example is 16.45, which has a chi-square distribution with two degrees of freedom and gives a p-value <0.001.

The overall p-value of the association between having a myocardial infarction and alcohol consumption can also be determined using the likelihood ratio test. To do this, the −2 log likelihood of the logistic regression model without any independent variables must be compared to the −2 log likelihood of the logistic regression model, which includes the two dummy variables for alcohol consumption. The −2 log likelihood of the logistic regression model with alcohol consumption is 260.0, while the −2 log likelihood of the logistic regression model without any independent variables is 277.2. The difference between the two −2 log likelihoods is, therefore, 17.2 and based on a chi-square distribution with two degrees of freedom, the p-value is <0.001. The chi-square distribution has two degrees of freedom, because in the logistic regression model with alcohol consumption, two additional parameters are estimated, i.e. the regression coefficients for the two dummy variables. So, also in this situation (i.e. the relationship between a dichotomous outcome variable and a categorical independent variable), there are three test statistics that can be used to obtain a p-value. One obtained from the chi square test (16.97), one obtained from the overall Wald test (16.45) and one obtained from the likelihood ratio test (17.2). Although the question answered by the three test statistics is the same, the numbers are slightly different, because the three methods are slightly different approximations.

5.5.5 *Logistic Regression Analysis with a Continuous Independent Variable*

In the previous two sections, logistic regression analysis was used for an analysis with a dichotomous independent variable (smoking) and a categorical independent variable (alcohol consumption). In this section the analysis of the relationship between a dichotomous outcome variable and a continuous independent variable will be discussed. In the case-control study in which the relationship between having a myocardial infarction and a number of possible risk factors is investigated, body mass index is a continuous possible risk factor. Output 5.11 shows the result of the logistic regression analysis to analyse the relationship between having a myocardial infarction and body mass index.

In Output 5.11 it can be seen that the regression coefficient for body mass index is 0.24, that the corresponding standard error is 0.06 and that therefore the Wald statistic is 17.13 with a corresponding p-value <0.001. Furthermore, it can be seen that the odds ratio for body mass index is 1.27 and that the 95% confidence interval around the odds ratio ranges between 1.13 and 1.42.

In the previous sections, the interpretation of the odds ratio was fairly simple, but with a continuous independent variable, the interpretation is slightly more difficult. As with linear regression analysis (see Sect. 4.4.4), the odds ratio for body mass index is the odds ratio for a one-unit difference in body mass index. When for a particular subject the body mass index is one unit higher than for another subject, the odds to have a myocardial infarction for that subject is 1.27 times higher. Because a linear relationship between having a myocardial infarction and body mass index is assumed, the odds ratio applies to two subjects with a body mass index of 21 and 20, but also to two subjects with a body mass index of 31 and 30, and so on. The assumption that there is a linear relationship between having a myocardial infarction and body mass should, of course, be evaluated (see Sect. 5.5.5.1).

One of the problems that can arise when interpreting the odds ratio of a continuous independent variable is that the magnitude of the odds ratio depends on the unit in which the continuous independent variable is measured. In the example, the odds ratio for a difference of one unit of body mass index is calculated. Of course, one unit of body mass index is not that much and therefore the corresponding odds ratio is not that high (despite the fact that the corresponding p-value is very low). In this situation, for example, the odds ratio for a difference of five units would yield a (clinically) more interpretable effect estimate. The question then is: how can an odds ratio (and the corresponding 95% confidence interval) for five units of body mass index be calculated using Output 5.11? When a difference of one unit of body mass index is related to a difference of 0.24 units in the outcome variable, then a difference of five units of body mass index is related to a difference of $5 \times 0.24 = 1.2$ units in the outcome variable. By taking the e-power of this number, the odds ratio for a

Output 5.11 Result of the logistic regression analysis to analyse the relationship between having a myocardial infarction and body mass index

							95% confidence interval	
	Coefficient	se	Wald	df	p-value	Odds ratio	Lower	Upper
bmi	0.24	0.06	17.13	1	<0.001	1.27	1.13	1.42
Constant	−5.72	1.39	16.99	1	<0.001			

se standard error, *df* degrees of freedom, *bmi* body mass index

Output 5.12 Result of the logistic regression analysis to analyse the relationship between having a myocardial infarction and body mass index where all body mass index values are divided by 5

							95% confidence interval	
	Coefficient	se	Wald	df	p-value	Odds ratio	Lower	Upper
bmi_5	1.20	0.29	17.13	1	<0.001	3.29	1.87	5.77
Constant	−5.72	1.39	16.99	1	<0.001			

se standard error, *df* degrees of freedom, *bmi* body mass index

difference of five units in body mass index is 3.29. For the 95% confidence interval around the odds ratio of 3.29, the same procedure can be followed. This means that the standard error of the regression coefficient must also be multiplied by five. Each step is accompanied by a certain error, and five of those steps are therefore accompanied by five times that error. The 95% confidence interval for the odds ratio for five steps in body mass index, therefore, ranges between 1.87 and 5.77. This result can also be obtained from a logistic regression analysis when all body mass index values in the dataset are divided by 5 (see Output 5.12).

It should be noted that the Wald statistic and the p-value shown in Output 5.12 are (of course) identical to the Wald statistic and p-value reported in Output 5.11, where the relationship is analysed for one unit of body mass index. There is also a more mathematical method to calculate an odds ratio for more than one unit in the continuous independent variable. To calculate the odds ratio for five units body mass index, the odds ratio for one unit body mass index can be raised to the fifth power. This can also be done for the lower and upper limit of the 95% confidence interval. Although this method can be used to calculate the odds ratio and the corresponding 95% confidence interval for more than one unit of a continuous independent variable, it can only be used when the outcome variable is measured on a logarithmic scale.

To answer the question whether having a myocardial infarction is associated with body mass index, many researchers probably will use an independent t-test (see Sect. 4.2). After all, there is a continuous variable (body mass index) that is compared between two groups (the cases and the controls). Although the independent t-test will give a proper answer of the research question, it should be realized that in this case the independent t-test is a reverse analysis, i.e. the outcome variable having a myocardial infarction is treated as a dichotomous independent variable, while the independent variable body mass index is treated as a continuous outcome variable.

5.5.5.1 Evaluation of the Linear Relationship with a Continuous Independent Variable

In the previous section, the relationship between having a myocardial infarction and the continuous independent variable body mass index was investigated. The result of this analysis was an odds ratio for a difference of one unit in body mass index.

Because the analysis assumes a linear relationship, the assumption is that this odds ratio applies to any difference of one unit of body mass index. Of course, like all other analyses with a continuous independent variable, the question is to what extent this assumption holds.

To obtain an impression of the shape of the relationship between having a myocardial infarction and body mass index, it is not possible to make a scatterplot, because a scatterplot is only informative when a continuous outcome variable is analysed (see Sect. 4.4.1). With a dichotomous outcome variable, one possibility to gain insight into the shape of the relationship is to divide the continuous independent variable (in this example) body mass index into a number of groups. For example, the variable can be divided into four groups based on quartiles. For each group, the number of subjects with (in this example) a myocardial infarction can be examined. Table 5.18 shows the numbers for the four body mass index quartiles.

In Table 5.18 it can be seen that the relationship between having a myocardial infarction and body mass index does not seem to be linear. In the first three quartiles, there seems to be a more or less linear increase in the proportion of subjects with a myocardial infarction, but for the last body mass index quartile, there is a small decrease in the proportion of subjects with a myocardial infarction. To confirm this observation statistically, the same procedures can be used as has been described for a continuous outcome variable (see Sect. 4.4.4.1). The first possibility, therefore, is not to analyse a linear relationship but to use a different mathematical function, for example a quadratic relationship. Output 5.13 shows the result of the logistic regression analysis in which both body mass index and body mass index squared are included in the analysis.

In Output 5.13 it can be seen that the p-value of the regression coefficient for body mass index squared is <0.001; in other words, the addition of body mass index

Table 5.18 Number of subjects with and without a myocardial infarction in the body mass index quartiles

	Myocardial infarction	No myocardial infarction
Quartile 1	10	40
Quartile 2	23	27
Quartile 3	36	14
Quartile 4	31	19

Output 5.13 Result of the logistic regression analysis to analyse the relationship between having a myocardial infarction and body mass index including body mass index squared

							95% confidence interval	
	Coefficient	se	Wald	df	p-value	Odds ratio	Lower	Upper
bmi	2.30	0.82	12.93	1	<0.001	18.71	3.79	92.35
bmi squared	−0.05	0.02	11.23	1	<0.001	0.95	0.92	0.98
Constant	−38.71	10.18	14.47	1	<0.001			

se standard error, *df* degrees of freedom, *bmi* body mass index

Table 5.19 Dummy coding for the variable body mass index

	Dummy 1	Dummy 2	Dummy 3
Quartile 1	0	0	0
Quartile 2	1	0	0
Quartile 3	0	1	0
Quartile 4	0	0	1

Output 5.14 Result of the logistic regression analysis to analyse the relationship between having a myocardial infarction and body mass index as a categorical variable

							95% confidence interval	
	Coefficient	se	Wald	df	p-value	Odds ratio	Lower	Upper
Dummy 1	1.23	0.45	7.31	1	0.007	3.41	1.40	8.29
Dummy 2	2.33	0.47	23.23	1	<0.001	10.29	4.07	26.02
Dummy 3	1.88	0.46	16.77	1	<0.001	6.53	2.66	16.02
Constant	−1.39	0.35	15.37	1	<0.001			

se standard error, *df* degrees of freedom

squared to the logistic regression analysis seems to be important. Of course, the importance of adding body mass index squared can also be evaluated with the likelihood ratio test. To do this, the −2 log likelihood of the model with only body mass index must be compared to the −2 log likelihood of the model with body mass index and body mass index squared. The two −2 log likelihoods are respectively 257.56 and 235.37. The difference between the two values is 22.19, which has a chi-square distribution with one degree of freedom and is, therefore, statistically significant ($p < 0.001$). So, it can be concluded that analysing the relationship between having a myocardial infarction and body mass index with a quadratic relationship is better than analysing a linear relationship. The odds ratio for body mass index of 1.27, which was obtained from the logistic regression analysis assuming a linear relationship should, therefore, not be used. One of the biggest problems with analysing a relationship with a continuous independent variable with a different mathematical function is that the regression coefficients are very difficult to interpret. Besides that, with this method, it can only be concluded that analysing a quadratic relationship is better than analysing a linear relationship. However, it cannot be concluded that analysing a quadratic relationship is the best way of analysing the relationship. Because of this, a different procedure is often used to evaluate whether there is a linear relationship. Similar to linear regression analysis, the continuous independent variable can be divided into a number of groups (e.g. four equal groups based on quartiles). Then, using dummy variables (see Table 5.19), this categorical variable is analysed with a logistic regression analysis. Output 5.14 shows the result of the analysis to analyse the relationship between having a myocardial infarction and body mass index as a categorical variable. In the analysis, body mass index is divided into quartiles and the coding of the dummy variables is used with the lowest quartile as reference group.

The interpretation of the regression coefficients for the three dummy variables is, of course, the same as in all the other analyses with dummy variables. The regression coefficient for the first dummy variable indicates the difference in outcome variable (the natural logarithm of the odds to have a myocardial infarction) between the second quartile of body mass index and the reference group, i.e. the first quartile of body mass index. This regression coefficient is 1.23 and the odds ratio is 3.41. In other words, subjects in the second quartile of the body mass index distribution have a 3.41 times higher odds to have a myocardial infarction compared to subjects in the lowest quartile. The corresponding p-value is 0.007. For the second dummy variable, a regression coefficient of 2.33 is observed and an odds ratio of 10.29. So subjects with a body mass index in the third quartile of the body mass index distribution have a 10.29 times higher odds to have a myocardial infarction compared to subjects in the lowest quartile. Finally, the regression coefficient for the third dummy variable is 1.88 and the odds ratio is 6.53. So subjects in the highest quartile of the body mass index distribution have a 6.53 times higher odds to have a myocardial infarction than subjects in the lowest quartile. The p-values for the latter two differences are both <0.001.

When there is an increasing or decreasing trend in the regression coefficients for the different dummy variables, the average body mass index values of the four quartiles are necessary to properly evaluate whether the relationship is linear or not (see also Sect. 4.4.4.1). However, in the present example, there is no increasing or decreasing trend in the regression coefficients, so the result immediately shows that there is no linear relationship between having a myocardial infarction and body mass index. To describe this relationship, it is therefore better to report the result of the analysis with the categorical body mass index variable than the result of the analysis with the continuous body mass index variable. To obtain a proper interpretation of the three regression coefficients, however, it is necessary to relate the regression coefficients and corresponding odds ratios to the mean body mass index values of the four quartiles. Table 5.20 shows these values.

In the analysis performed, the continuous independent variable body mass index was arbitrarily divided into four groups based on quartiles. Of course, when it is possible, it is better to use biological relevant groups for the categorization. In the case of body mass index, for example, the variable can be divided into normal weight (body mass index <25), overweight (body mass index between 25 and 30) and obese (body mass index >30). Although this would make the result easier to interpret, in the example this categorization is not really possible because in the dataset only five subjects are classified as obese.

So far, two possibilities are discussed to evaluate whether the relationship with a continuous independent variable is linear or not. First, a different mathematical function was used and second, the continuous independent variable was divided into groups (i.e. quartiles). A third possibility to evaluate whether the relationship with a continuous independent variable is linear is the use of splines (see Sect. 4.4.4.1). It was already mentioned that the general idea of the use of splines is that the continuous independent variable is divided into separate parts in which a different relationship between the outcome variable and the independent variable is estimated.

Table 5.20 Body mass index values of the four quartiles used in the logistic regression analysis

	Mean body mass index	Range in body mass index
Quartile 1	20.57	16.65–21.83
Quartile 2	23.04	21.87–24.01
Quartile 3	24.91	24.01–25.94
Quartile 4	27.78	25.95–32.02

Table 5.21 Part of the dataset that is used in the linear spline logistic regression analysis to analyse the relationship between having a myocardial infarction and body mass index

Id	Myocardial infarction	bmi	bmi1	bmi2	bmi3
1	1	24.7	23	1.7	0
2	1	25.1	23	2.1	0
3	1	26.4	23	3	0.4
.					
6	0	22	22	0	0
9	0	28.9	23	3	2.9
.					
200	0	28.2	23	3	2.2

bmi body mass index

It has also been mentioned that a distinction can be made between linear spline regression analysis and cubic spline regression analysis, although the latter leads to non-interpretable regression coefficients. Linear spline regression analysis within a logistic regression analysis, on the other hand lead to easily interpretable effect estimates (i.e. odds ratios). Suppose that in the example with body mass index, the independent variable is divided into three parts. In the linear spline regression analysis with two knots, the knots are chosen to be at a body mass index of 23 and a body mass index of 26. So, three regression lines for body mass index are estimated: one for the lowest body mass index values (≤23), one for the body mass index values between 23 and 26 and one for the highest body mass index values (>26). Table 5.21 shows part of the dataset that is used in the linear spline logistic regression analysis to analyse the relationship between having a myocardial infarction and body mass index.

Output 5.15 shows the results of the linear spline logistic regression analysis with two knots to analyse the relationship between having a myocardial infarction and body mass index.

In Output 5.15 it can be seen that for the first body mass index variable, the odds ratio is 1.75. This odds ratio indicates that when body mass index is ≤23, each difference of one unit in body mass index is associated with a 1.75 times higher odds to have a myocardial infarction. When body mass index is between 23 and 26, the odds ratio is 1.49 and when body mass index is >26, the odds ratio is 0.77. Based on the three regression coefficients derived from the linear spline logistic regression analysis, it can (also) be concluded that there is no linear relationship between having a myocardial infarction and body mass index (see Sect. 4.4.4.1). It should be realized that the reported odds ratios are expressed for one unit difference in body

Output 5.15 Result of the linear spline logistic regression analysis with two knots to analyse the relationship between having a myocardial infarction and body mass index

							95% confidence interval	
	Coefficient	se	Wald	df	p-value	Odds ratio	Lower	Upper
bmi1	0.56	0.21	7.29	1	0.007	1.75	1.17	2.63
bmi2	0.40	0.17	5.29	1	0.02	1.49	1.06	2.10
bmi3	−0.26	0.16	2.86	1	0.09	0.77	0.57	1.04
Constant	−12.97	4.58	8.01	1	0.005			

se standard error, *df* degrees of freedom, *bmi* body mass index

mass index within a particular body mass index range. This is different from the method in which body mass index was divided into quartiles. When that method is used, the odds ratios are expressed for the difference between the mean values of the different body mass index groups.

Although the use of splines is a nice alternative for evaluating whether a relationship with a continuous independent variable is linear, it is often difficult to define where the knots should be placed. In the present example, the knots are arbitrary placed at 23 and 26. However, mostly the knots are based on percentile points, but also that is rather arbitrary.

5.6 Confounding and Effect Modification

5.6.1 Introduction

As has been discussed in Sect. 4.5, in order to properly interpret the relationship between an outcome variable and a particular independent variable, it is necessary to adjust for possible confounding and to evaluate effect modification. When there is effect modification the relationship observed is different for different values of the effect modifier. For example, the relationship is different for males and females, different for young people and old people, and so on. Confounding has to do with the fact that the relationship observed is totally or partly caused by something else, i.e. the confounder. Although logistic regression analysis can be used to adjust for confounding and to evaluate effect modification when analysing a dichotomous outcome variable, in some cases it is also possible to do it in a somewhat simpler way using stratified analysis.

5.6.2 Confounding and Effect Modification Using Stratified Analysis

To illustrate how stratified analysis can be used to adjust for confounding and to evaluate effect modification, Example 5.1 will be used, i.e. the randomized controlled trial investigating the effect of an activity program on recovery in patients with low back pain. Table 5.22 shows the 2 × 2 table with the result of this randomized controlled trial.

In Sects. 5.1 and 5.4 three effect estimates have been calculated from this 2 × 2 table, i.e. the relative risk, the risk difference and the odds ratio. Although in a randomized controlled trial the relative risk and the risk difference can be used, in this example the odds ratio will be used as effect estimate. This has to do with the fact that certain methods that can be used to adjust for confounding and to evaluate effect modification using stratified analysis are only applicable to the odds ratio. In Sect. 5.4 it was already mentioned that the odds ratio for recovery for intervention compared to usual care is 2.67. Around this odds ratio of 2.67 a 95% confidence interval can be calculated with ranges between 1.42 and 5.02.

Now suppose that there are more females than males in the intervention group and also suppose that in general females recover more often than males. Then it could be that (part of) the effect of the intervention is caused by sex differences between the intervention and the control group. In that case, sex is a confounder in the relationship between recovery and the intervention. When these sex differences are not taken into account, the effect of the intervention is overestimated. Of course, the other way around is also possible: Suppose that there are more males than females in the intervention group and that, again, in general females recover more often than males. In that case, the effect of the intervention is underestimated when the sex differences are not taken into account.

These two examples directly imply that when there are equal numbers of males and females in both groups, sex can never be a confounder in the investigated relationship, regardless the magnitude of the relationship between sex and the outcome variable. On the other hand, it also directly implies that when sex is not related to the outcome variable, i.e. when there are equal proportions of males and females recovering, sex cannot be a confounder in the investigated relationship as well. These two aspects together are prerequisites for confounding: The possible confounder must have a relationship with the outcome variable and with the independent variable. In addition, the possible confounder may not be in the causal pathway between the outcome variable and the independent variable (see also Sect. 11.2). To evaluate whether sex is a confounder in the present example it can be

Table 5.22 2 × 2 table with the result of the randomized controlled trial

	Recovered	Not recovered	Total
Intervention	40	60	100
Usual care	20	80	100
Total	60	140	200

Table 5.23 2 × 2 tables stratified for males and females with the result of the randomized controlled trial

Females	Recovered	Not recovered	Total
Intervention	16	14	30
Regular care	14	56	70
Total	30	70	
Odds ratio	4.57 (1.81–11.54)		
Males	Recovered	Not recovered	Total
Intervention	24	46	70
Regular care	6	24	30
Total	30	70	
Odds ratio	2.09 (0.75–5.80)		

analysed to what extent sex is associated with the intervention variable and to what extent sex is associated with recovery. However, the question is: What is meant by being associated with? Many researchers assume that this question can be answered by evaluating whether the association is statistically significant or not. However that assumption is not correct. It is, for instance, possible that a statistically non-significant relationship is obtained between a possible confounder and the independent variable, but that the variable in question is still a (relevant) confounder. This has everything to do with the relationship between the possible confounder and the outcome variable. It is therefore not really advisable to evaluate confounding in this indirect way.

A much better possibility to adjust for confounding is to stratify the original 2 × 2 table by the possible confounder. A 2 × 2 table with recovery and intervention is then created for males and females separately. In addition to confounding, this stratification can also be used to investigate effect modification by sex. By stratifying the 2 × 2 table, it can be evaluated whether the effect of the intervention is different for males and females. Table 5.23 shows both 2 × 2 tables and the corresponding odds ratios.

In Table 5.23 it can be seen that for females the odds ratio is 4.57 (95% confidence interval ranges between 1.81 and 11.54), while for males the odds ratio is 2.09 (95% confidence interval ranges between 0.75 and 5.98). So, it can be concluded that there is effect modification, because the effect of the intervention is stronger for females than for males. However, in different groups of a possible effect modifier always a different effect will be observed and it should be questioned whether the observed difference between the effects is so relevant that both effects must be reported separately. The answer to this last question is difficult. Intuitively, an odds ratio of 4.57 seems to be much higher than an odds ratio of 2.09 and that, therefore, both odds ratios should be reported separately. On the other hand, the difference is not as big as it seems, because the odds ratio is measured on a logarithmic scale. Furthermore, it can be seen that the 95% confidence intervals around both odds ratios overlap to a large extent (or better: the odds ratios for both groups are within the 95% confidence intervals for the other group). It can, therefore, be concluded that the two odds ratios do not differ statistically significant from each other and that they should not be reported separately. In principle, both conclusions

Table 5.24 Result of the test for homogeneity of the two odds ratios for males and females shown in Table 5.23

Statistic	Chi-square	Degrees of freedom	Asymptotic p-value
Breslow-Day	1.26	1	0.26
Tarone	1.24	1	0.28

are correct. The only advantage of the conclusion that there is no effect modification is that it is partly based on a relatively objective criterion, i.e. the overlap in the odds ratios and 95% confidence intervals. Some statistical software provides the result of a statistical test that compares the two odds ratios with each other. This test is called the test for homogeneity and Table 5.24 shows the result of this test in the present example.

Table 5.24 shows two alternatives to test the homogeneity of the two odds ratios (i.e. Breslow-Day and Tarone). The tests use a slightly different approach but, in practice, the results will not differ much from each other. In Table 5.24 it can be seen that the p-values of both tests are 0.26 and 0.28 respectively. That is, the null hypothesis, which implies that both odds ratios are homogeneous, should not be rejected. Thus, the statistical test for homogeneity indicates that the two odds ratios do not differ statistically significant from each other and confirms the conclusion drawn based on the overlap in the odds ratios and 95% confidence intervals. So the odds ratios for males and females do not have to be reported separately. Again, it is not wrong to ignore these relatively objective indicators and still conclude that there is relevant effect modification. It should be realized that decisions based on p-values and the overlap of odds ratios and 95% confidence intervals are always very dependent on the number of subjects in the different groups of the possible effect modifier.

When it is concluded that there is relevant effect modification by sex, separate odds ratios are reported for males and females. In that case, confounding by sex is no longer a relevant issue. However, when the conclusion is that there is no relevant effect modification, then the next step in the analysis can be to evaluate whether sex is a confounder in the relationship between recovery and the intervention. As mentioned before, this question can also be answered with stratified analysis.

The general idea of using stratified analysis to evaluate possible confounding is that the weighted average of the two calculated odds ratios is an indication of the adjusted odds ratio. So, in the present example, the weighted average of the two odds ratios is an indication of the intervention effect adjusted for sex. The weighted average of the two odds ratios is known as the Mantel-Haenszel pooled odds ratio (see Eq. 5.29).

Table 5.25 Example of a stratified 2 × 2 table

	Outcome variable +	Outcome variable −	Total
Independent variable +	a_i	b_i	
Independent variable −	c_i	d_i	
Total			t_i

Table 5.26 Mantel-Haenszel pooled odds ratio and 95% confidence interval

Odds ratio	p-value	95% confidence interval
3.12	0.001	1.56–6.24

$$OR_{MH} = \frac{\sum\left(a_i \times \frac{d_i}{t_i}\right)}{\sum\left(b_i \times \frac{c_i}{t_i}\right)} \tag{5.29}$$

where OR_{MH} = Mantel-Haenszel pooled odds ratio, a_i, b_i, c_i, d_i = number of subjects in the cells of a stratified 2 × 2 table, and t_i = total number of subjects in a stratified 2 × 2 table (see Table 5.25).

When the Mantel-Haenszel pooled odds ratio is calculated with the numbers from the stratified 2 × 2 tables shown in Table 5.22, the pooled odds ratio is 3.12.

$$OR_{MH} = \frac{\left(56 \times \frac{16}{100}\right) + \left(24 \times \frac{24}{100}\right)}{\left(14 \times \frac{14}{100}\right) + \left(6 \times \frac{46}{100}\right)} = 3.12$$

The 95% confidence interval around this pooled odds ratio can be calculated manually using a complicated equation, but of course this can be performed by statistical software as well. Table 5.26 shows the result of the stratified analysis in which the pooled odds ratio with the corresponding 95% confidence interval is calculated.

So, the odds ratio for recovery for intervention compared to usual care, adjusted for sex is 3.12. It was already mentioned that the unadjusted odds ratio for recovery for intervention compared to usual care is 2.67. Both odds ratios are not equal, so there is some confounding by sex. Again, the question is whether the difference between the two odds ratios is relevant. Again, no answer is wrong, as long as the arguments are valid. In this example, the difference between the two odds ratios is so small that the confounding does not seem to be relevant, so reporting the unadjusted odds ratio is probably sufficient. It should again be realized that in this example the odds ratio has been used as effect estimate, while in the analysis of a randomized controlled trial a relative risk or a risk difference is also possible and maybe more appropriate. However, the test for homogeneity and the Mantel-Haenszel pooled effect estimate are only available for odds ratios.

Although the procedure to adjust for confounding and to evaluate effect modification using stratified analysis is fairly simple, it has a number of limitations. When there are multiple possible confounders and effect modifiers, many different (2 × 2) tables have to be made, leading to a small number of subjects in the different (2 × 2) tables. Furthermore, the method is mainly suitable for dichotomous confounders and effect modifiers, less suitable for categorical confounders and effect modifiers and not suitable for continuous confounders and effect modifiers. In these situations, the use of logistic regression analysis is necessary.

5.6.3 Confounding and Effect Modification Using Logistic Regression Analysis

The way to adjust for confounding and to evaluate effect modification with logistic regression analysis is identical to the way this was done with linear regression analysis (see Sect. 4.5). To illustrate the use of logistic regression analysis to adjust for confounding and to evaluate effect modification, again Example 5.1 will be used. In this example the effect of an activity program in patients with low back pain is investigated. The first step is to perform a logistic regression including only the intervention variable. Output 5.16 shows the result of this analysis.

To evaluate whether sex is a confounder in this relationship, sex can be added to the logistic regression analysis. Output 5.17 shows the result of this analysis.

As indicated earlier in Sect. 4.5, to evaluate confounding it is necessary to compare the regression coefficient from the unadjusted analysis (Output 5.16) with the regression coefficient from the adjusted analysis (Output 5.17). In the unadjusted analysis, the regression coefficient for the intervention variable is 0.98 and in the

Output 5.16 Result of the logistic regression analysis to analyse the relationship between recovery and the intervention

							95% confidence interval	
	Coefficient	se	Wald	df	p-value	Odds ratio	Lower	Upper
Intervention	0.98	0.32	9.24	1	0.002	2.67	1.42	5.02
Constant	−1.39	0.25	30.75	1	<0.001			

se standard error, *df* degrees of freedom

Output 5.17 Result of the logistic regression analysis to analyse the relationship between recovery and the intervention including sex

							95% confidence interval	
	Coefficient	se	Wald	df	p-value	Odds ratio	Lower	Upper
Intervention	1.19	0.36	10.83	1	<0.001	3.27	1.62	6.63
Sex	−0.49	0.35	1.89	1	0.17	0.62	0.31	1.23
Constant	−1.26	0.27	22.48	1	<0.001			

se standard error, *df* degrees of freedom

Output 5.18 Result of the logistic regression analysis to analyse the relationship between recovery and the intervention including sex and the interaction between the intervention and sex

							95% confidence interval	
	Coefficient	se	Wald	df	p-value	Odds ratio	Lower	Upper
Intervention	1.52	0.47	10.35	1	0.001	4.57	1.81	11.54
Sex	0.00	0.55	0.00	1	1.00	1.00	0.34	2.91
intervention*sex	−0.78	0.70	1.23	1	0.27	0.46	0.12	1.81
Constant	−1.39	0.30	21.52	1	<0.001			

se standard error, *df* degrees of freedom

adjusted analysis, the regression coefficient for the intervention variable is 1.19. In other words, there is confounding by sex, because when sex is not taken into account, the effect of the intervention is slightly underestimated. It has been suggested that confounding should be considered relevant when the regression coefficient changes by more than 10% when a possible confounder is added to the regression analysis. Of course, this is a very arbitrary cut-off value, but in the example, the change in the regression coefficient is about 20%. So, based on the arbitrary cut-off value, it can be concluded that there is relevant confounding by sex.

This is a different conclusion than the one based on the stratified analysis (see Sect. 5.6.2), in which it was concluded that the pooled (i.e. adjusted) odds ratio of 3.12 did not differ much from the unadjusted odds ratio of 2.7. The adjusted odds ratio derived from the logistic regression analysis adjusted for sex is 3.27, which differs slightly from the adjusted odds ratio obtained from the stratified analysis. It should be noted that, in practice, the result from the logistic regression analysis is mostly used.

Effect modification can also be evaluated using logistic regression analysis. Suppose the question is whether or not the intervention effect is different for males and females, or in other words, whether or not sex is an effect modifier in the relationship between intervention and recovery. To analyse effect modification, an interaction term must be made that consists of a multiplication of the intervention variable and the possible effect modifier, i.e. sex. Next, a logistic regression analysis is performed including three variables: the intervention variable, sex, and the interaction between the intervention variable and sex. Output 5.18 shows the result of this analysis.

To understand the interpretation of the regression coefficients from Output 5.18, the regression equation can best be written out.

$$ln(odds(recovery)) = -1.39 + 1.52 \times I + 0.00 \times S - 0.78 \times I \times S$$

The intervention effect for females can be calculated by entering 0 for sex in the regression equation (sex is coded 0 for females). For usual care (intervention = 0), the outcome variable is:

$$ln\,(odds(recovery))_{0,0} = -1.39 + 1.52 \times 0 + 0.00 \times 0 - 0.78 \times 0 \times 0 = -1.39$$

For intervention = 1, for females the outcome variable is:

$$ln\,(odds(recovery))_{1,0} = -1.39 + 1.52 \times 1 + 0.00 \times 0 - 0.78 \times 1 \times 0 = -1.39 + 1.52$$

The difference in outcome variable between intervention and usual care for females is therefore 1.52, which is exactly the regression coefficient for the intervention variable shown in Output 5.18. The corresponding odds ratio for the intervention for females is EXP[1.52] = 4.57. In a similar way, the intervention effect for males can be calculated.

$$ln\,(odds(recovery))_{0,1} = -1.39 + 1.52 \times 0 + 0.00 \times 1 - 0.78 \times 1 \times 0 = -1.39 + 0.00$$

$$ln\,(odds(recovery))_{1,1} = -1.39 + 1.52 \times 1 + 0.00 \times 1 - 0.78 \times 1 \times 1 = -1.39 + 1.52 + 0.00 - 0.78$$

The difference in outcome variable between intervention and usual care for males is therefore equal to 1.52–0.78 = 0.74. In other words, the difference in outcome variable between intervention and usual care for males is equal to the sum of the regression coefficient for the intervention variable (1.52) and the regression coefficient for the interaction term (−0.78). The odds ratio for the intervention for males is EXP[0.74] = 2.09.

It is, of course, no surprise that both odds ratios are equal to the odds ratios calculated using stratified analysis. Basically, exactly the same analysis has been performed. The conclusion is therefore again that there appears to be effect modification. The odds ratio for the intervention is higher for females than for males, so the intervention seems to work better in females than in males. The question is again to what extent this difference is relevant. For a relatively objective evaluation of effect modification, the magnitude of the regression coefficient for the interaction between the intervention variable and sex can be used, because that is the magnitude of the difference in regression coefficient between males and females. In many cases, therefore, the p-value of the regression coefficient for the interaction term is used to define whether the observed effect modification is relevant. In Output 5.18 it can be seen that the p-value for the interaction term is 0.27. Thus, the null hypothesis (the regression coefficient is 0; there is no difference between the regression coefficients for males and females) cannot be rejected. Based on this p-value, the conclusion is that no statistically significant effect modification is observed and that, therefore, one odds ratio for the intervention can be reported and no different odds ratios for males and females have to be reported.

Output 5.19 Result of the logistic regression analysis to analyse the relationship between recovery and the intervention including sex and the interaction between the intervention and sex recoded

							95% confidence interval	
	Coefficient	se	Wald	df	p-value	Odds ratio	Lower	Upper
Intervention	0.74	0.52	1.99	1	0.16	2.09	0.75	5.80
Sex_recoded	0.00	0.55	0.00	1	1.00	1.00	0.34	2.91
Intervention*sex_recoded	0.78	0.70	1.23	1	0.27	2.19	0.55	8.70
Constant	-1.39	0.46	9.23	1	0.002			

se standard error, *df* degrees of freedom

The p-value of 0.27 is, of course, similar to the p-values which were obtained from the tests for homogeneity of the two odds ratios (see Table 5.24). It should be noted that in practice, a somewhat higher cut-off value (e.g. $p < 0.10$) is often used to assess the relevance of effect modification. This is done because the standard error for an interaction term is relatively high. This is due to the fact that when effect modification is analysed, the population under study is divided into subgroups, in which the number of subjects is always lower than in the total population. Therefore, an effect modifier has to produce (very) large differences to be statistically significant. However, it should be noted that, given the limitations of statistical significance testing, it is rather strange that the p-value of the interaction term is mostly used to evaluate effect modification.

As has been mentioned before, the odds ratio for the intervention for females can be obtained directly from Output 5.18, while for the odds ratio for the intervention for males, two regression coefficients must be added together. The 95% confidence interval around the odds ratio for females can also be directly obtained from Output 5.18. The 95% confidence interval ranges between 1.81 and 11.54 and the corresponding p-value is 0.001. For males, however, the standard error for the sum of the two regression coefficients cannot be obtained directly from the output. In order to be able to obtain the 95% confidence interval around the odds ratio for males, the variable sex must be recoded and the data must be reanalysed with the recoded sex variable. Output 5.19 shows the result of this analysis.

In Output 5.19 it can be seen that, for males, the odds ratio for the intervention is 2.09 and the 95% confidence interval ranges between 0.75 and 5.80. The corresponding p-value is 0.16. So, looking at the two odds ratios, an interesting phenomenon occurs. For females, the odds ratio for intervention compared to usual care is statistically significant, while for males the odds ratio is not statistically significant. Based on this difference, many researchers conclude that there is a significant difference between the two odds ratios, which is a misinterpretation and, again, nicely shows the limitations of statistical significance testing.

Table 5.27 Illustration of the problem of non-collapsibility

A	Intervention	Control
Females	30	30
Males	30	30
Equal numbers for females and males in the intervention and control group		
B	Intervention	Control
Outcome variable = 1	50	30
Outcome variable = 0	10	30
Odds ratio for intervention compared to control to have the outcome variable = 5		
C	Outcome variable = 1	Outcome variable = 0
Females	30	30
Males	10	50
Odds ratio for females compared to males to have the outcome variable = 5		

5.6.4 *Non-collapsibility*

Evaluating confounding using logistic regression analysis when a dichotomous outcome variable is analysed is a bit more problematic than evaluating confounding using linear regression analysis when a continuous outcome variable is analysed. This has to do with the problem of non-collapsibility. This phenomenon, which is not known by most researchers, is illustrated in Table 5.27. In this illustration it can be seen that there is no relationship between the intervention variable and sex (i.e. the intervention group and the control group have equal numbers for males and females.). The unadjusted effect of the intervention (i.e. without adjusting for sex) is an odds ratio of 5. It can also be seen that sex is highly related to the outcome variable (the corresponding odds ratio is also 5). Because the numbers for males and females are exactly the same for both the intervention and control group an adjustment for sex should not change the magnitude of the treatment effect. However, when a logistic regression analysis is performed adjusting for sex, the adjusted odds ratio will be around 6.7; much higher than the expected odds ratio of 5.

So, when confounding is evaluated using logistic regression analysis it should be realized that confounding is mixed up with non-collapsibility. The change in regression coefficient when a possible confounder is added to a logistic regression analysis is not only caused by confounding, but also by non-collapsibility. It should, however, also be realised that the influence of non-collapsibility is, in general, very small.

Chapter 6
The Analysis of Survival Data

Abstract Survival data is characterised by a dichotomous outcome variable (the event) and the time till the event occurs. The analysis of survival data is specifically developed for analysing mortality data, but it is also used in other situations, such as time to recovery, etc. To describe survival data and to compare survival data between groups, Kaplan-Meier curves are normally used, while the log-rank test can be used to compare Kaplan-Meier curves with each other. To obtain effect estimates, Cox regression analysis can be used. Cox regression analysis is comparable to linear regression analysis and logistic regression analysis, in a way that the regression coefficients have the same interpretation, only the outcome variable is different. In Cox regression analysis, the outcome variable is the natural log of the hazard function. Because of that the regression coefficient of an independent variable can be transformed into a hazard ratio, i.e. a relative risk on average over time. Because the effect estimate is on average over time, this is only a good effect estimate when the hazards are proportional over time. Cox regression analysis is, therefore, also known as Cox proportional hazards regression analysis. Whether the hazards are proportional can, for instance, be investigated with a Cox regression analysis with a time-dependent covariate. In this chapter, furthermore, the evaluation of linearity of the relationship with a continuous independent variable, the adjustment for confounding and the investigation of effect modification are discussed. The way this is done in Cox regression analysis is exactly the same as in linear and logistic regression analysis.

6.1 Introduction

In Chap. 5 the analysis of a dichotomous outcome variable was discussed. It was shown that when comparing two groups, a 2×2 table can be used to show the results. Suppose that in an observational prospective cohort study investigating the relationship between mortality and smoking, 600 males aged 65 years and older are followed for 15 years. The outcome variable is mortality and Table 6.1 shows the 2×2 table with the result of this study.

J. W. R. Twisk, *Basic Principles of Applied Medical Statistics*,
https://doi.org/10.1007/978-3-031-86278-6_6

Table 6.1 2 × 2 Table to show the relationship between mortality and smoking

	Mortality yes	Mortality no	Total
Smoking	50	50	100
Non-smoking	50	450	500
Total	100	500	600

Table 6.2 2 × 2 Table to show the relationship between mortality and smoking

	Mortality yes	Mortality no	Total
Smoking	99	1	100
Non-smoking	450	50	500
Total	550	50	600

Because the result shown in Table 6.1 are from a prospective cohort study, the probability of mortality for smoking and non-smoking can be compared to each other. The probability of mortality for smoking is 0.50, while the probability of mortality for non-smoking is 0.10. Based on these probabilities, the risk difference (i.e. 0.50–0.10 = 0.40) and the relative risk (i.e. 0.50/0.10 = 5) can be calculated. Both effect estimates indicate that smoking is a strong risk factor for mortality.

Suppose now that the prospective cohort study is continued for another 15 years and that after these 15 years a new 2 × 2 table is made with the result of the study (see Table 6.2).

Table 6.2 shows that the probability of mortality for smoking is now 0.99 while the probability of mortality for non-smoking is also 0.99. So, the risk difference between smoking and non-smoking is 0 and the relative risk is 1.

Based on the result shown in Table 6.1 it can be concluded that smoking is a strong risk factor for mortality, but based on the result shown in Table 6.2 it can be concluded that smoking is not a risk factor for mortality at all. The problem here is the fact that a dichotomous outcome variable is being analysed (i.e. mortality) that always will occur. When the study continues long enough, everyone in the study eventually will die.

Does this mean that smoking is not a risk factor for mortality? On the one hand, yes, because smokers and non-smokers all die, but on the other hand, no, because the risk of smoking is that smokers die earlier than non-smokers. Therefore, one of the problems in analysing a dichotomous outcome variable discussed in Chap. 5 is that the time until the outcome variable occurs is not included in the analysis. Because mortality research is the classic example in this case, the statistical methods that take into account the time until the dichotomous outcome variable occurs are called survival analyses.

6.2 Comparing Two Groups—Incidence Densities

When a study result is presented in a 2 × 2 table, the probability of having a dichotomous outcome variable in one group is compared to the probability of having the same dichotomous outcome variable in the other group. Because in a prospective study, the probability of having a dichotomous outcome variable is known as a cumulative incidence, in principle, two cumulative incidences are compared with each other. When the time until the dichotomous outcome variable occurs is taken into account, no longer the cumulative incidences are compared to each other, but the incidence densities.

When an incidence density is calculated in a mortality study, the number of subjects being dead is divided not only by the number of subjects in the study population, i.e. the number of subjects who were alive at the start of the study, but also by the total time those subjects had the opportunity to die. The latter is known as time at risk. Suppose a small-scale prospective cohort study is performed with 10 subjects with a maximal follow-up time of 10 years and with mortality as dichotomous outcome variable. Figure 6.1 shows the survival data.

Within survival data, two possibilities can be distinguished: the subject has the dichotomous outcome variable, in the example this means that the subject dies, or the subject does not have the dichotomous outcome variable, in the example this means that the subject stays alive. In survival terminology, not having the dichotomous outcome variable is known as censoring. Censoring can take place in two ways: first, at the end of the study. When a particular subject does not have the dichotomous outcome variable at the end of the study, the subject is censored. The second possibility is that a subject is no longer willing or able to participate in the study at a certain time point. In that case, the subject is also censored, which means that the last available information of that particular subject indicates that the subject does not have the dichotomous outcome variable, but after that particular

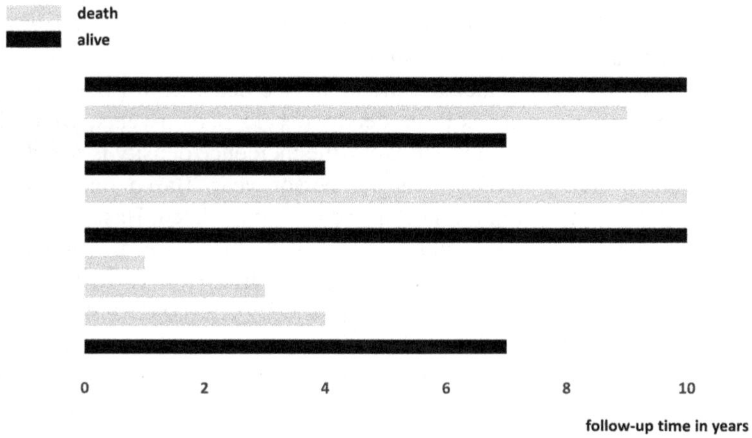

Fig. 6.1 Illustration of survival data; each bar represents a subject

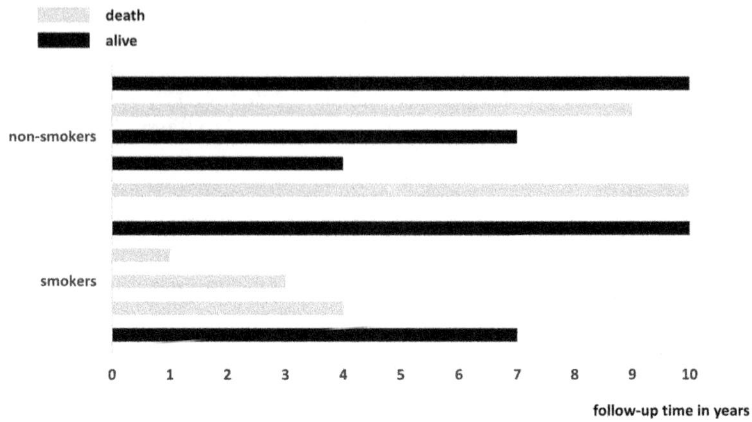

Fig. 6.2 Illustration of survival data; comparing smokers and non-smokers; each bar represents a subject

measurement there is no information available. In Fig. 6.1 it can be seen that five out of 10 subjects died and that the other five subjects were censored: two at the end of the study and three during the study. From Fig. 6.1 it is easy to calculate the incidence density of mortality for the study population. To do this, the number of deaths (i.e. five) must be divided by the total time that the subjects in the study were at risk of dying. For this purpose, the time at risk for all subjects is added together. For example, the first subject in the study has been at risk for 7 years, the second person for 1 year, the third person for 3 years, and so on. The total population has been at risk for 65 years; a number which is also known as the number of person-years. So, the incidence density of mortality in the total study population is five deaths divided by 65 years at risk, which is 0.077 deaths per person-year. Although the incidence density of a particular study population can provide interesting information, it becomes much more interesting when the incidence densities of different groups are compared to each other. Figure 6.2 divides the study population into a group of smokers and a group of non-smokers.

Figure 6.2 can be used to calculate the incidence densities for both groups. For smokers, the incidence density is three deaths per 25 person-years, which is 0.12 deaths per person-year, and for non-smokers, the incidence density is two deaths per 40 person-years, which is 0.05 deaths per person-year. Based on the incidence densities, the effect of smoking on mortality can be calculated. Basically two effect estimates are available, i.e. the incidence density difference and the incidence density ratio. In the example, the incidence density difference is 0.12–0.05 = 0.07 deaths per person-year. The incidence density ratio is 0.12/0.05 = 2.4. Although the latter is often interpreted as a relative risk, it is not the same. In a relative risk, only the number of subjects having the dichotomous outcome variable are compared to each other. In an incidence density ratio, the time until the dichotomous outcome variable occurs is also taken into account. To illustrate the difference between the two effect estimates, in the example shown in Fig. 6.2, the relative risk is 1.5 (the probability of mortality for smokers is 0.6 and for non-smokers 0.4), which is much lower than the incidence density ratio of 2.4.

By comparing the relative risk and the incidence density ratio, the importance of the time until the dichotomous outcome variable occurs can be evaluated. In the example, the incidence density ratio is higher than the relative risk, so the effect of smoking on mortality is not only based on the fact that more smokers die than non-smokers (after all, the relative risk is greater than 1), but also on the fact that they die faster.

The incidence density difference and the incidence density ratio are effect estimates. In order to estimate the uncertainty of the observed result in the generalization to the source population, 95% confidence intervals have to calculated around the effect estimates. Equation 6.1 specifies how to calculate the standard error of the incidence density difference.

$$se(idd) = \sqrt{a_1/P_1^2 + a_2/P_2^2} \tag{6.1}$$

where *se(idd)* = standard error of the incidence density difference, a_1, a_2 = number of subjects having the dichotomous outcome variable in both groups and P_1, P_2 = person-time in both groups.

When the numbers of the example are entered into Eq. 6.1, the standard error of the incidence density difference is 0.078.

$$se(idd) = \sqrt{3/25^2 + 2/40^2} = 0.078$$

Using this standard error, the 95% confidence interval around the incidence density difference can be calculated (see Eq. 6.2).

$$idd \pm z_{(1-\alpha/2)} \times se(idd) \tag{6.2}$$

where *idv* = incidence densities difference, $z_{(1-\alpha/2)}$ = value of the standard normal distribution for which $(1 - \alpha/2)\%$ of the distribution is below that value and *se(idv)* = standard error of the incidence density difference.

When the numbers of the example are entered into Eq. 6.2, the 95% confidence interval around the incidence density difference ranges between −0.08 and 0.22 deaths per person-year.

$$0.07 \pm 1.96 \times 0.078 = [-0.08 - 0.22]$$

Based on this confidence interval, it can also be concluded that the observed incidence density difference of 0.07 deaths per person-year is not statistically significant. The value of the null hypothesis (i.e. 0) is within the 95% confidence interval.

For the calculation of the standard error of the incidence density ratio a log transformation must be applied. This is comparable to what was done for the relative risk (see Sect. 5.1.2). The standard error of the natural logarithm of the incidence density ratio is very easy to calculate (see Eq. 6.3).

$$se[ln(idr)] \pm \sqrt{1/a_1 + 1/a_2} \tag{6.3}$$

where $se[ln(idr)]$ = standard error of the natural logarithm of the incidence density ratio and a_1, a_2 = number of subjects having the dichotomous outcome variable in both groups.

When the numbers of the example are entered into Eq. 6.3, the standard error of the natural logarithm of the incidence density ratio is 0.91.

$$se[ln(idr)] \pm \sqrt{1/3 + 1/2} = 0.91$$

Next, a 95% confidence interval around the natural logarithm of the incidence density ratio can be calculated with Eq. 6.4.

$$ln(idr) \pm z_{(1-\alpha/2)} \times se[ln(idr)] \tag{6.4}$$

where $ln\ (idr)$ = natural logarithm of the incidence density ratio, $z_{(1-\alpha/2)}$ = value of the standard normal distribution for which $(1-\alpha/2)\%$ of the distribution is below that value and $se[ln(idr)]$ = standard error of the natural logarithm of the incidence density ratio.

When the numbers of the example are entered into Eq. 6.4, the 95% confidence interval around the natural logarithm of the incidence density ratio ranges between − 0.91 and 2.66 deaths per person-year.

$$ln(2.4) \pm 1.96 \times 0.91 = 0.88 \pm 1.72 = [-0.91 - 2.66]$$

Of course, the limits of this 95% confidence interval must be transformed back to the original data. Analogous to the situation described for the relative risk (see Sect. 5. 1.2), the e-power of both limits has to be taken. This leads to a 95% confidence interval around the incidence density ratio which ranges between 0.40 and 14.30. First, it can be seen that the 95% confidence interval is very wide, which is due to the small number of subjects in the study population and second it can be seen that the observed incidence density ratio of 2.4 is not statistically significant. This is due to the fact that the value of the null hypothesis (i.e. 1) is inside the limits of the 95% confidence interval.

6.3 Comparing Two Groups—Kaplan-Meier Survival Curves

In the previous section, the incidence density has been used to describe a dichotomous outcome variable and the time until the dichotomous outcome variable occurs. To illustrate this combined outcome variable the Kaplan-Meier survival curve can be used. To make a Kaplan-Meier survival curve, the follow-up time is divided into small periods and the probability of survival for each of these periods is calculated. This probability is based on the fact that a person is still alive at the beginning of that particular period. Equation 6.5 shows the way in which these probabilities can be calculated (this equation is also known as the Kaplan-Meier equation).

$$S(t) = S(t-1) \times \mathit{survival\ fraction} \quad (6.5)$$

where $S(t)$ = probability of survival in period t, given the probability that period t is started alive.

The way in which the Kaplan-Meier survival curve can be made is illustrated by the example shown in Fig. 6.1. In this example a group of 10 subjects is followed for 10 years. First of all, the survival probability at the beginning of the study is 1, because all subjects are alive at the beginning of the study. At time point 1, one of the 10 subjects is dead. The survival probability at 1 year is then equal to 1 multiplied by the survival fraction (1×0.9) = 0.9. So the 1-year survival probability is 0.9. At time point 2 nothing happens and at time point 3 another subject died. The survival probability over the third period is the probability that a subject will survive this period, given the probability to start that period alive, which is 0.9. This probability is multiplied by the survival fraction over the third period (8/9), which gives a 3-year survival probability of 0.8. In the fourth period one subject died and one subject is censored (which, by the way, does not affect the survival probability at this time point because it is assumed that the subject is still alive when censored). The survival probability over the fourth period is 0.8 (the probability of starting this period alive) multiplied by 7/8 (the survival fraction over this period) = 0.7. So the 4-year survival probability is 0.7. Because the next death occurs in the ninth period, all survival probabilities in the in-between periods are 0.7. The survival probability over the ninth period is therefore 0.7 (the probability of starting this period alive) multiplied by 3/4 (the survival fraction over this period) = 0.53. So the 9-year survival probability is 0.53. The survival probability over the last period is 0.53 (the probability of starting this period alive) multiplied by 2/3 (the survival fraction over this period) = 0.35. This means that the 10-year survival probability in this cohort is 0.35. Table 6.3 shows the calculation of the survival probabilities.

Figure 6.3 shows the Kaplan-Meier survival curve based on the survival probabilities shown in Table 6.3.

Although the Kaplan-Meier survival curve of a study population can provide interesting descriptive information, it becomes more interesting when the

Table 6.3 Calculation of survival probabilities based on the data shown in Fig. 6.1

S(0)	1	
S(1)	1 × 9/10	0.9
S(2)	0.9	
S(3)	0.9 × 8/9	0.8
S(4)	0.8 × 7/8	0.7
S(5)	0.7 × 6/6	0.7
S(6)	0.7	
S(7)	0.7	
S(8)	0.7 × 4/4	0.7
S(9)	0.7 × 3/4	0.53
S(10)	0.53 × 2/3	0.35

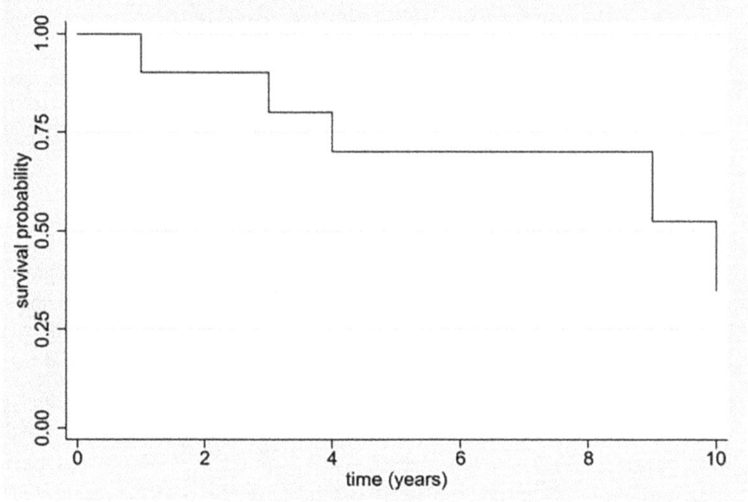

Fig. 6.3 Kaplan-Meier survival curve based on the survival probabilities shown in Table 6.3

Kaplan-Meier survival curves of two groups are compared to each other. This can be illustrated with the data shown in Fig. 6.2, in which a group of smokers and a group of non-smokers were followed over a period of 10 years. For both groups, a Kaplan-Meier survival curve can be made using the Kaplan-Meier equation. Figure 6.4 shows the Kaplan-Meier survival curves for both groups.

Comparing the Kaplan-Meier survival curves for smokers and non-smokers, it is obvious that the Kaplan-Meier survival curve for non-smokers is better than the Kaplan-Meier survival curve for smokers. Not only the number of deaths among smokers is higher than the number of deaths among non-smokers, also smokers die faster than non-smokers (which can be seen from the fact that the Kaplan-Meier survival curve for smokers decreases much faster than the Kaplan-Meier survival curve for non-smokers). The next question, of course, is how much worse the

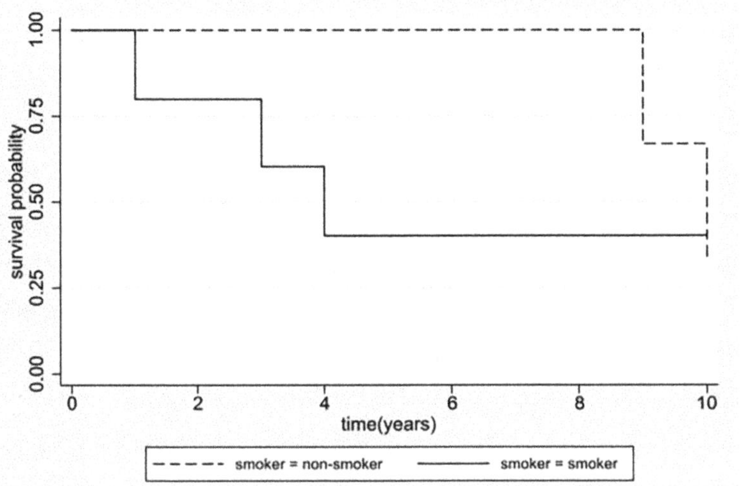

Fig. 6.4 Kaplan-Meier survival curves for smokers and non-smokers based on the data shown in Fig. 6.2

Kaplan-Meier survival curve for smokers is compared to the Kaplan-Meier survival curve for non-smokers.

As has been discussed before, for 2 × 2 tables, in which only the number of deaths for both groups are compared, three effect estimates can be calculated; the relative risk, the risk difference and the odds ratio (see Sects. 5.1 and 5.4). However, the comparison of the two Kaplan-Meier survival curves does not directly lead to an effect estimate. To obtain an effect estimate, a regression method must be used (see Sect. 6.6). However, a p-value can be calculated for the difference between the two Kaplan-Meier survival curves. The statistical test that can be used in this situation is the log-rank test.

The idea behind the log-rank test is quite simple. Similar to the chi-square test, the log-rank test compares the number of observed subjects having the dichotomous outcome variable with the expected number of subjects having the dichotomous outcome variable when the null hypothesis is true. The difference between the log-rank test and the chi-square test is that the log-rank test compares the number of observed and expected subjects at each time point, while the chi-square test only compares the number of observed and expected subjects at the end of the study. The basic principle of the log-rank test can best be explained by Table 6.4.

Table 6.4 shows the 10 time points of the study. The six columns show the observed number of deaths for both groups, the number of subjects at risk for both groups and the expected number of deaths when the null hypothesis is true for both groups. When the null hypothesis is true in this case means that the probability of dying is the same in both groups. In Fig. 6.2 it can be seen that at the first time point one person (a smoker) died; so one death is observed. In both groups, five subjects are at risk of dying at that time. So the probability of dying, when the null hypothesis

Table 6.4 Basic principle of the log rank test based on the Kaplan-Meier survival curves shown in Fig. 6.4

Time	Observed		Number at risk		Expected[a]	
	Smoking	Non-smoking	Smoking	Non-smoking	Smoking	Non-smoking
1	1	0	5	5	0.50	0.50
2	0	0	5	5		
3	1	0	4	5	0.44	0.56
4	1	c	3	5	0.375	0.625
5	0	0	2	4		
6	0	0	2	4		
7	c	c	2	4		
8	0	0	1	3		
9	0	1	1	2	0.25	0.75
10	c	1 c			0.33	0.67
Total	3	2			1.895	3.105

c censored
[a] Expected when the null hypothesis is true

is true, is 0.50 for smokers and 0.50 for non-smokers (after all, the null hypothesis states that the probability of dying is the same in both groups). Since one death is observed, the number of expected deaths (when the null hypothesis is true) is the same in both groups, i.e. 0.5 deaths in both groups are expected. Figure 6.2 also shows that at the third time point one subject (again a smoker) died. However, the number of subjects at risk in both groups is no longer the same. Since one smoker died at the first time point, there are now only four smokers at risk of dying. Because when the null hypothesis is true the probabilities of dying are the same, the expected number of deaths for smokers is equal to the ratio of subjects at risk in both groups multiplied by the number of deaths observed. For smokers, the ratio of subjects at risk is 4/9. When this is multiplied by the one death, it leads to 0.44 expected deaths. For non-smokers, 0.56 deaths (5/9 times 1) are expected. This same calculations can be applied to all time points (see Table 6.4).

The next step in the log-rank test is to sum the expected number of deaths for both groups. For smokers a total of 1.895 deaths are expected and for non-smokers a total of 3.105 deaths are expected. Using Eq. 6.6, the test statistic of the log rank test can be calculated.

$$X^2 = \sum \frac{(O - E)^2}{E} \tag{6.6}$$

where χ^2= chi-square test statistic, O = observed number of subjects having the dichotomous outcome variable and E = expected number of subjects having the dichotomous outcome variable when the null hypothesis is true.

When the numbers from Table 6.4 are entered into Eq. 6.6, the test statistic is 1.04.

$$X^2 = \frac{(3-1.895)^2}{1.895} + \frac{(2-3.105)^2}{3.105} = 1.04$$

This test statistic has a chi-square distribution with a number of degrees of freedom equal to the number of groups that are compared - 1. In the example with two groups, the chi-square distribution has one degree of freedom, and the value 1.04 corresponds to a p-value of 0.31. This p-value indicates that the probability of finding the Kaplan-Meier survival curves from Fig. 6.3 (or even further away from the null hypothesis) when the null hypothesis is true (i.e. when the Kaplan-Meier survival curves for smokers and non-smokers are the same) is 0.31. Since this probability is >0.05, the difference between the Kaplan-Meier survival curves is not statistically significant.

6.4 Another Example

It has to be noted that survival analysis is not only used in mortality research; there are many other examples in which a survival analysis is useful. One of such an example is Example 6.1, which is an extension of Example 5.1. In the example, a randomised controlled trial is performed on patients with low back pain. The dichotomous outcome variable is perceived recovery. In the study an activity program is compared to usual care and for both groups 100 patients are included. The difference between Example 6.1 and Example 5.1 is that in Example 6.1 information is also available at what time a patient reported recovery. This information can be used to calculate the incidence density for both groups (see Table 6.5).

In Table 6.5 it can be seen that the time at risk for the usual care group is 405 months and for the intervention group 297 months. Time at risk is a bit strange in this situation because recovery is a positive outcome variable, but within survival analysis, time at risk is normally used. To calculate the incidence density for both groups, the number of patients recovered must be divided by the time at risk. The incidence density in the usual care group is 0.049 (20/405), and in the intervention group 0.135 (40/297). Because the time at risk is measured in months, these numbers can be interpreted as the number of recoveries per person-month.

So, in the intervention group, not only the number of patients reporting recovery is higher than in the usual care group (40 versus 20), but also the time at risk is shorter. For both incidence densities, the difference and the ratio can be calculated, and using Eqs. 6.2 and 6.4, the corresponding 95% confidence intervals can be calculated around these effect estimates. In the example, the incidence density

Table 6.5 Incidence density for the intervention group and usual care group

	Patients recovered	Total time at risk (months)	Incidence density
Intervention	40	297	0.135
Usual care	20	405	0.049

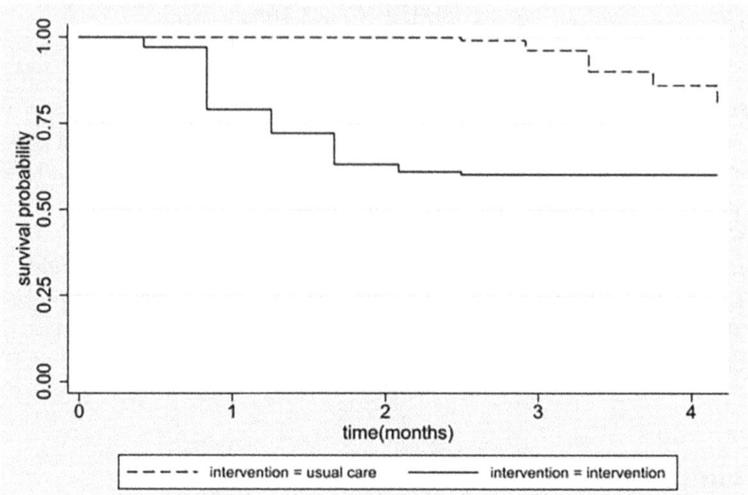

Fig. 6.5 Kaplan-Meier survival curves for recovery for the intervention group and the usual care group

difference between the intervention group and the usual care group is 0.086 patient per person month and the incidence density ratio is 2.76. The corresponding 95% confidence intervals range between 0.038 and 0.134 patients per person-month for the incidence density difference and between 1.61 and 4.72 for the incidence density ratio.

For both the intervention group and the usual care group a Kaplan-Meier survival curve can be made, which can be compared to each other using the log rank test. Figure 6.5 shows both Kaplan-Meier survival curves.

In Fig. 6.5 it can be seen that the Kaplan-Meier survival curve for the intervention group is much lower and also decreases much faster than for the usual care group. For the interpretation of the Kaplan-Meier survival curves, again it must be realized that the outcome variable of the study (i.e. recovery) is positive. In the case of a positive outcome variable, a low and/or rapidly decreasing Kaplan-Meier survival curve indicates a favourable course, in contrast to the earlier example with mortality as outcome variable.

Based on the Kaplan-Meier survival curves, a log-rank test can be performed. The test statistic of the log rank test is 13.53, which has a chi-square distribution with one degree of freedom, which gives a p-value <0.001. This p-value can be interpreted as the probability of finding the observed Kaplan-Meier survival curves (or more extreme away from the null-hypothesis) when the null-hypothesis is true, i.e. when the Kaplan-Meier survival curves are exactly the same.

Again, it should be noted that no effect measure can be calculated directly from the comparison of the Kaplan-Meier survival curves. To obtain an effect estimate, the incidence density difference or the incidence density ratio can be calculated, or a regression method can be used (see Sect. 6.6).

6.5 Comparing More than Two Groups

In Sect. 6.4 data from a randomized controlled trial were analysed in patients with low back pain. The intervention is an activity program, which is compared to usual care. In this randomized controlled trial, however, also a second intervention group is involved. In addition to the activity program, this second intervention group also received behavioural therapy. This study is the same as the study described in Chap. 5 in which the number of patients who reported recovery in the different groups were compared to each other (see Example 5.1a). In the present example, not only the numbers, but also the time at which recovery was reported is available (Example 6.1a). In Sect. 6.4, the incidence densities of the first intervention group and the usual care group were calculated, but now, also the incidence density of the second intervention group is calculated (see Table 6.6).

In Table 6.6, it can be seen that the incidence density of the second intervention group is 0.216 (50/232) recovery per person-month. When this incidence density is compared to the incidence density of the first intervention group, it appears that the number of patients who reported recovery is higher in the second intervention group and that the time to recovery is shorter. To obtain effect estimates for the second intervention group, the incidence density differences and/or the incidence density ratios can be calculated. For the comparison of the two intervention groups, for example, the incidence density difference is 0.081 recovery per person-month (in favour of the second intervention group) and the incidence density ratio is 1.6 (again in favour of the second intervention group). Using Eqs. 6.2 and 6.4, the corresponding 95% confidence intervals can be calculated. For the incidence density difference, the 95% confidence interval ranges between 0.01 and 0.15 recovery per person-month and for the incidence density ratio between 1.06 and 2.42.

For both effect estimates, therefore, there is a statistically significant difference between the two intervention groups (for both the incidence density difference and the incidence density ratio, the value of the null hypothesis is outside the 95% confidence interval). Of course, for the three groups that are compared in this study, the Kaplan-Meier survival curves can be made and the corresponding log rank test can be performed. Figure 6.6 shows the three Kaplan-Meier survival curves.

In Fig. 6.6 it can be seen that in the second intervention group not only most patients report recovery but also that the patients recover the fastest. In this example, the log-rank test gives a chi-square value of 28.51, which has a chi-square distribution with two degrees of freedom (the number of groups - 1). The corresponding p-value is <0.001. So, the probability of finding the observed Kaplan-Meier survival

Table 6.6 Incidence density for the three groups

	Patients recovered	Total time at risk (in moths)	Incidence density
Intervention 1	40	297	0.135
Intervention 2	50	232	0.216
Usual care	20	405	0.049

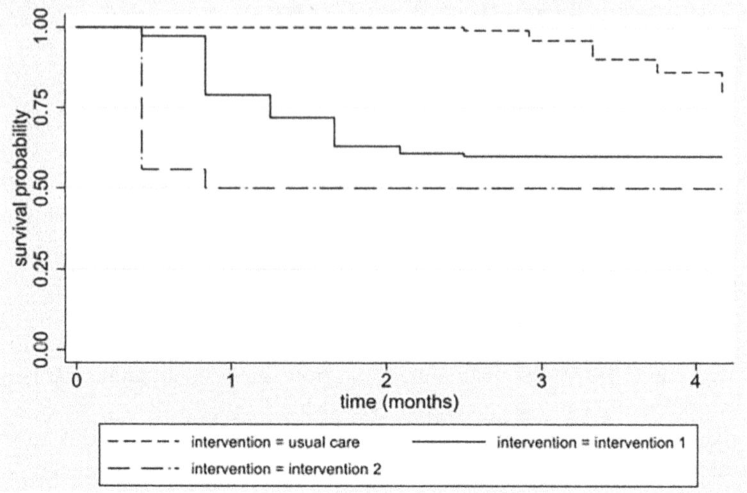

Fig. 6.6 Kaplan-Meier survival curves for recovery for the two intervention groups and the usual care group

Table 6.7 Result of the pairwise log-rank tests for the differences in recovery between the three groups

	Chi-square value	p-value
Control—Intervention 1	13.53	<0.001
Control—Intervention 2	24.61	<0.001
Intervention 1—Intervention 2	5.50	0.02

curves (or even further away from the null hypothesis) when the null hypothesis is true is <0.001. The null hypothesis in this case indicates that the three Kaplan-Meier survival curves are the same.

As has been mentioned before for the analysis of variance (for comparing more than two groups for a continuous outcome variable, see Sect. 4.3) and the chi-square test for a 2 × 3 table (for comparing more than two groups for a dichotomous outcome variable, see Sect. 5.3), the p-value of the log rank test does not say anything about which Kaplan-Meier survival curves differ statistically significant from each other. To evaluate this, a manual post-hoc procedure can be applied (as with the 2 × 3 table) in which the three groups are pairwise compared to each other. Table 6.7 shows the result of the three pairwise comparisons.

The results shown in Table 6.7 are not really surprising. Both intervention groups are statistically significant different from the usual care group, and both intervention groups are also statistically significant different from each other. However, it should be realized that in this analysis no correction has been made for multiple testing (see Sect. 4.3).

6.6 Cox Regression Analysis

6.6.1 *Introduction*

Analogous to studies with a continuous outcome variable (see Sect. 4.4) and a dichotomous outcome variable (see Sect. 5.5), there is regression method available that can be used to analyse the relationship between survival data and all kinds of independent variables. Instead of linear regression analysis (for a continuous outcome variable) or logistic regression analysis (for a dichotomous outcome variable), Cox regression analysis can be used. Similar to logistic regression analysis, the idea behind Cox regression analysis is to transform the outcome variable in such a way that a kind of linear regression analysis can be performed. With survival data it turns out that the natural logarithm of the hazard function is an outcome variable that can be used. The hazard can be seen as the inverse of survival. The mathematical details will not be discussed any further, because they are complicated and the understanding of the mathematics is not necessary for the application of the method and the interpretation of the results, (see for details, for example, Kleinbaum, 1996).

There is, however, a difference between Cox regression analysis on the one hand and linear and logistic regression analysis on the other, and that is that the result of a Cox regression analysis does not include an intercept value. This has to do with the fact that the intercept in a Cox regression analysis is not a single number, but a function over time. The intercept (i.e. the baseline hazard) changes over time and is therefore not shown in the output of a Cox regression analysis. Equation 6.7 shows the Cox regression equation.

$$ln(hazard) = ln(h_0) + b_1 x \tag{6.7}$$

where h_0= baseline hazard function, b_1 = regression coefficient for the independent variable and x = independent variable.

6.6.2 *Cox Regression Analysis with a Dichotomous Independent Variable*

To illustrate the use of Cox regression analysis, Example 6.1 will be used. In the randomized controlled trial, an intervention (i.e. an activity program) is compared to a control condition (i.e. usual care). In the previous sections, the incidence density difference, the incidence density ratio and the log-rank test were all in favour of the intervention. Output 6.1 shows the result of the Cox regression analysis to obtain the effect of the intervention.

In Output 6.1 it can be seen that the regression coefficient for the intervention is 0.95. The interpretation is identical to that of the regression coefficient in linear and logistic regression analysis, i.e. the difference in the outcome variable between the

Output 6.1 Result of the Cox regression analysis to analyse the relationship between recovery and the intervention

	Coefficient	se	Wald	df	p-value
Intervention	0.95	0.28	11.99	1	<0.001

se standard error, *df* degrees of freedom

intervention group and the usual care group. Since the outcome variable in Cox regression analysis is the natural logarithm of the hazard for recovery, this means that the difference in the natural logarithm of the hazard for recovery between both groups is 0.95. To better interpret this number, (as in logistic regression analysis) the rule can be used that the difference of two logarithms with the same base is equal to the logarithm of the ratio of the two numbers. By taking the e-power of the regression coefficient, the ratio between two hazards is obtained (see Eqs. 6.8a, 6.8b and 6.8c).

$$b_1 = ln\,(hazard)_{int} - ln\,(hazard)_{cont} \tag{6.8a}$$

$$b_1 = \left[\frac{ln\,(hazard)_{int}}{ln\,(hazard)_{cont}}\right] \tag{6.8b}$$

$$EXP(b_1) = \frac{ln\,(hazard)_{int}}{ln\,(hazard)_{cont}} \tag{6.8c}$$

The e-power of the regression coefficient gives a hazard ratio and its interpretation is identical to that of the incidence density ratio. In the example, the regression coefficient for the intervention is 0.95, the e-power of which gives a hazard ratio of 2.59. This hazard ratio is a combination of the difference in the number of patients recovered and the difference in time to recovery. The hazard ratio indicates that the probability of recovery in the intervention group is 2.59 times as high as in the usual care group on average over time. The addition on average over time distinguishes the interpretation of the hazard ratio from the interpretation of the relative risk. Cox regression analysis is also referred to as Cox proportional hazards regression analysis. The assumption is that the hazard ratio should not differ too much over time, i.e. the hazard ratio must be proportional over time (see Sect. 6.8).

In Output 6.1 it can also be seen that the Wald statistic is used for statistical testing. As with logistic regression analysis, the Wald statistic is defined as the regression coefficient divided by the standard error squared (see Eq. 6.9).

$$Wald = \left({}^{b_1}\!/_{se(b_1)}\right)^2 \tag{6.9}$$

where $Wald$ = Wald statistic, b = regression coefficient and $se(b)$= standard error of the regression coefficient.

When the results from Output 6.1 are entered into Eq. 6.9, the Wald-statistic is 11.99.

Output 6.2 Result of the Cox regression analysis to analyse the relationship between recovery and the intervention

							95% confidence interval	
	Coefficient	se	Wald	df	p-value	Hazard ratio	Lower	Upper
Intervention	0.95	0.28	11.99	1	<0.001	2.59	1.51	4.44

se standard error, *df* degrees of freedom

$$Wald = \left({}^{0.95}\!/_{0.29} \right)^2 = 11.99$$

The Wald statistic has a chi-square distribution with one degree of freedom, and the corresponding p-value is <0.001. The uncertainty of the effect estimate can, of course, be quantified using a 95% confidence interval. To calculate a 95% confidence interval around the hazard ratio of 2.59, the 95% confidence interval around the regression coefficient must first be calculated (the same as in logistic regression analysis) (see Eq. 6.10).

$$b_1 \pm z_{\left(1 - \alpha/2\right)} \times se(b_1) \tag{6.10}$$

where b_1= regression coefficient, $z_{\left(1 - \alpha/2\right)}$ = value of the standard normal distribution for which $\left(1 - \alpha/2\right)$ % of the distribution is before that value and $se(b_1)$ = standard error of the regression coefficient.

When the results from Output 6.1 are entered into Eq. 6.10, the 95% confidence interval ranges between 0.41 and 1.49.

$$0.95 \pm 1.96 \times 0.28 = [0.41 - 1.49]$$

Next, the e-power of both limits must be taken to obtain the 95% confidence interval around the hazard ratio. In the example, the 95% confidence interval ranges between 1.51 and 4.44. Of course, this confidence interval can also be obtained using statistical software (see Output 6.2).

As has been mentioned before, the interpretation of the hazard ratio is similar to the interpretation of the incidence density ratio. However, when the hazard ratio obtained from the Cox regression analysis is compared to the incidence density ratio, they are not exactly the same. The incidence density ratio is 2.72, with a 95% confidence interval ranging between 1.59 and 4.65, while the hazard ratio is 2.59 with a 95% confidence interval ranging between 1.51 and 4.44. The main reason for the difference is that the incidence density ratio is based on observed data and that the result of the Cox regression analysis is based on modelled data assuming proportional hazards.

Within Cox regression analysis, the magnitude of the regression coefficient and the corresponding standard error are estimated using maximum likelihood, which is comparable to logistic regression analysis (see Sect. 5.5.3). In Cox regression

Table 6.8 Result of three statistical tests to obtain a p-value for the difference in recovery between the intervention group and the usual care group

	Chi-square value	p-value
Log rank test	13.53	<0.001
Wald test	11.99	<0.001
Likelihood ratio test	12.86	<0.001

analysis, the likelihood ratio test can, therefore, also be used to compare two models. This is done by comparing the −2 log likelihood of the model without the intervention variable (i.e. 606) to the −2 log likelihood of the model with the intervention variable (i.e. 619). The difference between the two (i.e. 13) has a chi-square distribution with one degree of freedom and has a p-value <0.001. As with logistic regression analysis, the absolute value of the −2 log likelihood is not informative and only relevant for the likelihood ratio test (see also Sect. 5.5.3). The p-value derived from the likelihood ratio test has the same interpretation as the p-value associated with the Wald test derived from the Cox regression analysis and the log rank test based on the Kaplan-Meier survival curves. As with logistic regression analysis, the numbers are comparable but not exactly the same (see Table 6.8).

It is important to realize that the log-rank test is fundamentally different from the Wald test and the likelihood ratio test. This is because the log-rank test is based on observed data, while the Wald test and the likelihood-ratio test are based on modelled data assuming proportional hazards (see Sect. 6.8).

6.6.3 Cox Regression Analysis with a Categorical Independent Variable

In Sect. 6.5 it was mentioned that a log rank test can be used to compare three or more groups with each other. To illustrate this, the example of the randomised controlled trial with three groups was used (Example 6.1a). The differences between the three groups can of course also be analysed using Cox regression analysis. As with linear and logistic regression analysis, this requires the three group categorical independent variable to be represented by two dummy variables (see Table 6.9).

The coding for the dummy variables indicates that in the analysis the usual care group is used as reference group. Therefore, the regression coefficient for the first dummy variable indicates the difference in the outcome variable between the first intervention group and the usual care group and the regression coefficient for the second dummy variable indicates the difference in the outcome variable between the second intervention group and the usual care group. Output 6.3 shows the result of this analysis.

In Output 6.3 it can be seen that the hazard ratio for the first intervention group compared to the usual care group is 2.33 and the hazard ratio for the second intervention group compared to the usual care group is 3.61. It should be noted

Table 6.9 Dummy coding for the intervention variable

	Dummy 1	Dummy 2
Usual care	0	0
Intervention 1	1	0
Intervention 2	0	1

Output 6.3 Result of the Cox regression analysis to analyse the relationship between recovery and the two interventions

							95% confidence interval	
	Coefficient	se	Wald	df	p-value	Hazard ratio	Lower	Upper
Dummy 1	0.85	0.27	9.52	1	0.002	2.33	1.36	3.99
Dummy 2	1.28	0.27	23.27	1	<0.001	3.61	2.14	6.09

se standard error, *df* degrees of freedom

that the hazard ratio for the first intervention group and the usual care group is different from the one shown in Output 6.1. The difference between the two (which basically should be the same) is caused by the difference in the analysis of three groups simultaneously and the analysis of two groups.

In some statistical software, the output of a Cox regression analysis with a categorical independent variable also includes the so-called overall Wald test. The overall Wald test gives a Wald statistic and a corresponding p-value, which is comparable to the p-value obtained from the log rank test comparing the three groups with each other. The test statistic of the overall Wald test is 23.38, which has a chi-square distribution with two degrees of freedom and gives a p-value <0.001. Again, it should be realized that the log-rank test is based on observed data, while the overall Wald test is based on modelled data assuming proportional hazards.

The question of whether there is a statistically significant difference between the three groups can of course also be answered using the likelihood ratio test. The -2 log likelihood of the model with the two dummy variables is 1193.00, while the -2 log likelihood of the model without the two dummy variables is 1219.64, which leads to a difference of 26.64. This difference has a chi-square distribution with two degrees of freedom and has a p-value <0.001.

6.6.4 Cox-Regression Analysis with a Continuous Independent Variable

In the previous sections, Cox regression analyses with a dichotomous and a categorical independent variable were discussed. Basically, with these analyses, the same questions were answered as with incidence densities and log-rank tests. The added value of a Cox regression analysis in these situations is, for example, the possibility of adjusting for confounding and the evaluation of effect modification (see Sect. 6.7). However, when there is a continuous independent variable, it is no longer possible to calculate incidence densities or to perform a log-rank test. When the relationship between survival data and a continuous independent variable is analysed, Cox regression analysis must be used. To illustrate the use of Cox regression analysis with a continuous independent variable, Example 6.2 is used. In this example a cohort of 288 elderly subjects is followed for a period of 8 years. The dichotomous outcome variable of interest is having a stroke, which occurred in 45 subjects. The continuous independent variable is cholesterol measured at the start of the study, Output 6.4 shows the result of the Cox-regression analysis to analyse the relationship between having a stroke and cholesterol.

The interpretation of the regression coefficient for cholesterol is of course identical to the interpretation of the regression coefficient for continuous independent variables in linear and logistic regression analysis. The regression coefficient shown in Output 6.4 (i.e. 0.98) is the difference in the outcome variable for a one-unit difference in the independent variable. In Cox regression analysis this means that the natural logarithm of the hazard for having a stroke (on average over time) differs by 0.98 units between two subjects who differ one unit in cholesterol. In Output 6.4 it can further be seen that the hazard ratio for a one unit difference in cholesterol is 2.66 and that the corresponding 95% confidence interval ranges between 1.45 and 4.89. Finally, it can be seen that the relationship between having a stroke and cholesterol has a p-value of 0.002, which is based on the Wald statistic of 9.97.

Similar to linear and logistic regression analysis with a continuous independent variable, Cox regression analysis with a continuous independent variable assumes that there is a linear relationship between having a stroke and cholesterol. Again, of course, the question is whether this assumption is justified. It should be realized that the fact that the linear relationship with cholesterol is statistically significant does not mean that a linear relationship is the most appropriate way to describe this relationship.

6.6.4.1 Evaluation of the Linear Relationship with a Continuous Independent Variable

It is clear that the regression analyses discussed so far (linear, logistic and Cox regression analysis) are very similar. Only the outcome variable is different in the three regression methods. It is therefore obvious that the evaluation of the linear

Output 6.4 Result of the Cox regression analysis to analyse the relationship between having a stroke and cholesterol

							95% confidence interval	
	Coefficient	se	Wald	df	p-value	Hazard ratio	Lower	Upper
Cholesterol	0.98	0.31	9.97	1	0.002	2.66	1.45	4.89

se standard error, *df* degrees of freedom

relationship with a continuous independent variable in Cox regression analysis can be done in the same three ways as has been discussed for linear (see Sect. 4.4.4.1) and logistic (see Sect. 5.5.5.1) regression analysis. So, either a different mathematical function can be used, the continuous independent variable can be divided into groups and analysed as a categorical variable using dummy variables, or spline functions can be used. First, a different mathematical function (i.e. a quadratic relationship) is analysed. Output 6.5 shows the result of the Cox regression analysis with cholesterol and cholesterol squared.

In Output 6.5 it can be seen that the regression coefficient for cholesterol squared has a p-value of 0.03, which is statistically significant. So, the quadratic relationship between having a stroke and cholesterol is a better way of analysing this relationship than the linear relationship shown in Output 6.4. It has already been mentioned that the problem of analysing the relationship with a different mathematical function is that the regression coefficients are difficult to interpret. Therefore, in practice, mostly a more pragmatic method is used to evaluate whether the relationship with a continuous independent variable is linear. In this more pragmatic method the continuous independent variable is divided into groups and then an analysis is performed with the categorical independent variable. As with the examples for linear and logistic regression analysis, the continuous independent variable cholesterol is divided into four groups based on quartiles. Table 6.10 shows the dymmy coding for the four groups based on quartiles and Output 6.6 shows the result of the Cox regression analysis with the three dummy variables with the lowest cholesterol quartile as reference group.

Output 6.6 clearly shows that there is no linear relationship between having a stroke and cholesterol. It can be seen that the hazard for having a stroke is higher in the second and fourth quartile than in the third quartile. In Output 6.6 it can also be seen that the standard errors of the three regression coefficients are relatively high, which leads to wide 95% confidence intervals around the hazard ratios for the different quartiles. This has to do with the relative low number of subjects having a stroke in the reference group. In the first quartile only one subject has a stroke. So, the estimated hazard ratios have to be interpreted with caution. A possible solution to deal with this problem is to use one of the other quartiles as reference group.

Output 6.5 Result of the Cox regression analysis to analyse the relationship between having a stroke and cholesterol including cholesterol squared

							95% confidence interval	
	Coefficient	se	Wald	df	p-value	Hazard ratio	Lower	Upper
Cholesterol	−5.12	2.71	3.59	1	0.06	0.01	0.00	1.19
Cholesterol squared	0.61	0.27	5.00	1	0.03	1.85	1.08	3.16

se standard error, *df* degrees of freedom

Table 6.10 Dummy coding for the variable cholesterol

	Dummy 1	Dummy 2	Dummy 3
Quartile 1	0	0	0
Quartile 2	1	0	0
Quartile 3	0	1	0
Quartile 4	0	0	1

Output 6.6 Result of the Cox regression analysis to analyse the relationship between having a stroke and cholesterol as a categorical variable

							95% confidence interval	
	Coefficient	se	Wald	df	p-value	Hazard ratio	Lower	Upper
Dummy 1	2.23	1.03	4.70	1	0.03	9.34	1.24	70.41
Dummy 2	1.25	1.10	1.29	1	0.26	3.48	0.41	29.77
Dummy 3	2.91	1.02	8.13	1	0.004	18.43	2.49	136.51

se standard error, *df* degrees of freedom

Table 6.11 Dummy coding for the variable cholesterol with the last quartile as reference group

	Dummy 1	Dummy 2	Dummy 3
Quartile 1	1	0	0
Quartile 2	0	1	0
Quartile 3	0	0	1
Quartile 4	0	0	0

Output 6.7 Result of the Cox regression analysis to analyse the relationship between having a stroke and cholesterol as a categorical variable using the last quartile as reference group

							95% confidence interval	
	Coefficient	se	Wald	df	p-value	Hazard ratio	Lower	Upper
Dummy 1	−2.92	1.02	8.13	1	0.004	0.05	0.007	0.402
Dummy 2	−0.68	0.33	4.36	1	0.04	0.51	0.27	0.96
Dummy 3	−1.67	0.49	11.42	1	<0.001	0.19	0.07	0.50

se standard error, *df* degrees of freedom

Table 6.11 shows the dummy coding using the last quartile as reference group and Output 6.7 shows the result of the corresponding Cox regression analysis.

In Output 6.7 it can be seen that the standard error for the regression coefficients for the second and the third quartile (the regression coefficients for dummy 2 and dummy 3) using the last quartile as reference group are much lower than in the results of the Cox regression analysis using the first quartile as reference group. It can further be seen that all regression coefficients are negative and the corresponding hazard ratios are below 1. This is, of course, not a surprise because in this analysis, the fourth quartile is used as a reference group and in that quartile the risk of having a stroke is the highest.

Table 6.12 Mean and range for cholesterol of the four quartiles used in the Cox regression analysis

	Mean	Range
Quartile 1	4.0	2.9–4.4
Quartile 2	4.7	4.5–4.9
Quartile 3	5.2	5.0–5.4
Quartile 4	5.7	5.5–6.4

Table 6.13 Part of the dataset that is used in the linear spline Cox regression analysis to analyse the relationship between having a stroke and cholesterol

Id	Stroke	Cholesterol	Cholesterol1	Cholesterol2
1	1	5.6	5.2	0.4
2	1	5.8	5.2	0.6
3	1	5.8	5.2	0.6
4	0	2.9	2.9	0
5	0	3.4	3.4	0
.				
288	9	5.8	5.2	0.6

Because there is no increasing or decreasing trend in the regression coefficients it is not necessary to compare the trend in the regression coefficients to the trend in the mean values of the quartiles. However, for an appropriate interpretation of the regression coefficients and corresponding hazard ratios shown in Output 6.7, it necessary to relate them to the mean values. Table 6.12 shows the mean values of the four quartiles.

It must be realized that it is not necessary to divide the continuous independent variable into four groups. Basically, any number of groups can be chosen, but the choice depends to a large extent on the number of subjects in the study population. Furthermore, it is (always) preferable to divide the continuous independent variable into groups based on biologically relevant cut-off values instead of arbitrary cut-off values (see Sect. 5.5.5.1).

The third possibility to evaluate whether the relationship with a continuous independent variable is linear is the use of splines (see Sects. 4.4.4.1 and 5.5.5.1). It has already been mentioned that the general idea of using splines is that the continuous independent variable is divided into separate parts in which a different relationship between the outcome variable and the independent variable is estimated. It has also been mentioned that a distinction can be made between linear spline regression analysis and cubic spline regression analysis, and that the latter leads to non-interpretable regression coefficients. Linear spline regression analysis within a Cox regression analysis, on the other hand lead to easily interpretable regression coefficients and corresponding hazard ratios. In the present example, the use of linear spline Cox regression analysis is illustrated using one knot for cholesterol at 5.2 (a value which is often used to define moderate cardiovascular risk). Table 6.13 shows part of the dataset used for this analysis.

Output 6.8 shows the results of the linear spline Cox regression analysis with one knot to analyse the relationship between having a stroke and cholesterol.

Output 6.8 Result of the linear spline Cox regression analysis with one knot to analyse the relationship between having a stroke and cholesterol

							95% confidence interval	
	Coefficient	se	Wald	df	p-value	Hazard ratio	Lower	Upper
Cholesterol1	−0.23	0.42	0.31	1	0.58	0.79	0.35	1.81
Cholesterol2	2.86	0.60	22.85	1	<0.001	17.53	5.42	56.74

se standard error, *df* degrees of freedom

In Output 6.8 it can be seen that the regression coefficient for cholesterol1 is −0.23. This coefficient indicates that when cholesterol is ≤5.2, one unit difference in cholesterol is related to −0.23 units difference in the outcome variable, i.e. the natural logarithm of the hazard for having a stroke. The regression coefficient for cholesterol2 has te same interpretation, but then for cholesterol concentrations >5.2. So, only for cholesterol values >5.2 a strong positive relationship between having a stroke and cholesterol is obtained. It should be realized that for both parts a linear relationship is assumed, which is, of course, also questionable. Regarding the evaluation of a linear relationship between having a stroke and cholesterol, based on the result shown in Output 6.8, it can be concluded that the relationship is not linear (see Sect. 4.4.4.1).

6.7 Confounding and Effect Modification

As has been mentioned before, one of the added values of Cox regression analysis is the fact that an adjustment can be made for confounding and that effect modification can be evaluated. Again, this is done in exactly the same way as with linear and logistic regression analysis. For the adjustment for confounding, the possible confounder has to be added to the Cox regression analysis and to evaluate the relevance of the confounding, the unadjusted analysis can be compared to the adjusted analysis. To illustrate this, Example 6.1a will be used and it will be evaluated whether the relationship between recovery and the two intervention groups is confounded by age. Output 6.9 shows the results of the unadjusted analysis and Output 6.10 shows the result of the analysis adjusted for age.

In order to evaluate possible confounding by age, the regression coefficients for the two dummy variables must be compared between the unadjusted analysis and the adjusted analysis. For the first dummy variable, which indicates the difference between the first intervention group and the usual care group, the regression coefficient in the unadjusted analysis is 0.85 and in the adjusted analysis 0.79. So, age has a small confounding effect on the difference between the first intervention group and the usual care group. Also within Cox regression analysis the arbitrary cut-off value of 10% change in the regression coefficient can be used to determine whether the confounding is relevant or not. So, in this case, the confounding effect of age can

Output 6.9 Result of the Cox regression analysis to analyse the relationship between recovery and the two interventions

							95% confidence interval	
unadjusted	Coefficient	se	Wald	df	p-value	Hazard ratio	Lower	Upper
Dummy 1	0.85	0.27	9.52	1	0.002	2.33	1.36	3.99
Dummy 2	1.28	0.27	23.27	1	<0.001	3.61	2.14	6.09

se standard error, *df* degrees of freedom

Output 6.10 Result of the Cox regression analysis to analyse the relationship between recovery and the two interventions including age

							95% confidence interval	
	Coefficient	se	Wald	df	p-value	Hazard ratio	Lower	Upper
Dummy 1	0.79	0.28	8.29	1	0.004	2.21	1.29	3.79
Dummy 2	1.27	0.27	22.48	1	<0.001	3.55	2.10	6.00
Age	−0.07	0.01	23.68	1	<0.001	0.93	0.91	0.96

se standard error, *df* degrees of freedom

be considered not relevant. For the second dummy variable, which indicates the difference between the second intervention group and the usual care group, the regression coefficient in the unadjusted analysis is 1.28 and in the adjusted analysis 1.27. So, age has an even smaller confounding effect on the difference between the second intervention group and the usual care group. Because the dummy variables only have a proper interpretation when they are both analysed at the same time in a regression analysis, it is irrelevant whether the possible confounder affects both regression coefficients or only one. Suppose that one of the two regression coefficients shows a large difference between the unadjusted and adjusted analysis, while the other regression coefficient remains more or less the same, the confounding is considered to be relevant.

For evaluating effect modification, also the same procedure can be used as has been described for linear and logistic regression analysis. To evaluate effect modification, an interaction term has to be made by multiplying the independent variable of interest with the possible effect modifier. In the example in which two intervention groups are compared to the usual care group, there are two independent variables of interest and therefore, there are two interaction terms. Output 6.11 shows the result of a Cox regression analysis in which possible effect modification by sex is investigated.

Interpreting the different regression coefficients of Output 6.11 is not easy. Basically, the interpretation of the result of the analysis with interaction terms is similar to the interpretation described for linear regression analysis (see Sect. 4.5) and logistic regression analysis (see Sect. 5.6.3). The difference with the other examples is that in the present example a categorical independent variable is analysed, which makes it slightly more complicated. Therefore, the different

Output 6.11 Result of the Cox regression analysis to analyse the relationship between recovery and the two intervention groups including the interaction with sex

							95% confidence interval	
	Coefficient	se	Wald	df	p-value	Hazard ratio	Lower	Upper
Dummy 1	1.22	0.37	11.01	1	<0.001	3.38	1.65	6.94
Dummy 2	1.97	0.31	39.75	1	<0.001	7.15	3.88	13.18
Sex	−0.21	0.49	0.002	1	0.97	0.98	0.38	2.55
Dummy 1*sex	−0.53	0.59	0.81	1	0.37	0.59	0.19	1.86
Dummy 2*sex	−2.15	0.66	10.72	1	0.001	0.12	0.03	0.42

se standard error, *df* degrees of freedom

regression coefficients shown in Output 6.11 will be discussed one by one. The regression coefficient for the first dummy variable (1.22) is the difference in the outcome variable between the first intervention group and the usual care group. However, because the interaction term with sex is also included in the Cox regression analysis, this regression coefficient only applies for sex = 0, i.e. only for females. So, the corresponding hazard ratio (3.38) is the hazard ratio for the first intervention group compared to the usual care group for females. The regression coefficient for the second dummy variable (1.97) is the difference in outcome variable between the second intervention group and the usual care group for females. The regression coefficient for sex is not interesting in the example, because the effect of sex on the outcome variable is not relevant in light of the estimation of the intervention effect. Nevertheless, the regression coefficient for sex can be interpreted as the difference in outcome variable between males and females, but only for the usual care group, because for the usual care group, the two interaction terms are 0. The regression coefficients for the two interaction terms are important in the context of the research question. The regression coefficient for the interaction term between the first dummy variable and sex (−0.53) is the difference between males and females in the difference in outcome variable between the first intervention group and the usual care group. The regression coefficient for the interaction between the second dummy variable and sex (−2.15) is the difference between males and females in the difference in outcome variable between the second intervention group and the usual care group. This last difference is not only large, but also statistically significant ($p = 0.001$) and, therefore, the conclusion of the Cox regression analysis is that there is significant effect modification by sex. As a result, the effects of the interventions (and the corresponding 95% confidence intervals) should be reported separately for males and females. For females, these effect estimates can be taken directly from Output 6.11 (i.e. hazard ratios of 3.38 and 7.15 respectively). For males, the regression coefficients and, therefore, the hazard ratios can be calculated from the regression coefficients shown in Output 6.11, i.e. the regression coefficients for the two dummy variables must be added to the regression coefficients for the two interaction terms. So, the difference in outcome variable between the first intervention group and the usual care group for males is

Output 6.12 Result of the Cox regression analysis to analyse the relationship between recovery and the two intervention groups including the interaction with sex recoded

							95% confidence interval	
	Coefficient	se	Wald	df	p-value	Hazard ratio	Lower	Upper
Dummy 1	0.69	0.46	2.30	1	0.13	2.00	0.82	4.89
Dummy 2	−0.18	0.58	0.10	1	0.76	0.84	0.27	2.59
Sex_recode	0.21	0.49	0.002	1	0.97	1.02	0.39	2.66
Dummy 1*sex_recode	0.53	0.59	0.81	1	0.37	1.69	0.54	5.23
Dummy 2*sec_recode	−2.15	0.66	10.72	1	0.001	8.56	2.37	30.95

se standard error, *df* degrees of freedom

Table 6.14 Overview of the results of the Cox regression analyses for males and females separately

	Hazard ratio	95% confidence interval	p-value
Females			
Intervention 1	3.38	1.65–6.94	<0.001
Intervention 2	7.15	3.88–13.18	<0.001
Males			
Intervention 1	2.00	0.82–4.89	0.13
Intervention 2	0.84	0.27–2.59	0.84

1.22–0.53 = 0.69, which leads to a hazard ratio of 1.99. The difference in outcome variable between the second intervention group and the usual care group for males is 1.97–2.15 = −0.18, which leads to a hazard ratio of 0.84. It is, however, not possible to obtain the corresponding 95% confidence intervals from Output 6.11. Therefore, a similar analysis must be performed in which sex is recoded. Output 6.12 shows the result of this Cox regression analysis and Table 6.14 summarizes the results for males and females separately. Based on these results, it can be concluded that both interventions are very successful for females, but not so much for males.

6.8 Evaluation of the Proportional Hazards Assumption

In discussing Cox regression analysis it was stated that the hazard ratio represents a relative risk on average over time. This is only a valid effect estimate when the hazard ratio remains more or less the same over time. Hence, Cox regression analysis is also known as Cox proportional hazards regression analysis. The fact that reporting a hazard ratio on average over time can sometimes lead to problems is

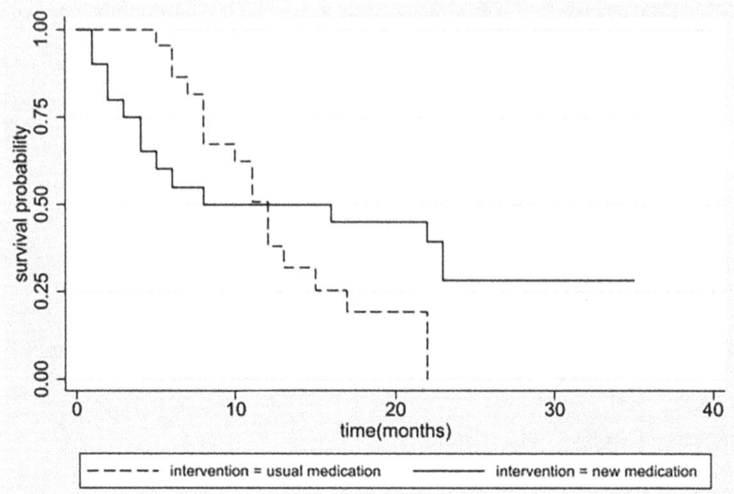

Fig. 6.7 Kaplan-Meier survival curves for mortality for the usual medication group and the new medication group

Output 6.13 Result of the Cox regression analysis to analyse the relationship between mortality and the new medication

							95% confidence interval	
	Coefficient	se	Wald	df	p-value	Hazard ratio	Lower	Upper
Medication	−0.29	0.40	0.53	1	0.47	0.75	0.34	1.64

se standard error, *df* degrees of freedom

illustrated by Example 6.3, in which the effect of a new medication for lung cancer patients is investigated.

The new medication is compared to the usual medication and the outcome variable is mortality. The study involves 42 patients, 20 of whom received the new medication, 22 received the usual medication. First, Kaplan-Meier survival curves are made for both groups and the log rank test is performed (see Fig. 6.7). The chi-square value of the log rank test is 0.56 which leads to a p-value of 0.46.

What can be seen directly in Fig. 6.7 is that the new medication has an unfavourable effect on survival at the beginning of the follow-up period (the Kaplan-Meier survival curve decrease faster). However, in the second part of the follow-up period, the new medication has a beneficial effect on survival (the Kaplan-Meier survival curve stays much flatter). With a Cox regression analysis a hazard ratio and a 95% confidence interval can be calculated. Output 6.13 shows the result of this analysis.

In Output 6.13 it can be seen that the hazard ratio for mortality for the new medication compared to the usual medication is 0.75 and that the corresponding 95% confidence interval ranges between 0.34 and 1.64. The p-value is 0.47. In short, based on the Cox regression analysis, it can be concluded that although the new medication has a beneficial effect on mortality, this beneficial effect is not statistically significant. However, the hazard ratio indicates an average over time and looking at the Kaplan-Meier survival curves (Fig. 6.7), it appears that the average over time does not really reflects what is going on, i.e. the hazards are definitely not proportional over time. In other words, the assumption of proportional hazards does not hold.

Visual inspection of the Kaplan-Meier survival curves is undoubtedly the best way to evaluate whether the hazard ratio on average over time is a good reflection of what is going on. The problem, however, is that with a Kaplan-Meier survival curve, the influence of other variables cannot be taken into account and when a continuous independent variable is analysed, Kaplan-Meier survival curves cannot be made. Therefore, in addition to the Kaplan-Meier survival curve, there are a number of other possibilities to evaluate whether the proportional hazards assumption holds. Some researchers think that this assumption can also be evaluated by investigating the estimated survival curves from the Cox regression analysis. However, this is a misconception, because the estimated survival curves from the Cox regression analysis are estimated under the assumption of proportional hazards and can, therefore, not be used to evaluate whether or not the proportional hazards assumption holds.

One approach to evaluate whether the proportional hazards assumption holds is the log-minus-log plot. In the log-minus-log plot, the influence of other variables can be taken into account. Besides that, the log-minus-log plot also has the advantage that it is relative easy to evaluate whether the proportional hazards assumption holds. The assumption holds when in the log-minus-log plot the lines of the groups to be compared are parallel (for a detailed explanation, see e.g. Kleinbaum, 1996). Another possibility to evaluate whether the proportional hazards assumption holds, is to test the Schoenfeld residuals. This statistical test uses a chi-square value and when the test provides a significant p-value it indicates that the proportional hazards assumption does not hold. In the present example, the chi-square value of the Schoenfeld residuals test is 10.28, and based on a chi-square distribution with one degree of freedom, the corresponding p-value is 0.001, which means that the proportional hazards assumption does not hold. Another way to evaluate whether the proportional hazards assumption holds is to use a method which is known as Cox regression analysis with a time-dependent covariate. This is basically a strange name because it is really only about analysing an interaction between the independent variable and a dichotomous time variable, which divides the follow-up period into two periods. In the present example, for example, it makes sense to divide the follow-up period in a period before 10 months and a period after 10 months; 10 months is the point where the two Kaplan-Meier survival curves cross. Output 6.14 shows the result of the Cox regression analysis in which the interaction between the new medication variable and the dichotomous time variable has been added to the analysis. It is important to realize that the dichotomous time variable itself is not added to the Cox regression analysis. This is different from regular interaction terms, where in addition to the interaction term, the two components of the interaction must

Output 6.14 Result of the Cox regression analysis to analyse the relationship between mortality and the new medication including the interaction with a dichotomous time variable

							95% confidence interval	
	Coefficient	se	Wald	df	p-value	Hazard ratio	Lower	Upper
Medication	0.75	0.49	2.30	1	0.13	2.12	0.80	5.57
Medicaton*time	−3.08	0.96	10.22	1	0.001	0.046	0.007	0.30

se standard error, *df* degrees of freedom

Output 6.15 Result of the Cox regression analysis to analyse the relationship between mortality and the new medication including the interaction with a recoded dichotomous time variable

							95% confidence interval	
	Coefficient	se	Wald	df	p-value	Hazard ratio	Lower	Upper
Medication	−2.33	0.83	7.93	1	0.005	0.10	0.02	0.49
Medicaton*time_recoded	3.08	0.96	10.22	1	0.001	21.78	3.29	144.07

se standard error, *df* degrees of freedom

also be added separately to the regression analysis. Furthermore, it is important to know that in the present example the dichotomous time variable is coded 1 for the time period after 10 months and 0 for the time period before 10 months.

In Output 6.14 it can be seen that the p-value for the interaction term is 0.001. So, the interaction between the new medication variable and the dichotomous time variable is statistically significant. This indicates that the proportional hazards assumption does not hold, which means that separate hazard ratios must be reported for the different time periods. Since the dichotomous time variable is coded 0 for the period before 10 months, the hazard ratio for that period can be obtained directly from Output 6.14, i.e. 2.12 with a 95% confidence interval ranging between 0.80 and 5.57. When the value 1 is entered for the dichotomous time variable, the regression coefficient for the new medication variable in the period after 10 months can be calculated, i.e. 0.75–3.08 = −2.33. From this regression coefficient, the e-power can be taken to obtain the hazard ratio for the new medication compared to the usual medication for the period after 10 months. This hazard ratio is 0.10. The new medication therefore has a strong protective effect from 10 months onwards. However, based on Output 6.14, it is not possible to directly calculate the 95% confidence interval around the hazard ratio for the period after 10 months; To do this, the dichotomous time variable has to be recoded. Output 6.15 shows the result of the Cox regression analysis after recoding the dichotomous time variable.

In Output 6.15 it can indeed be seen that the hazard ratio for the new medication is 0.10. It can also be seen that the 95% confidence interval ranges between 0.02 and 0.49 and the p-value is 0.005.

Using the dichotomous time variable, the follow-up period is divided into two parts and (if necessary) separate hazard ratios are estimated for both periods. Using the p-value of the interaction term, it can be concluded that the hazard ratios for both periods differ statistically significant from each other. The disadvantage of this procedure is that the choice of the cut-off value is slightly arbitrary, although the Kaplan-Meier survival curves can give a good indication for the cut-off value.

A Cox regression analysis with a time-dependent covariate does not necessarily have to be limited to two time periods, but can be extended to three or more time periods as needed. Of course, it is important to keep in mind whether the hazard ratios for the different time periods are estimated in a reliable way, which depends mainly on the number of subjects having the dichotomous outcome variable in a particular time period.

6.9 Limitations of Cox Regression Analysis

Although Cox regression analysis is widely used to analyse survival data, it has a number of important limitations. In Sect. 6.8 the assumption of proportional hazards was discussed. The hazard ratio derived from a Cox regression analysis is an average over the entire follow-up period and it is questionable whether this average over time is a good reflection of what is going on.

A second limitation of Cox regression analysis is the fact that the independent variables are treated as time-independent. Suppose that the relationship between the onset of cardiovascular disease and several risk factors is analysed. When Cox regression analysis is used, mostly the risk factors are measured at the start of the study and the cohort is followed for a certain amount of time to investigate whether subjects develop cardiovascular disease and when they develop cardiovascular disease. Whether the estimated hazard ratio really indicates the risk of a particular risk factor is questionable, because changes in risk factors are not taken into account. For example, when smoking is analysed as a possible risk factor for cardiovascular disease, a subject can quit smoking during the follow-up period. Quitting smoking is not taken into account in a Cox regression analysis and, therefore, the hazard ratio for smoking will not (totally) indicate the real risk of smoking. There are, however, extensions of Cox regression analysis available in which independent variables can be treated as time-dependent. Because of the complexity of these analyses, a detailed description of these methods is beyond the scope of this book (see for more details, for example, Kleinbaum, 1996).

A third limitation of Cox regression analysis is that the dichotomous outcome variable (which is also known as the event) is irreversible. When the outcome variable is mortality, then the irreversible nature is of course no problem, but when Cox regression analysis is used for dichotomous outcome variables such as low back pain, absenteeism from work, or sport injuries, the irreversibility is ignored in the Cox regression analysis. However, there is a possibility to deal with this limitation using Cox regression analysis for recurrent events. Suppose that a study is performed investigating the effect of a new intervention for patients with low back pain. The new intervention is compared to usual care and the study continues for a

Table 6.15 Example of a dataset with a reversible dichotomous outcome variable

		Recovery				
Id	Intervention	3 weeks	6 weeks	12 weeks	24 weeks	52 weeks
1	1	0	1	1	0	0
2	0	0	0	1	1	1
3	0	0	0	0	0	1
4	1	1	1	0	0	1
n	0	1	1	1	1	1

Intervention 0 = usual care, 1 = intervention
Recovery 0 = not recovered, 1 = recovered

Table 6.16 Restructured dataset generated from the dataset shown in Table 6.15

Id	Intervention	Recovery	Time (weeks)
1	1	0	3
1	1	1	6
1	1	1	12
1	1	0	24
1	1	0	52
2	0	0	3
2	0	0	6
2	0	1	12
2	0	1	24
2	0	1	52

Intervention 0 = usual care, 1 = intervention
Recovery 0 = not recovered, 1 = recovered

year with measurements at 3, 6, 12, 24 and 52 weeks. The dichotomous outcome variable of the study is perceived recovery, which is basically a reversible outcome variable because patients that report recovery at a certain time point can report complaints again at another time point. Table 6.15 shows part of the dataset that could be observed in this study.

In Table 6.15 it can be seen that, for example, patient 1 reports recovery after 6 weeks, but has a relapse at 24 weeks which continues till the end of the study. Because with a Cox regression analysis, a subject can only have one event and one time variable, patient 1 will have an event at 6 weeks. The analysis will ignore the fact that this patient has a relapse at 24 weeks, so it will not give a valid estimate of the effect of the intervention. To include all observations at all time points in the analysis, the data can be restructured (see Table 6.16).

With a Cox regression analysis, all time intervals can be analysed separately, but it is not possible to take into account the fact that some observations belong to the same patient and are, therefore, not independent anymore. To take this dependency into account, Cox regression analysis for recurrent events can be used. This is in fact a Cox regression analysis on the dataset shown in Table 6.16, but with an additional correction for the fact that some observations belong to the same patient (see also

Sect. 9.5). The detailed explanation of Cox regression analysis for recurrent events is beyond the scope of this book (see for more details, for example, Twisk et al., 2005).

6.10 Competing Risk Analysis

Another assumption of Cox regression analysis is that censoring is non-informative. This assumption is, for example, violated when subjects in the intervention group of a randomised controlled trial are censored more often than subjects in the control group. Another situation in which the assumption of non-informative censoring is violated is the presence of a competing risk or competing event. For example, suppose the relationship between having a myocardial infarction and smoking is analysed. In that study death before having a myocardial infarction can be considered as a competing event, because it is expected that smokers will die earlier due to other causes. Censoring these subjects at the time of death is not only problematic because the assumption of non-informative censoring is violated, but also because the probability of experiencing the event of interest (i.e. myocardial infarction) is estimated in a hypothetical setting in which the competing event cannot occur, which has very little clinical relevance. In that case the estimated hazard ratio for smoking compared to non-smoking to have a myocardial infarction is highly influenced by the competing risk of death. The best way to deal with the competing risk is to estimate cause specific hazard ratios, which means that besides the hazard ratio for having a myocardial infarction also the hazard ratio for the competing event has to be estimated. In the analysis to estimate the hazard ratio for having a myocardial infarction, the subjects who die (before having a myocardial infarction) are censored, while in the analysis to estimate the hazard ratio for death the subjects who have a myocardial infarction (before death) are censored. Both hazard ratios should be combined to obtain a proper answer to the research question. The problem of competing risks is also the reason why researchers interested in risk factors for cause specific mortality (e.g. cardiovascular disease mortality) always report the results of the analysis with all-cause mortality as outcome variable as well. For more details about competing risk analysis, one is referred to Schuster et al. (2020).

Chapter 7
Multiple Regression Analysis—Association Models and Prediction Models

Abstract When more than one independent variable is analysed in a regression analysis, a multiple regression analysis is performed. Regarding multiple regression analysis a distinction has to be made between association models and prediction models. The aim of an association model is to estimate the relationship between a main independent variable and a particular outcome variable as good as possible. The latter means that confounding has to be taken into account and that effect modification has to be investigated. The aim of a prediction model on the other hand is to predict a particular outcome variable as good as possible by a set of independent variables. For both the building of an association model and a prediction model different procedures are available and different procedures can lead to different results and conclusions. The final part of this chapter deals with a discussion of quality indicators for a prediction model. Regarding the quality of a prediction model a distinction is made between internal quality, i.e. how good the model fits the data and external validity, i.e. how good the model behaves in an external dataset.

7.1 Introduction

In the previous three chapters, linear regression analysis, logistic regression analysis, and Cox regression analysis have been discussed. The choice which method to use, depends on the outcome variable: linear regression analysis is used for a continuous outcome variable, logistic regression analysis is used for a dichotomous outcome variable, and Cox regression analysis is used for survival data.

In all three chapters, examples were given with one independent variable. An analysis with only one independent variable is known as a univariable analysis. Mostly, however, more than one independent variable is analysed. When more than one independent variable is analysed, the regression analysis is known as multivariable or multiple regression analysis. In the previous chapters, multiple regression analysis was, for example, used when a possible confounder or effect modifier was added to the regression analysis. Multiple regression analysis should not be confused with multivariate regression analysis. In the latter, not multiple independent

J. W. R. Twisk, *Basic Principles of Applied Medical Statistics*,
https://doi.org/10.1007/978-3-031-86278-6_7

variables but multiple outcome variables are analysed. Multivariate regression methods are (mathematically) complicated and the results are often difficult to interpret. A detailed explanation of multivariate regression methods is therefore beyond the scope of this book.

Multiple regression analyses are used to build statistical models. In this context, a distinction must be made between association models and prediction models. The aim of an association model is to estimate the relationship between a certain outcome variable and one main independent variable (the independent variable of interest) as good as possible. The aim of a prediction model is to predict a certain outcome variable as good as possible with a set of independent variables. Both association models and prediction models can be built for all types of outcome variables and can be applied within every regression analysis.

7.2 Association Models

The general idea of building an association model will be discussed using Example 7.1. The aim of this cross-sectional cohort study is to estimate the relationship between cholesterol and body mass index as good as possible. In addition to cholesterol and body mass index, age, sex and a number of lifestyle variables (i.e. physical activity, alcohol consumption and smoking) are measured in 200 subjects (see Table 7.1). It should be noted that in this example it is assumed that the relationship between cholesterol and the continuous independent variables body mass index and age is linear. Furthermore, both physical activity and alcohol consumption are categorical independent variables represented by two dummy variables in which the lowest category is used as reference group (i.e. inactive and non-drinker). The dummy variables are shown as activity 1 and 2 and alcohol 1 and 2.

Table 7.1 Descriptive information of the variables used in Example 7.1

	Mean	Standard deviation		Number of subjects
Cholesterol (mmol/l)	6.3	0.8		
Body mass index	28.2	3.0		
Age (years)	61.9	6.3		
Sex			Males Females	82 118
Smoking			Smoker Non-smoker	70 130
Physical activity			Inactive Moderate active Very active	66 77 57
Alcohol consumption			Non-drinker Moderate drinker Heavy drinker	81 85 34

Output 7.1 Result of the linear regression analysis to analyse the relationship between cholesterol and body mass index

					95% confidence interval	
	Coefficient	se	t-value	p-value	Lower	Upper
bmi	0.086	0.018	4.69	<0.001	0.050	0.122
Constant	3.87	0.52	7.45	<0.001	2.84	4.89

se standard error, *bmi* body mass index

Output 7.2 Result of the linear regression analysis to analyse the relationship between cholesterol and body mass index adjusted for all possible confounders

					95% confidence interval	
	Coefficient	se	t-value	p-value	Lower	Upper
bmi	0.167	0.020	8.27	<0.001	0.127	0.207
Age	0.035	0.008	4.20	<0.001	0.019	0.052
Sex	0.51	0.27	1.94	0.054	−0.01	1.04
Smoking	0.38	0.10	3.80	<0.001	0.18	0.58
Activity 1	−0.03	0.11	−0.27	0.79	−0.25	0.19
Activity 2	−0.01	0.13	−0.08	0.93	−0.26	0.24
Alcohol 1	−0.47	0.27	−1.73	0.09	−1.00	0.06
Alcohol 2	0.16	0.25	0.65	0.51	−0.33	0.65
Cons	0.78	0.58	−1.35	0.18	−1.92	0.36

se standard error, *bmi* body mass index

In the example, an association model is built with cholesterol as the outcome variable and body mass index as the independent variable of interest. In order to estimate the relationship between cholesterol and body mass index as good as possible, it is necessary to adjust for possible confounders and to evaluate effect modification between body mass index and possible effect modifiers. Although various procedures are available to build an association model, the first step in all association models is a to perform a so called crude analysis in which the univariable relationship between cholesterol and body mass index is analysed. Because the outcome variable is continuous, this relationship is analysed with linear regression analysis. Output 7.1 shows the result of this analysis.

In Output 7.1 it can be seen that the regression coefficient for the relationship between cholesterol and body mass index is 0.086, so a difference of one unit in body mass index corresponds to a difference of 0.086 in cholesterol. Furthermore, it can be seen that the p-value associated with this relationship is <0.001 and that the 95% confidence interval around the regression coefficient ranges between 0.050 and 0.122.

The mostly used procedure to build an association model is relatively simple. After reporting the crude result, a fully adjusted result is reported (see Output 7.2). The adjustment for possible confounders is irrespective whether the adjustment for a possible confounder is necessary or not, i.e. irrespective whether a possible

Table 7.2 Crude and adjusted result for the relationship between cholesterol and body mass index

	Regression coefficient	95% confidence interval	p-value
Crude	0.086	0.050–0.122	<0.001
Adjusted[a]	0.167	0.127–0.207	<0.001

[a] Adjusted for age, sex, smoking, physical activity and alcohol consumption

Output 7.3 Result of the linear regression analysis to analyse the relationship between cholesterol and body mass index adjusted for age and sex

					95% confidence interval	
	Coefficient	se	t-value	p-value	Lower	Upper
bmi	0.108	0.018	6.02	<0.001	0.073	0.144
Age	0.042	0.008	5.24	<0.001	0.026	0.058
Sex	0.51	0.11	4.51	<0.001	0.28	0.73
Cons	0.41	0.59	0.69	0.49	−0.76	1.58

se standard error, *bmi* body mass index

Table 7.3 Crude and adjusted results for the relationship between cholesterol and body mass index

	Regression coefficient	95% confidence interval	p-value
Crude	0.086	0.050–0.122	<0.001
Adjusted 1[a]	0.108	0.073–0.144	<0.001
Adjusted 2[b]	0.167	0.127–0.207	<0.001

[a] Adjusted for age and sex
[b] Adjusted for age, sex, smoking, physical activity and alcohol consumption

confounder leads to a relevant change in the regression coefficient of the independent variable of interest (i.e. body mass index).

Table 7.2 shows the results as they could be reported in a scientific paper. It is important to realise that only the results for body mass index are reported and not the coefficients, 95% confidence intervals and p-values for the possible confounders. The results for the possible confounders have nothing to do with the research question, so they must not be reported.

It is also possible to distinguish between different types or groups of possible confounders. In Example 7.1, age and sex are so-called demographic independent variables and are, therefore, different from the lifestyle independent variables smoking, physical activity and alcohol consumption. In this case, three analyses can be performed. A crude analysis (see Output 7.1), an analysis adjusted for age and sex (see Output 7.3) and an analysis also adjusted for the lifestyle independent variables (i.e. a fully adjusted analysis; see Output 7.2).

Table 7.3 shows the results as they could be reported in a scientific paper.

Building an association model adjusting for all possible confounders is, of course, only possible in situations where either the number of possible confounders is relatively low and/or the number of subjects in the study population is relatively high. When there are many possible confounders and/or a relatively low number of subjects in the study population, it is impossible to adjust for all possible

Table 7.4 Results of the step-by-step procedure to detect relevant confounders in the relationship between cholesterol and body mass index

	Model 1	Model 2	Model 3
	bmi	bmi adjusted for alcohol	bmi adjusted for alcohol and age
Age	21%	18%	
Sex	60%	2%	<1%
Smoking	1%	<1%	3%
Activity	0%	0%	1%
Alcohol	141%		

bmi body mass index, % percent change in regression coefficient for body mass index

confounders at the same time. In that situation, a step-by-step procedure must be used. In this step-by-step procedure, first, each possible confounder is added separately to a regression model, which only includes the independent variable of interest. For each possible confounder it is evaluated how much the regression coefficient for the independent variable of interest changes due to the possible confounder. The possible confounder that causes the largest change in regression coefficient is then added to the model as first relevant confounder. Next, the procedure is repeated with the remaining possible confounders until none of the remaining possible confounders causes a relevant change in the regression coefficient for the independent variable of interest anymore. Mostly this arbitrary cut-off value is set at a change of 10% in the regression coefficient for the independent variable of interest. It should be realized that the arbitrary cut-off value is only used in a situation when a choice has to be made which of the possible confounders has to be adjusted for. When this step-by-step procedure is performed in the present example, an analysis adjusted for alcohol consumption and age seemed to be the most appropriate. The regression coefficient for body mass index adjusted for alcohol consumption and age is 0.171 with a 95% confidence interval ranging between 0.131 and 0.212. The corresponding p-value is <0.001. Table 7.4 shows the details of the step-by-step procedure.

In the building of an association model described so far, effect modification is ignored. So, first the result for the whole study population is reported. However, mostly, in an additional analysis, effect modification is evaluated for the (biologically plausible) effect modifiers. This is usually done in the (fully) adjusted model. In this procedure the (biologically plausible) interaction terms are added separately to the model. Next, for statistically significant interaction terms, either separate regression coefficients are reported for the groups of the statistically significant effect modifier or the direction of the effect modification is interpreted without reporting the separate regression coefficients. The latter is mostly used when a significant effect modification is found with a continuous effect modifier (see Sect. 4.5). In the present example, for example, effect modification between body mass index and sex can be investigated. Output 7.4 shows the result of this analysis.

The most interesting part of Output 7.4 is the p-value for the interaction term (i.e. bmi*sex), because that p-value indicates whether there is statistically significant

Output 7.4 Result of the linear regression analysis to analyse the relationship between cholesterol and body mass index adjusted for all possible confounders including the interaction between body mass index and sex

					95% confidence interval	
	Coefficient	se	t-value	p-value	Lower	Upper
bmi	0.193	0.024	7.93	<0.001	0.145	0.241
Age	0.034	0.008	4.01	<0.001	0.017	0.050
Sex	2.52	1.10	2.30	0.03	0.36	4.69
Smoking	0.37	0.10	3.67	<0.001	0.17	0.57
Activity 1	−0.03	0.11	−0.23	0.82	−0.24	0.19
Activity 2	0.01	0.13	0.09	0.93	−0.24	0.26
Alcohol 1	−0.56	0.27	−2.06	0.04	−1.10	−0.02
Alcohol 2	0.19	0.25	0.78	0.44	−0.30	0.68
bmi*sex	−0.075	0.040	−1.88	0.06	−0.153	0.004
Cons	−1.38	0.66	−2.10	0.04	−2.68	−0.09

se standard error, *bmi* body mass index

effect modification between body mass index and sex. The p-value for the interaction term is 0.06 and this is higher than the arbitrary cut-off value of 0.05 for statistical significance. However, in many situations a slightly higher cut-off value is used for interaction terms (see Sect. 4.5). When a slightly higher cut-off value is used (e.g. 0.10) the p-value 0.06 can be considered statistically significant. In that case, separate results can be reported for males and females. Because females are coded 0, the result for females can be directly derived from Output 7.4. The regression coefficient for body mass index for females is 0.193 with a 95% confidence interval ranging between 0.145 and 0.241 and a p-value <0.001. For males, the regression coefficient for body mass index can also be directly derived from Output 7.4. This regression coefficient is equal to $0.193 - 0.075 = 0.118$. To obtain the standard error of this coefficient and, therefore, to obtain the 95% confidence interval and the p-value, the analysis should be repeated with sex coded differently, i.e. males coded 0 and females coded 1. Output 7.5 shows the result of this analysis.

In Output 7.5 it can be seen that the regression coefficient for body mass index for males is indeed 0.118. It can also be seen that the 95% confidence interval ranges between 0.053 and 0.183 and that the p-value is <0.001. Although the interest of the analyses is only in the regression coefficient for body mass index, a few other remarks about Outputs 7.4 and 7.5 must be made. Firstly, it can be seen that the regression coefficients for all the added confounders are not influenced by the recoding of sex. Only the magnitude of the regression coefficient for body mass index has changed. The regression coefficients for sex and for the interaction term are also changed, but only in the sign. Secondly, it should be realised that the regression coefficient for sex in Outputs 7.4 and 7.5 has a rather strange interpretation, i.e. the difference in cholesterol between males and females when body mass index is 0.

The procedure for building an association model described before, is by far the mostly used procedure. However, there are of course other procedures available.

Output 7.5 Result of the linear regression analysis to analyse the relationship between cholesterol and body mass index adjusted for all possible confounders including the interaction between body mass index and sex recoded

					95% confidence interval	
	Coefficient	se	t-value	p-value	Lower	Upper
bmi	0.118	0.032	3.60	<0.001	0.053	0.183
Age	0.034	0.008	4.01	<0.001	0.017	0.050
Sex_recoded	−2.52	1.10	−2.30	0.03	−4.69	−0.36
Smoking	0.37	0.10	3.67	<0.001	0.17	0.57
Activity 1	−0.03	0.11	−0.23	0.82	−0.24	0.19
Activity 2	0.01	0.13	0.09	0.93	−0.24	0.26
Alcohol 1	−0.56	0.27	−2.06	0.04	−1.10	−0.02
Alcohol 2	0.19	0.25	0.78	0.44	−0.30	0.68
bmi*sex_recoded	0.075	0.040	1.88	0.06	−0.004	0.153
Cons	1.14	0.95	1.20	0.23	−0.74	3.02

se standard error, *bmi* body mass index

One of the procedures is to start the analysis with the evaluation of effect modification with body mass index for all independent variables. The interaction terms for the different possible effect modifiers are evaluated separately and the interaction term with the lowest p-value is selected first. After selecting the effect modifier with the lowest p-value for the interaction term, the procedure is repeated within the subgroups of the selected effect modifier and again the interaction with the lowest p-value is selected. For both groups, this can be the same independent variable, but it can also be a different independent variable. The procedure is repeated until no significant effect modifications are observed anymore. The crude result of the analysis is then the regression coefficient for the independent variable of interest in the different subgroups. When this procedure is performed in the example dataset, the first interaction term which is selected is the interaction between body mass index and smoking. The p-value for this interaction is 0.004. In the next step, for smokers and for non-smokers, the second most important effect modifier is physical activity. The interaction term between body mass index and one of the dummy variables for physical activity has the lowest p-value and is statistically significant in both smokers and non-smokers. So, it makes sense to report the crude relationship between cholesterol and body mass index for the subgroups defined by smoking and physical activity. Table 7.5 shows the results for the different subgroups.

In Table 7.5 it can be seen that the strongest relationships between cholesterol and body mass index are found for the smokers and then especially for the inactive and the moderate active smokers. It can also be seen that a statistically significant relationship between cholesterol and body mass index is found for very active non-smokers. It should, however, be realised that basically the relationship between cholesterol and body mass index for the inactive non-smokers is stronger than the relationship between cholesterol and body mass index for the very active non-smokers (0.08 versus 0.07), but due to the lower number of subjects in the

Table 7.5 Results of the linear regression analyses to analyse the relationship between cholesterol and body mass index in different subgroups for smoking and physical activity

		Regression coefficient	95% confidence interval	p-value
Non-smoker				
	Inactive	0.08	−0.05–0.21	0.22
	Moderate active	−0.11	−0.17–0.02	0.12
	Very active	0.07	0.05–0.17	0.001
Smoker				
	Inactive	0.27	0.16–0.38	<0.001
	Moderate active	0.16	0.07–0.15	0.001
	Very active	0.04	−0.12–0.20	0.62

inactive non-smokers group, the stronger relationship for this group has a much higher p-value (0.22 versus 0.001).

It should be noted that the results reported in Table 7.5 are crude results. In the next step of the analyses, the analyses should be adjusted for the remaining independent variables, i.e. sex, age and alcohol consumption.

7.3 Prediction Models

7.3.1 Introduction

In the previous section, a few possible strategies were discussed to build an association model. The aim of an association model is to estimate the relationship between a certain outcome variable and one main independent variable as good as possible. The aim of a prediction model is totally different. The aim of a prediction model is to predict a certain outcome variable as good as possible with a set of independent variables. For example, in Example 7.1, the research question can be whether cholesterol can be predicted by body mass index, age, sex, smoking, alcohol consumption and physical activity. This seems to be quite simple: the best way to do this is to use all the variables from the dataset. However, the purpose of building a prediction model is to make the best prediction with the simplest model, i.e. without the variables that do not contribute much to the prediction of cholesterol. In statistical terminology, building a prediction model has to do with building the most parsimonious model to predict a particular outcome variable.

To decide whether or not a certain independent variable contributes (much) to the prediction of the outcome variable, the p-value is mostly used. In the literature, there are several options provided for the best cut-off p-values, but mostly a p-value of 0.05 is used. When the number of subjects is relatively low, also a p-value of 0.10 is often used as cut-off value. The last years, also higher cut-off p-values are used. One of the most intriguing cut-off values is a p-value of 0.157 (Steyerberg, 2019), and it is even suggested that a p-value of 0.50 should be used for selection (Harrell &

Frank, 2015). In the present examples, cut-off p-values of 0.05 and 0.10 are used, but the principles behind building a prediction model do not depend on the choice of a cut-off p-value.

It should be realised that although variable selection is a very popular way to build a prediction model, it is also highly criticized (Harrell & Frank, 2015). The most important criticism is that the selection is based on an arbitrary cut-off value and that the method is highly data driven, which reduces the external validity of the prediction model (see Sect. 7.5).

Comparable to building an association model, there are also different procedures available for building a prediction model. In the next sections, backward selection and forward selection will be discussed.

7.3.2 Backward Selection

The simplest procedure that can be used to build a prediction model is backward selection. The starting point of backward selection is the biggest possible model. Then, step-by-step, variables are removed from the model leading to a final model in which all independent variables make a relevant contribution to the prediction of the outcome variable. In the example, a p-value of 0.05 is used as a cut-off value for deciding whether an independent variable makes a relevant contribution to the prediction. Output 7.6 shows the starting point of the backward selection, i.e. the result of a linear regression analysis with all possible independent variables. As has been mentioned before, in the example it is assumed that the relationship between cholesterol and continuous independent variables (i.e. age and body mass index) is linear. Furthermore, both physical activity and alcohol consumption are categorical independent variables represented by two dummy variables in which the lowest category is used as reference group (i.e. inactive and non-drinker). Again, the dummy variables are shown as activity 1 and 2 and alcohol 1 and 2.

Output 7.6 Result of the linear regression analysis to predict cholesterol including all independent variables

					95% confidence interval	
	Coefficient	se	t-value	p-value	Lower	Upper
bmi	0.167	0.020	8.27	<0.001	0.127	0.207
Age	0.035	0.008	4.20	<0.001	0.019	0.052
Sex	0.51	0.27	1.94	0.054	−0.01	1.04
Smoking	0.38	0.10	3.80	<0.001	0.18	0.58
Activity 1	−0.03	0.11	−0.27	0.79	−0.25	0.19
Activity 2	−0.01	0.13	−0.08	0.93	−0.26	0.24
Alcohol 1	−0.47	0.27	−1.73	0.09	−1.00	0.06
Alcohol 2	0.16	0.25	0.65	0.51	−0.33	0.65
Cons	0.78	0.58	−1.35	0.18	−1.92	0.36

se standard error, *bmi* body mass index

Output 7.7 Result of the linear regression analysis to predict cholesterol without physical activity

					95% confidence interval	
	Coefficient	se	t-value	p-value	Lower	Upper
bmi	0.167	0.020	8.47	<0.001	0.128	0.207
Age	0.035	0.008	4.53	<0.001	0.020	0.050
Sex	0.51	0.26	1.94	0.054	−0.01	1.03
Smoking	0.39	0.10	3.90	<0.001	0.19	0.58
Alcohol 1	−0.48	0.27	−1.78	0.08	−1.00	0.05
Alcohol 2	0.17	0.24	0.70	0.49	−0.31	0.64
Cons	−0.79	0.57	−1.39	0.17	−1.92	0.34

se standard error, *bmi* body mass index

Output 7.6 is exactly the same as Output 7.2. The only difference is that the research question to be answered is totally different. The analysis, which result is shown in Output 7.2, was performed to analyse the relationship between cholesterol and body mass index and all other independent variables were added to the model as possible confounders. The analysis, which result is shown in Output 7.6 is performed as a starting point to build a prediction model for cholesterol.

In Output 7.6 it can be seen that the p-values for the two dummy variables for physical activity are the highest (0.79 and 0.93, respectively) and both are above the cut-off value of 0.05. So, physical activity seems to contribute the least to the prediction of cholesterol, and the first step will be to remove the two dummy variables for physical activity from the model. It is important to realize that the dummy variables for an independent variable always belong together and that one of the dummy variables should not be removed from the model. As soon as only one of a set of dummy variables is removed from the model, the regression coefficient for the remaining dummy variable has a completely different interpretation. Output 7.7 shows the result of the linear regression analysis in which the two dummy variables for physical activity are removed from the linear regression model.

In Output 7.7 it can be seen that the second dummy variable for alcohol consumption has the highest p-value, which is also higher than the cut-off value of 0.05. Because alcohol consumption is a categorical variable represented by two dummy variables, the importance of alcohol consumption should be evaluated by the lowest p-value for the two dummy variables. The p-value for the first dummy variable for alcohol consumption is 0.08 and is the second highest p-value in the model (behind the p-value for the second dummy variable for alcohol consumption). Because this p-value is also higher than the cut-off value of 0.05, alcohol consumption should be removed from the model. However, the regression coefficients for the dummy variables for alcohol consumption have a different sign. Due to the negative sign of the regression coefficient for the first dummy variable, it can be seen that moderate drinkers have lower cholesterol than non-drinkers. Due to the positive sign of the regression coefficient for the second dummy variable, it can also be seen that heavy drinkers have higher cholesterol than non-drinkers. Combining these findings, it can be concluded that the difference in cholesterol between moderate drinkers and heavy

Output 7.8 Result of the linear regression analysis to predict cholesterol without physical activity, using heavy drinkers as reference group for alcohol consumption

					95% confidence interval	
	Coefficient	se	t-value	p-value	Lower	Upper
bmi	0.167	0.020	8.47	<0.001	0.128	0.207
Age	0.035	0.008	4.53	<0.001	0.020	0.050
Sex	0.51	0.26	1.94	0.054	−0.01	1.03
Smoking	0.39	0.10	3.90	<0.001	0.19	0.58
Alcohol 1	−0.17	0.24	−0.70	0.49	−0.64	0.31
Alcohol 2	−0.64	0.16	−4.15	<0.001	−0.95	−0.34
Cons	−0.62	0.58	−1.08	0.28	−1.76	0.51

se standard error, *bmi* body mass index

drinkers is bigger than the differences indicated by the regression coefficients for the two dummy variables. The difference in cholesterol between moderate drinkers and heavy drinkers equals −0.47−0.17 = −0.64. The problem, however, is that this difference is not presented in the result of the regression analysis and therefore, also no p-value for this difference is provided. In order to get a more appropriate evaluation whether alcohol consumption makes a relevant contribution to predict cholesterol, the analysis should be performed with a different reference group for alcohol consumption. Output 7.8 shows the result of a linear regression analysis to predict cholesterol in which heavy drinkers are used as reference group for alcohol consumption.

In Output 7.8, the regression coefficient for the first dummy variable for alcohol consumption now indicates the difference in cholesterol between non-drinkers and heavy drinkers. This regression coefficient is the same the regression coefficient for the second dummy variable shown in Output 7.7; it only has a different sign. The regression coefficient for the second dummy variable in Output 7.8 indicates the difference in cholesterol between moderate drinkers and heavy drinkers and that regression coefficient is indeed −0.64. It can also be seen that the p-value belonging to the difference in cholesterol between moderate drinkers and heavy drinkers is <0.001. Based on this p-value it can be concluded that alcohol consumption makes a relevant contribution to predict cholesterol and, therefore, it should not be removed from the model. Instead of alcohol consumption, sex has to be removed from the model. Sex has the highest p-value (0.054), which is just above the cut-off value of 0.05. Output 7.9 shows the result of the linear regression analysis in which the two dummy variables for physical activity and sex are removed from the regression model.

In Output 7.9 it can be seen that only the regression coefficient for the first dummy variable for alcohol consumption has a p-value higher than 0.05, but it has already been mentioned that a set of dummy variables has to be evaluated using the lowest p-value for the regression coefficients for the dummy variables. So in this example, the importance of alcohol consumption has to be evaluated by the p-value for the regression coefficient for the second dummy variable for alcohol

Output 7.9 Result of the linear regression analysis to predict cholesterol without physical activity and sex, using heavy drinkers as reference group for alcohol consumption

					95% confidence interval	
	Coefficient	se	t-value	p-value	Lower	Upper
bmi	0.166	0.020	8.35	<0.001	0.127	0.206
Age	0.041	0.007	5.57	<0.001	0.026	0.055
Smoking	0.33	0.10	3.46	0.001	0.14	0.52
Alcohol 1	0.23	0.13	1.75	0.08	−0.03	0.48
Alcohol 2	−0.71	0.15	−4.66	<0.001	−1.01	−0.41
Cons	−0.83	0.57	−1.45	0.15	−1.95	0.30

se standard error, *bmi* body mass index

consumption, which is much lower than 0.05. So, none of the remaining variables used in the prediction model have a p-value higher than the cut-off value of 0.05, and, therefore, Output 7.9 shows the final prediction model for cholesterol, which looks as follows:

$$cholesterol = -0.83 + 0.166 \times bmi + 0.041 \times age + 0.33 \times smoking$$
$$+0.23 \times non\ drinking - 0.0711 \times moderate\ drinking$$

With this prediction model, cholesterol can be predicted for each subject given the values of the independent variables in the model. When, for example, the data of the first subject of Example 7.1 (a subject with a body mass index of 27.41, 66 years of age, who is non-smoker and non-drinker) are entered into the equation, the predicted cholesterol is 6.63. This is a huge underestimation, because for this particular subject the observed cholesterol is 7.90.

7.3.3 Forward Selection

A slightly more extensive procedure to build a prediction model is forward selection. With forward selection, first, the relationships between the outcome variable and all independent variables are analysed separately. Output 7.10 shows the results of these linear regression analyses. For alcohol consumption the dummy variable coding is used in which heavy drinkers are the reference group.

The idea of a forward selection procedure is first to select the best predictor. The best predictor usually means the independent variable with the lowest p-value. In Output 7.10 it can be seen that age has the lowest p-value. Body mass index and sex also have a p-value <0.001, but the value of the test statistic shows that the p-value for age is the lowest. So the first model in the forward selection procedure will be a model with age. All other independent variables are now added (separately) to the model with age. Output 7.11 shows the results of these linear regression analyses.

Output 7.10 Result of separate linear regression analyses to predict cholesterol with body mass index, age, sex, smoking, physical activity and alcohol consumption

					95% confidence interval	
	Coefficient	se	t-value	p-value	Lower	Upper
bmi	0.086	0.018	4.69	<0.001	0.050	0.122
Cons	3.86	0.52	7.45	<0.001	2.84	4.89
					95% confidence interval	
	Coefficient	se	t-value	p-value	Lower	Upper
Age	0.062	0.008	7.82	<0.001	0.046	0.077
Cons	2.45	0.49	5.00	<0.001	1.49	3.43
					95% confidence interval	
	Coefficient	se	t-value	p-value	Lower	Upper
Sex	0.40	0.11	3.57	<0.001	0.18	0.62
Cons	6.12	0.07	85.23	<0.001	5.98	6.26
					95% confidence interval	
	Coefficient	se	t-value	p-value	Lower	Upper
Smoking	0.182	0.12	1.54	0.125	−0.05	0.42
Cons	6.22	0.07	88.65	<0.001	6.08	6.36
					95% confidence interval	
	Coefficient	se	t-value	p-value	Lower	Upper
Active 1	−0.04	0.13	−0.28	0.78	−0.30	0.23
Active 2	0.13	0.15	0.90	0.37	−0.16	0.42
Cons	6.26	0.10	63.29	<0.001	6.07	6.46
					95% confidence interval	
	Coefficient	se	t-value	p-value	Lower	Upper
Alcohol 1	0.15	0.16	0.90	0.37	−0.17	0.46
Alcohol 2	−0.21	0.16	−1.30	0.19	−0.53	0.11
Cons	6.31	0.14	46.60	<0.001	6.05	6.58

se standard error, *bmi* body mass index

Output 7.11 shows that the next independent variable to be added to the prediction model is body mass index. After all, this independent variable now has the lowest p-value. The model with age and body mass index becomes the new model, and all other independent variables are added separately to this model. Output 7.12 shows the results of this third step.

In Output 7.12 it can be seen that in this step, the second dummy variable for alcohol consumption is the strongest predictor for cholesterol. The observed result may be difficult to assess, because the p-value for the first dummy variable for alcohol consumption is quite high. However, it has already been mentioned that dummy variables in a regression model belong together and should always be analysed together. So, the third model will be a model with age, body mass index, and the two dummy variables for alcohol consumption. Again, all other independent variables are added separately to this model to evaluate whether other independent

Output 7.11 Result of separate linear regression analyses (in a model including age) to predict cholesterol with body mass index, sex, smoking, physical activity and alcohol consumption

					95% confidence interval	
	Coefficient	se	t-value	p-value	Lower	Upper
Age	0.057	0.008	7.46	<0.001	0.042	0.072
bmi	0.068	0.016	4.16	<0.001	0.036	0.100
Cons	0.82	0.61	1.33	0.18	−0.39	2.03

					95% confidence interval	
	Coefficient	se	t-value	p-value	Lower	Upper
Age	0.058	0.008	6.96	<0.001	0.041	0.074
Sex	0.17	0.11	1.61	0.11	−0.04	0.38
Cons	2.65	0.61	5.26	<0.001	1.65	3.64

					95% confidence interval	
	Coefficient	se	t-value	p-value	Lower	Upper
Age	0.065	0.008	8.33	<0.001	0.050	0.081
Smoking	0.31	0.10	3.00	0.003	0.11	0.51
Cons	2.14	0.49	4.32	<0.001	1.16	3.11

					95% confidence interval	
	Coefficient	se	t-value	p-value	Lower	Upper
Age	0.066	0.008	7.90	<0.001	0.049	0.082
Activity 1	−0.17	0.12	−1.40	0.16	−0.40	0.07
Activity 2	−0.21	0.13	−1.56	0.12	−0.47	0.06
Cons	2.34	0.50	4.63	<0.001	1.34	3.33

					95% confidence interval	
	Coefficient	se	t-value	p-value	Lower	Upper
Age	0.059	0.008	7.34	<0.001	0.043	0.075
Alcohol 1	0.08	0.14	0.58	0.56	−0.20	0.37
Alcohol 2	−0.11	0.14	−0.77	0.44	−0.39	0.17
Cons	2.64	0.51	5.14	<0.001	1.62	3.66

se standard error, *bmi* body mass index

variables in the dataset make a relevant contribution to predict cholesterol. Output 7.13 shows the results of this fourth step.

In Output 7.13 it can be seen that now smoking is the most relevant predictor for cholesterol. Smoking is therefore added to the model. In the next step, the two remaining independent variables (i.e. sex and physical activity) are added separately to this model. Output 7.14 shows the results of these analyses.

Output 7.14 shows that the p-value for sex is very close to 0.05, but it is slightly higher, so both sex and physical activity are not added to the prediction model. The final prediction model, therefore, includes the independent variables age, body mass index, alcohol consumption, and smoking. This result was also found with backward selection (see Sect. 7.3.2). However, it should be realised that both procedures do not always lead to the same result.

Output 7.12 Result of separate linear regression analyses (in a model including age and body mass index) to predict cholesterol with sex, smoking, physical activity and alcohol consumption

					95% confidence interval	
	Coefficient	se	t-value	p-value	Lower	Upper
Age	0.042	0.008	5.24	<0.001	0.026	0.058
bmi	0.108	0.018	6.02	<0.001	0.073	0.143
Sex	0.51	0.11	4.51	<0.001	0.28	0.73
Cons	0.41	0.59	0.69	0.49	−0.76	1.58
					95% confidence interval	
	Coefficient	se	t-value	p-value	Lower	Upper
Age	0.061	0.008	7.96	<0.001	0.046	0.076
bmi	0.067	0.016	4.12	<0.001	0.035	0.098
Smoking	0.29	0.10	2.94	0.004	0.10	0.49
Cons	0.56	0.61	0.92	0.36	−0.64	1.76
					95% confidence interval	
	Coefficient	se	t-value	p-value	Lower	Upper
Age	0.061	0.008	7.59	<0.001	0.045	0.077
bmi	0.070	0.016	4.26	<0.001	0.037	0.102
Activity 1	−0.20	0.11	−1.72	0.09	−0.42	0.03
Activity 2	−0.22	0.13	−1.69	0.09	−0.47	0.04
Cons	0.67	0.62	1.08	0.28	−0.56	1.90
					95% confidence interval	
	Coefficient	se	t-value	p-value	Lower	Upper
Age	0.037	0.007	4.97	<0.001	0.022	0.051
bmi	0.171	0.020	8.40	<0.001	0.013	0.212
Alcohol 1	0.06	0.12	0.47	0.64	−0.19	0.30
Alcohol 2	−0.85	0.15	−5.62	<0.001	−1.15	−0.55
Cons	−0.49	0.58	−0.85	0.39	−1.64	0.65

se standard error, *bmi* body mass index

In most statistical software, forward and backward selection can be performed automatically. However, it is recommended to perform the selection manually, as this will give much more insight into the selection process. In some cases, it is even necessary to select the variables manually, for example when there are dummy variables in the prediction model. The automatic procedures often do not recognize that certain dummy variables belong together, which, for example, can lead to deletion of individual dummy variables. Furthermore, in some situations independent variables are forced into a prediction model. In intervention studies, for example, the intervention variable is very often included in the prediction model, regardless of the corresponding p-value.

Output 7.13 Result of separate linear regression analyses (in a model including age, body mass index and alcohol consumption) to predict cholesterol with sex, smoking and physical activity

					95% confidence interval	
	Coefficient	se	t-value	p-value	Lower	Upper
Age	0.034	0.008	4.29	<0.001	0.019	0.050
bmi	0.172	0.020	8.41	<0.001	0.132	0.212
Alcohol 1	−0.11	0.25	−0.42	0.67	−0.60	0.39
Alcohol 2	−0.83	0.15	−5.46	<0.001	−1.13	−0.53
Sex	0.20	0.26	0.76	0.45	−0.32	0.71
Cons	−0.39	0.59	−0.66	0.51	−1.56	0.78
					95% confidence interval	
	Coefficient	se	t-value	p-value	Lower	Upper
Age	0.041	0.007	5.57	<0.001	0.026	0.055
bmi	0.166	0.020	8.35	<0.001	0.127	0.206
Alcohol 1	0.23	0.13	1.75	0.08	−0.03	048
Alcohol 2	−0.71	0.15	−4.66	<0.001	−1.01	−0.41
Smoking	0.33	0.10	3.45	0.001	0.14	0.52
Cons	−0.83	0.57	−1.45	0.15	−1.95	0.30
					95% confidence interval	
	Coefficient	se	t-value	p-value	Lower	Upper
Age	0.038	0.008	4.72	<0.001	0.022	0.054
bmi	0.169	0.021	8.12	<0.001	0.128	0.210
Alcohol 1	0.10	0.14	0.70	0.48	−0.18	0.37
Alcohol 2	−0.80	0.17	−4.67	<0.001	−1.14	−0.46
Activity 1	−0.08	0.11	−0.73	0.47	−0.31	0.14
Activity 2	−0.06	0.13	−0.44	0.66	−0.31	0.20
Cons	−0.51	0.59	−0.87	0.39	−1.67	0.65

7.3.4 *Effect Modification and Prediction Models*

In the building of a prediction model discussed so far, effect modification is ignored. In practice, this is usually done, although some statisticians emphasize that the starting model for a backward selection, for example, has to include not only all the independent variables, but also all possible interactions. And not only all possible interactions between two independent variables (the two-way interactions), but also those between three independent variables (the three-way interactions), between four independent variables (the four-way interactions) and so on. It will be clear that with such a large number of independent variables the regression coefficients cannot be accurately estimated, and that this theoretical approach is impossible in practice.

One of the possibilities to include effect modification in a prediction model, which is often used in practice, is a priori stratification. For example, with an a priori stratification by sex, separate prediction models are built for males and females. There are no strict rules for this a priori stratification. Biological

Output 7.14 Result of separate linear regression analyses (in a model including age, body mass index, alcohol consumption and smoking) to predict cholesterol with sex and physical activity

					95% confidence interval	
	Coefficient	se	t-value	p-value	Lower	Upper
Age	0.035	0.008	4.53	<0.001	0.020	0.051
bmi	0.167	0.020	8.47	<0.001	0.128	0.207
Alcohol 1	−0.17	0.24	−0.70	0.49	−0.64	0.31
Alcohol 2	−0.64	0.16	−4.15	<0.001	−0.95	−0.34
Smoking	0.39	0.10	3.90	<0.001	0.19	0.58
Sex	0.51	0.26	1.94	0.054	−0.01	1.03
Cons	−0.62	0.58	−1.08	0.28	−1.76	0.51
					95% confidence interval	
	Coefficient	se	t-value	p-value	Lower	Upper
Age	0.041	0.008	5.18	<0.001	0.025	0.057
bmi	0.166	0.020	8.14	<0.001	0.125	0.206
Alcohol 1	0.24	0.14	1.68	0.09	−0.04	0.51
Alcohol 2	−0.69	0.17	−4.10	<0.001	−1.03	−0.36
Smoking	0.33	0.10	3.36	0.001	0.13	0.52
Activity 1	−0.02	0.11	−0.20	0.85	−0.24	0.20
Activity 2	−0.02	0.13	−0.17	0.87	−0.27	0.23
Cons	−0.83	0.58	−1.44	0.15	−1.98	0.31

plausibility, the nature and the number of subjects in the study population, and the available independent variables may play a role in the choice for an a priori stratification.

A second option that is sometimes used in practice is first to build a prediction model with the independent variables, without including interaction terms in the model. A few interaction terms are then added to the final prediction model to evaluate whether these interaction terms improve the prediction. Although this procedure is widely used, it often leads to a kind of fishing expedition: interaction terms are added to the model without really thinking about its biological plausibility.

7.3.5 Preselection in a Backward Selection Procedure

Although backward selection is the most efficient way to build a prediction model, it has the limitation that the starting model should not be too large. For example, when a dataset contains 50 independent variables while the study population consists of 200 subjects, then a backward selection procedure is not possible because there are far too many independent variables in relation to the number of subjects in the study population. In such a situation, the independent variables added to the starting model for the backward selection are sometimes preselected. In a preselection, first, the relationship between the outcome variable and all independent variables is analysed separately. Second, the backward selection procedure is not started with all available independent variables (after all, that is impossible because the study population does not have enough subjects), but with only those independent variables that had a p-value lower than a certain cut-off value in the separate analyses. For the cut-off value used for preselection there are several options. Some researchers use 0.10, while others use 0.15 or 0.20. Again, there are no strict rules for the cut-off value used for preselection. In fact, preselection is comparable to the first step in a forward selection procedure. The difference is that after the preselection, a backward selection procedure is performed with the selected variables to build the final prediction model.

When a preselection is performed In Example 7.1, with a cut-off p-value of 0.10, physical activity, alcohol consumption and smoking are not preselected (see Output 7.10). This is rather surprising, because smoking and alcohol consumption are present in the final prediction model. This example shows, therefore, nicely that the danger of preselection is that important variables do not pass the preselection. The lower the cut-off value used in the preselection, the greater the probability that this will occur. Because of this, preselection is not recommended by many statisticians.

7.3.6 Quality of a Prediction Model

After building a prediction model, it is necessary to indicate the quality of the final prediction model. For linear regression analysis, the R-square (i.e. explained variance) is often used as an indicator for the quality of the prediction model (see Sect. 4. 4.6). In the present example, the R-square of the prediction model for cholesterol including age, body mass index, alcohol consumption and smoking is 0.48. This means that 48% of the variance in cholesterol can be explained by the independent variables in the final prediction model. It is always difficult to indicate whether this percentage is high or low and whether the prediction model is good or bad. The interpretation depends highly on the type of study and the independent variables used. In a fully controlled laboratory study, only a very high explained variance indicates a good prediction model, while in an observational study in which many questionnaires have been used, an explained variance of 10 to 15% can be considered good. Besides the R-square most statistical software also report the adjusted R-square. The adjusted R-square takes into account the number of independent variables used in the final prediction model and is often considered as a more appropriate indicator for the quality of the prediction model. In the present example, the adjusted R-square is 0.47.

7.4 Dichotomous Outcome Variables

It is probably not surprising that association models and prediction models with a dichotomous outcome variable or survival data are built in the same way as has been described for continuous outcome variables (see Sects. 7.2 and 7.3). The difference is that for dichotomous outcome variables multiple logistic regression analysis is used and that for survival data multiple Cox regression analysis is used. Especially prediction models are often build for dichotomous outcomes. In medical practice, it is often important to use a number of simple independent variables to predict as good as possible whether or not a particular treatment will be effective, whether or not a patient has a particular disease, and so on. When a prediction model is built to predict whether a patient has a particular disease, the model is also known as a prognostic model. The way a prognostic model can be built is, of course, exactly the same as for a prediction model; in fact, a prognostic model is a special case of a prediction model.

One of the advantages of a prediction model with a dichotomous outcome variable is that the (predicted) probability of the outcome variable can be calculated for any subject in the study population, given the values of the independent variables used in the prediction model for that particular subject. Because prediction models are so often used with dichotomous outcome variables, Example 7.2 will be used to illustrate the building of a prediction model with a dichotomous outcome variable. The dataset is based on data from an intervention study in patients with low back pain. All 120 patients in this study received a new intervention and the question is whether it is possible to predict whether the patient recovers within 6 months based on a number of fairly easy to measure independent variables. Table 7.6 shows descriptive information of the variables used in Example 7.2.

Table 7.6 shows that after 6 months, about 40% of the 120 patients have recovered. Furthermore, the dataset contains a number of continuous independent variables (pain, score on a function test, duration of symptoms and age) and a number of dichotomous independent variables (sex, medication use and overweight). In the example, a prediction model will be built using a backward selection procedure. For the continuous independent variables, a linear relationship with recovery is assumed and effect modification will be ignored. Given the relatively

Table 7.6 Descriptive information of the variables used in Example 7.2

		Number of subjects	Mean	Standard deviation
Recovered	Yes/no	47/63		
Sex	Males/females	25/95		
Medication use	Yes/no	35/85		
Overweight	Yes/no	41/79		
Pain			3.9	1.5
Function score			22.3	3.6
Duration (weeks)			5.8	2.6
Age (years)			43.3	2.2

Output 7.15 Result of the logistic regression analysis to predict recovery including all independent variables

							95% confidence interval	
	Coefficient	se	Wald	df	p-value	Odds ratio	Lower	Upper
Sex	−0.98	0.56	3.07	1	0.08	0.38	0.13	1.12
Medication	−1.01	0.49	4.17	1	0.04	0.37	0.14	0.96
Overweight	0.08	0.44	0.03	1	0.86	1.08	0.45	2.59
Pain	−0.40	0.15	7.54	1	0.01	0.67	0.51	0.89
Function	−0.03	0.06	0.21	1	0.65	0.97	0.87	1.09
Duration	−0.22	0.09	6.47	1	0.01	0.80	0.67	0.95
Age	0.09	0.10	0.75	1	0.39	1.09	0.90	1.32
Cons	−0.34	4.61	0.01	1	0.94			

se standard error

Output 7.16 Result of the logistic regression analysis to predict recovery without overweight

							95% confidence interval	
	Coefficient	se	Wald	df	p-value	Odds ratio	Lower	Upper
Sex	−0.97	0.56	3.03	1	0.08	0.38	0.13	1.13
Medication	−1.01	0.49	4.23	1	0.04	0.36	0.14	0.95
Pain	−0.40	0.15	7.55	1	0.01	0.67	0.51	0.89
Function	−0.03	0.06	0.20	1	0.66	0.97	0.87	1.09
Duration	−0.22	0.09	6.44	1	0.01	0.80	0.67	0.95
Age	0.09	0.10	0.75	1	0.39	1.09	0.90	1.32
Cons	−0.31	4.61	0.01	1	0.95			

se standard error

small population of 120 patients, a p-value of 0.10 is used as cut-off value for selection. Output 7.15 shows the result of the multiple logistic regression analysis including all independent variables.

In Output 7.15 it can be seen that the first independent variable to be removed from the prediction model is overweight, because overweight has the highest p-value (0.86), which is also above the cut-off value of 0.10. So, a new logistic regression analysis is performed with all independent variables except overweight. Output 7.16 shows the result of this analysis.

In Output 7.16 it can be seen that the next independent variable to be removed from the prediction model is function. The p-value of this variable is 0.66, which is the highest p-value of all independent variables and which is also higher than the cut-off value of 0.10. Output 7.17 shows the result of the logistic regression analysis without function.

In Output 7.17, it can be seen that the next independent variable to be removed from the prediction model is age. This variable has the highest p-value of all independent variables in the prediction model (0.34), and which is still higher than the cut-off value of 0.10. Output 7.18 shows the result of the logistic regression analysis without age.

Output 7.17 Result of the logistic regression analysis to predict recovery without overweight and function

							95% confidence interval	
	Coefficient	se	Wald	df	p-value	Odds ratio	Lower	Upper
Sex	−0.98	0.56	3.10	1	0.08	0.37	0.13	1.12
Medication	−1.01	0.49	4.25	1	0.04	0.37	0.14	0.95
Pain	−0.41	0.15	7.82	1	0.01	0.67	0.50	0.89
Duration	−0.22	0.09	6.37	1	0.01	0.80	0.67	0.95
Age	0.09	0.10	0.90	1	0.34	1.10	0.91	1.33
Cons	−1.21	4.25	0.08	1	0.77			

se standard error

Output 7.18 Result of the logistic regression analysis to predict recovery without overweight, function and age

							95% confidence interval	
	Coefficient	se	Wald	df	p-value	Odds ratio	Lower	Upper
Sex	−0.85	0.54	2.53	1	0.11	0.43	0.15	1.22
Medication	−1.00	0.49	4.20	1	0.04	0.37	0.14	0.96
Pain	−0.40	0.14	7.80	1	0.01	0.67	0.51	0.89
Duration	−0.21	0.09	5.97	1	0.02	0.81	0.68	0.96
Cons	2.69	0.78	11.98	1	<0.001			

se standard error

Output 7.19 Result of the logistic regression analysis to predict recovery without overweight, function, age and sex

							95% confidence interval	
	Coefficient	se	Wald	df	p-value	Odds ratio	Lower	Upper
Medication	−0.90	0.48	3.60	1	0.06	0.41	0.16	1.03
Pain	−0.38	0.14	7.39	1	0.01	0.68	0.52	0.90
Duration	−0.21	0.09	6.05	1	0.01	0.81	0.68	0.96
Cons	2.44	0.75	10.59	1	<0.001			

se standard error

Output 7.18 shows that the next independent variable that can be removed from the prediction model is sex. Sex has the highest p-value (0.11), which is also higher than the cut-off value of 0.10. Output 7.19 shows the result of the logistic regression analysis without sex.

Because all the independent variables of the model shown in Output 7.19 have p-values below the cut-off value of 0.10, the final prediction model includes the independent variables medication, pain and duration. Because a logistic regression analysis is performed, in which the outcome variable is the natural logarithm of the odds of recovery, the final prediction model looks as follows:

Table 7.7 Descriptive information of the patients with the lowest and highest predicted probabilities to recover

Id	Medication	Pain	Duration	Predicted probability	Recovered
41	No	8	11	0.05	No
56	No	1	3	0.81	Yes

$$ln(odds(recovery)) = 2.44 - 0.90 \times medication - 0.38 \times pain - 0.21 \times duration$$

In Sect. 5.5.1 it was already indicated that this logistic regression equation can also be written in another way. In this way, the probability of recovery can be calculated for each patient in the dataset, given the value of the independent variables.

$$p(recovery) = \frac{1}{1 + e^{-(2.44 - 0.90 \times medication - 0.38 \times pain - 0.21 \times duration)}}$$

When, for example, the data of the first patient of Example 7.2 (a patient without medication use, with a pain score of 3 and with 4 weeks of complaints before the start of the intervention) are entered into the equation, the predicted probability to recover is 0.61. When the predicted probability is calculated for each patient in the dataset, it can be seen that the lowest predicted probability to recover in the dataset is 0.05, while the highest predicted probability to recover is 0.81 (see Table 7.7).

The range of predicted probabilities in a dataset is an indication how well the prediction model can discriminate between patients recovered and patients not recovered. Although it seems to be a nice quality indicator of the prediction model, it is not much used in practice. In Sect. 7.4.1, a number of quality indicators for a logistic prediction model will be discussed that are mostly used in practice. It should be realized that the explained variance, which is used as quality indicator in linear prediction models (see Sect. 7.3.6), is not directly available for logistic prediction models. There are, however, alternative approaches to obtain some sort of explained variance. All these alternative approaches use the difference between the -2 log likelihood of the final prediction model and the -2 log likelihood of the model without any independent variables to calculate an R-square value. In the present example the -2 log likelihood of the final prediction model is 140.5, while the -2 log likelihood of the model without any independent variable is 160.7. When the difference between the two is expressed as a percentage of the -2 log likelihood of the model without any independent variables an R-square is obtained. In the present example this R-square value is 0.13.

The above mentioned way to calculate the R-square for a logistic prediction model is known as the Hosmer-Lemeshow method. There are also other methods available to calculate an R-square for a logistic prediction model. Both the Cox & Schnell R-square and the Nagelkerke R-square are a bit higher than the Hosmer-Lemeshow R-square. In the present example, the Cox & Schnell R-square is 0.16, while the Nagelkerke R-square is 0.22. Despite the differences between the different methods to calculate the R-square, and despite the fact that the R-square is the square

Table 7.8 AIC values for different models to predict recovery

	AIC
Sex, medication, overweight, pain, function, duration, age	152.65
Sex, medication, pain, function, duration, age	150.69
Sex, medication, pain, duration, age	149.89
Sex, medication, pain, duration	147.80
Medication, pain, duration, age	148.49

AIC Akaike information criterion

of the multiple correlation coefficient, which is not really defined for dichotomous variables, the R-square is often used to determine the quality of a logistic prediction model. At least, the R-square should be interpreted with caution and it is probably better not to use the R-square as quality indicator for a logistic prediction model. Especially not, because there are better alternatives available to indicate the quality of a logistic prediction model (see Sect. 7.4.1).

As has been mentioned before, other cut-off values are sometimes used for building a prediction model and it has also been mentioned that one of the most intriguing cut-off values is a p-value of 0.157 (Steyerberg, 2019). The 0.157 cut-off value is based on the Akaike information criterion (AIC). The AIC is a model fit indicator which is calculated from the −2 log likelihood and which is adjusted for the number of independent variables in the model. The value itself is not informative, but the AIC can be used for model selection. In fact, the model with the lowest value of the AIC is the best (i.e. most parsimonious) model to predict a particular outcome and the lowest AIC seems to correspond with a cut-off p-value of 0.157. To illustrate the use of the AIC, Table 7.8 shows the AIC values for the different models to predict recovery. From Table 7.8 it can be seen that the best model to predict recovery based on the AIC is a model including sex, medication, pain and duration, which is the same model that is obtained when a cut-off p-value of 0.157 is used for selection.

7.4.1 Quality of a Logistic Prediction Model

The three mostly used methods to express the quality of a logistic prediction model are the Hosmer-Lemeshow test, the calibration curve and the C-statistic. All three methods are based on a comparison between the predicted probability and the occurrence or non-occurrence of the dichotomous outcome variable. The idea behind the Hosmer-Lemeshow test is that the study population is divided into 10 more or less equally sized groups, with the first group consisting of the subjects with the 10% lowest predicted probabilities, the next group consisting of the subjects with the next 10% lowest predicted probabilities, and so on. The last group consists of the subjects with the 10% highest predicted probabilities. The idea behind the Hosmer-Lemeshow test can best be explained with a small numerical example. Suppose

Table 7.9 Numerical example with predicted probabilities

Id	Predicted probability	Myocardial infarction
1	0.40	0
2	0.60	0
3	0.40	1
4	0.65	1
5	0.50	0
6	0.55	1
7	0.30	0
8	0.60	1
9	0.40	0
10	0.60	1

Table 7.10 Numerical example with predicted probabilities divided into two groups

Id		Predicted probability	Myocardial infarction
	Group 1		
1		0.40	0
3		0.40	1
5		0.50	0
7		0.30	0
9		0.40	0
	Group 2		
2		0.60	0
4		0.65	1
6		0.55	1
8		0.60	1
10		0.60	1

there are 10 subjects of whom it has been predicted whether or not they will have a myocardial infarction (see Table 7.9).

To illustrate the idea behind the Hosmer-Lemeshow test, the dataset can be divided in two groups. One group with the lowest predicted probabilities and one group with the highest predicted probabilities (see Table 7.10).

In the next step, the mean predicted probability of myocardial infarction is calculated for both groups. Then, based on the mean predicted probability, the expected number of subjects with myocardial infarction is calculated. In the last step, the expected number of subjects with myocardial infarction is compared to the observed number of subjects with myocardial infarction in each group. The smaller the difference between the expected number of subjects and the observed number of subjects, the higher the quality of the prediction model. In the numerical example, the mean predicted probability of having a myocardial infarction in the first group is 0.40 and in the second group 0.60. Because five subjects are present in both groups, in the first group, the expected number of subjects with myocardial infarction is two

Table 7.11 Numerical example with predicted probabilities divided into two groups including expected and observed number of subjects

Id	Predicted probability	Myocardial infarction	Expected	Observed
Group 1				
1	0.40	0	2 myocardial infarction	1 myocardial infarction
3	0.40	1		
5	0.50	0		
7	0.30	0	3 no myocardial infarction	4 no myocardial infarction
9	0.40	0		
Group 2				
2	0.60	0	3 myocardial infarction	4 myocardial infarction
4	0.65	1		
6	0.55	1		
8	0.60	1	2 no myocardial infarction	1 no myocardial infarction
10	0.60	1		

and in the second group, the expected number of subjects with myocardial infarction is three (see Table 7.11).

The final step of the Hosmer-Lemeshow test is to compare the expected number of subjects with and without myocardial infarction in the two groups with the observed number of subjects with and without myocardial infarction. Equation 7.1 shows the way the test statistic used in the Hosmer-Lemeshow test is calculated.

$$X^2 = \sum \frac{(O - E)^2}{E} \tag{7.1}$$

Where X^2= test statistic, O = observed number of subjects and E = expected number of subjects.

When the numbers shown in Table 7.11 are entered into Eq. 7.1, the test statistic is 1.67.

$$X^2 = \frac{(1-2)^2}{2} + \frac{(4-3)^2}{3} + \frac{(4-3)^2}{3} + \frac{(1-2)^2}{2} = 1.67$$

The test statistic of the Hosmer-Lemeshow test has a chi-square distribution with eight degrees of freedom. For the small numerical example, the Hosmer-Lemeshow test cannot be performed, but it can be performed for the final logistic prediction model to predict recovery in 120 patients with low back pain (Example 7.2). Table 7.12 shows the result of the Hosmer-Lemeshow test for the final prediction model.

Table 7.12 shows a table with the predicted and observed number of patients recovered, and the predicted and observed number of patients not recovered. For example, in the group with the lowest predicted probability of recovery, 12 patients

Table 7.12 Result of the Hosmer-Lemeshow test for the final prediction model to predict recovery

	No recovery		Recovery		
	Observed	Expected	Observed	Expected	Total
1	12	11.691	1	1.309	13
2	10	10.699	3	2.301	13
3	10	9.068	2	2.932	12
4	9	8.371	3	3.629	12
5	4	7.696	8	4.304	12
6	9	6.410	2	4.590	11
7	6	6.816	7	6.184	13
8	5	4.541	5	5.459	10
9	5	4.493	7	7.507	12
10	3	3.216	9	8.784	12

not recovered, while 11.691 patients were expected not to recover. It is clear that the smaller the difference between the predicted number of subjects and the observed number of subjects, the better the quality of the prediction model will be. The smaller the difference, the lower the test statistic and the higher the corresponding p-value. So, for a prediction model with good quality a high p-value is found. The null-hypothesis for the Hosmer-Lemeshow test is that the observed and expected numbers are equal. In the present example the chi-square value calculated with the numbers shown in Table 7.12 is 8.75 and based on a chi-square distribution with eight degrees of freedom, the corresponding p-value is 0.36. So, the Hosmer-Lemeshow test gives a non-significant p-value, which indicates that the null-hypothesis is not rejected. So based on the statistical test, the quality of the prediction model is good. However, although the Hosmer-Lemeshow test is developed as a statistical test, the p-value itself is mostly interpreted. The higher the p-value, the higher the quality of the prediction model. In this case, a p-value of 0.36 can be considered to indicate a moderate quality of the prediction model. It should be noted that depending on how particular statistical software deals with ties in the predicted probabilities, het Hosmer-Lemeshow test can give slightly different results.

The second quality indicator, the calibration curve, is based on the same numbers as has been used in the Hosmer-Lemeshow test. In the calibration curve the expected and observed probability of recovery are compared to each other in the same 10 groups as has been used for the Hosmer-Lemeshow test. Table 7.13 shows the observed and expected probabilities in the 10 groups, while Fig. 7.1 shows the calibration curve.

It is not easy to evaluate the quality of the prediction model based on the calibration curve. When the observed probabilities are exactly the same as the expected probabilities, the straight line goes through all the dots, which indicates a perfect fit, and therefore a prediction model with very high quality. The conclusion that can be drawn from the calibration curve shown in Fig. 7.1 is more or less the same as the conclusion that can be drawn from the Hosmer-Lemeshow test, i.e. moderate quality of the final prediction model.

Table 7.13 Data used for the calibration curve of the prediction model to predict recovery

	Numbers			Probabilities	
	Observed	Expected	Total	Observed	Expected
1	1	1.309	13	0.08	0.10
2	3	2.301	13	0.23	0.18
3	2	2.932	12	0.17	0.24
4	3	3.629	12	0.25	0.30
5	8	4.304	12	0.67	0.36
6	2	4.590	11	0.18	0.42
7	7	6.184	13	0.54	0.48
8	5	5.459	10	0.50	0.55
9	7	7.507	12	0.58	0.63
10	9	8.784	12	0.75	0.73

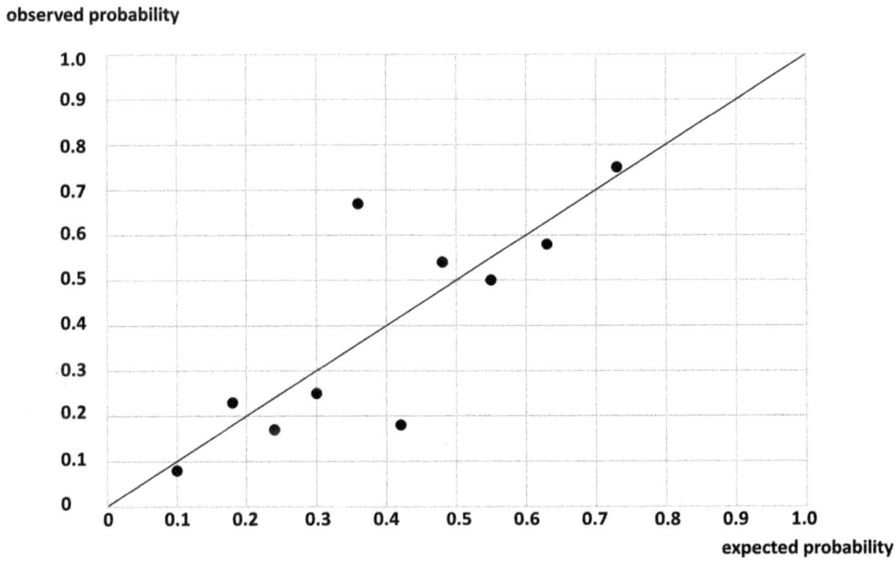

Fig. 7.1 Calibration curve of the prediction model to predict recovery

A third indicator to quantify the quality of a prediction model is based on the sensitivity and specificity of the prediction model. The sensitivity of a prediction model is the percentage of subjects who are correctly predicted to have the dichotomous outcome variable. The specificity is the percentage of subjects who are correctly predicted not to have the dichotomous outcome variable. The higher the sensitivity and specificity, the better the quality of the prediction model. The combination of sensitivity and specificity is often presented by an ROC curve (ROC stands for receiver operator characteristic, but that is not important in this context). In the ROC curve, the y-axis shows the sensitivity, while the x-axis shows the 1 - specificity. The indicator for the quality of the prediction model is the area

Table 7.14 Sensitivity and specificity of the prediction model to predict recovery with different cut-off values

	Cut-off 0.04				Cut-off 0.81		
Probability	Recovered	Not recovered	Total	Probability	Recovered	Not recovered	Total
< 0.04	0	0	0	< 0.81	47	73	120
≥ 0.04	47	73	120	≥ 0.81	0	0	0
Total	47	73		Total	47	73	
Sensitivity	47/47 = 100%			Sensitivity	0/47 = 0%		
Specificity	0/73 = 0%			Specificity	73/73 = 100%		
	Cut-off 0.25				Cut-off 0.50		
Probability	Recovered	Not recovered	Total	Probability	Recovered	Not recovered	Total
< 0.25	4	28	32	< 0.50	25	59	84
≥ 0.25	43	45	88	≥ 0.50	22	14	36
Total	47	73		Total	47	73	
Sensitivity	43/47 = 91%			Sensitivity	22/47 = 47%		
Specificity	28/73 = 38%			Specificity	59/73 = 81%		

under the ROC curve (AUC), and this AUC is also known as the C-statistic. The general idea of the calculation of the C-statistic, will be explained using the prediction model for recovery (Example 7.2).

The first step is, again, to calculate the predicted probabilities based on the final prediction model. It was already shown that the lowest predicted probability of recovery is 0.05 and the highest predicted probability is 0.81. Based on different cut-off values, the sensitivity and specificity of the prediction model can be calculated. Table 7.14 shows a few examples of the calculation of sensitivity and specificity of the prediction model with different cut-off values and Fig. 7.2 shows the ROC-curve based on these sensitivities and specificities.

In Fig. 7.2 it can be seen that the AUC (the C-statistic) is 0.73. Whether the C-statistic of 0.73 indicates a good or bad quality of the prediction model is (again) difficult to determine. The value of the C-statistic is theoretically between 0.5 and 1 and there is a rule of thumb which states that a C-statistic above 0.80 indicates a high quality prediction model, a C-statistic below 0.60 indicates a bad quality prediction model and a C-statistic between 0.60 and 0.80 indicate a moderate quality prediction model. In this example the C-statistic of 0.73, therefore, indicates a moderate quality of the final model to predict recovery. So, based on the three indicators for the quality of the logistic prediction model for recovery (i.e. the Hosmer-Lemeshow test, the calibration curve and the C-statistic) it can be concluded that the quality of the final prediction model to predict recovery is moderate.

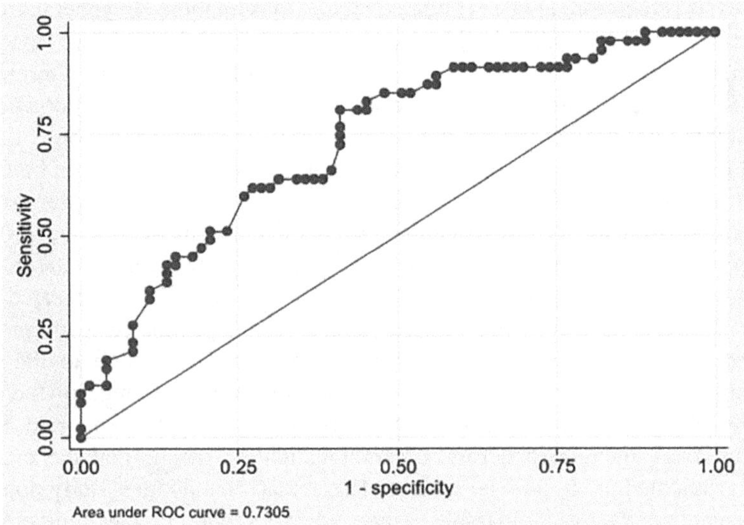

Fig. 7.2 ROC curve for the prediction model to predict recovery

7.5 Validity of a Prediction Model

Besides the fact that the quality of the prediction model is important, it is also important to report the validity of the prediction model. Because the prediction model is built with data from a certain study population it is important to have an indication of how well this prediction model behaves in other populations, such as a population of new patients. The different methods that can be used for the validation of a prediction model can be divided into methods used for internal validation and methods used for external validation. Internal validation means that the prediction model is validated within the data used to build the prediction model. External validation means that the prediction model is validated in an external dataset. A number of methods are available for internal validation of a prediction model. One of those methods is cross-validation. The idea behind cross-validation is that the dataset is randomly divided into two groups. One part of the dataset is used to build the prediction model (this part is called the derivation set or learning set) and the other part of the dataset is used to validate the prediction model (this part is therefore called the validation set or test set). It is common practice to report both the quality indicators of the original prediction model and those of the prediction model, applied to the validation set. It should be clear that cross-validation can only be used when the number of subjects in the study population is (very) large.

A second internal validation method is the so-called jack-knife method. Within this method, the prediction model is built in the total dataset. Then, one observation is removed from the dataset and with the new dataset (which now consists of n−1 observations) the prediction model is validated. This is repeated for all observations.

The analysis is therefore always validated on n - 1 observations. In general, the mean and/or range of the quality indicators obtained from the jack-knife analyses is reported, in addition to the quality indicators of the original prediction model.

The third commonly used internal validation method is bootstrapping. Bootstrapping is a method that is used for all kinds of purposes and one of them is the validation of a prediction model. First of all, a prediction model is built in the total dataset. A new dataset is then created by randomly drawing the same number of observations from the original dataset, but with replacement. So, the difference between the original dataset and the new dataset is that in the new dataset, certain observations can occur more than once. The bootstrap procedure is repeated a large number of times (e.g. 1000) and with the bootstrap samples, the prediction model is validated. In general, as with the jack-knife method, in addition to the quality indicators of the original prediction model, the mean and/or range of the quality indicators obtained from the analyses on the bootstrap samples is reported.

As has been mentioned before, external validation means that the prediction model is validated in an external dataset. This means that another study population must be available that is comparable to the study population in which the prediction model was built. For example, the same type of patients from another hospital. In light of the external validity of the prediction model, besides the quality indicators of the original prediction model, also the quality indicators of the prediction model applied in the external dataset are reported.

7.5.1 Number of Independent Variables in a Prediction Model

It is important to realize that the number of independent variables added to a prediction model is directly related to the validity of the prediction model. The more variables present in the final prediction model, the lower the validity of the model. In light of this, there is a rule of thumb that indicates that at least 15 subjects per variable should be present in the dataset in order to get a reasonable valid prediction model. When a prediction model is made for a dichotomous outcome variable, the rule of the thumb is related to the number of subjects with (or without) the dichotomous outcome variable. So, for example, in the final model to predict cholesterol, around 13 independent variables can be present, because the study population consist of 200 subjects. For the final prediction model for recovery, on the other hand, at the most, 3 independent variables can be present, because in the study population only 47 patients recovered.

As with all cut-off values and rule of thumbs in statistics, the rule of thumb for the maximal number of independent variables present in a final prediction model is highly arbitrary and also other rule of thumbs (e.g. 10 or 20 subjects per independent variable) are mentioned in the literature. It is important to note that all cut-off values and rule of thumbs used in statistics should be interpreted with caution.

Chapter 8
Machine Learning

Abstract In this chapter a short introduction is given in machine learning methods. First, classification and regression trees are introduced. Both are necessary to understand the use of more complicated methods such as bagging (e.g. random forest) and boosting (e.g. XGBoost). Furthermore, the bias-variance trade-off is discussed, which deals with the quality of a prediction model. When the internal quality is high, the external validity is often low. In machine learning terminology, the internal quality is often referred to as bias, while the external validity is often referred to as variance. The second part of this chapter deals with shrinkage methods. Shrinkage methods aim to shrink the regression coefficients of a prediction model in order to increase the external validity of the model.

8.1 Introduction

Machine learning is a general name for a lot of statistical methods. Basically, the multiple linear and logistic regression analyses discussed in Chap. 7 can also be seen as machine learning methods. Mostly, however, machine learning is used for other methods that can be used for building prediction models.

8.2 Classification and Regression Trees

8.2.1 Classification Tree Analysis

Classification tree analysis is a hierarchical method to build a prediction model for a dichotomous outcome variable, which is based on interactions. The general idea of classification tree analysis is first to find the most important interaction in the data. Based on the most important interaction, the study population is split into different parts and within these parts other interactions are analysed. It is important to note that within the classification tree analysis, interactions are not limited to dichotomous and categorical independent variables, also continuous independent variables

J. W. R. Twisk, *Basic Principles of Applied Medical Statistics*,
https://doi.org/10.1007/978-3-031-86278-6_8

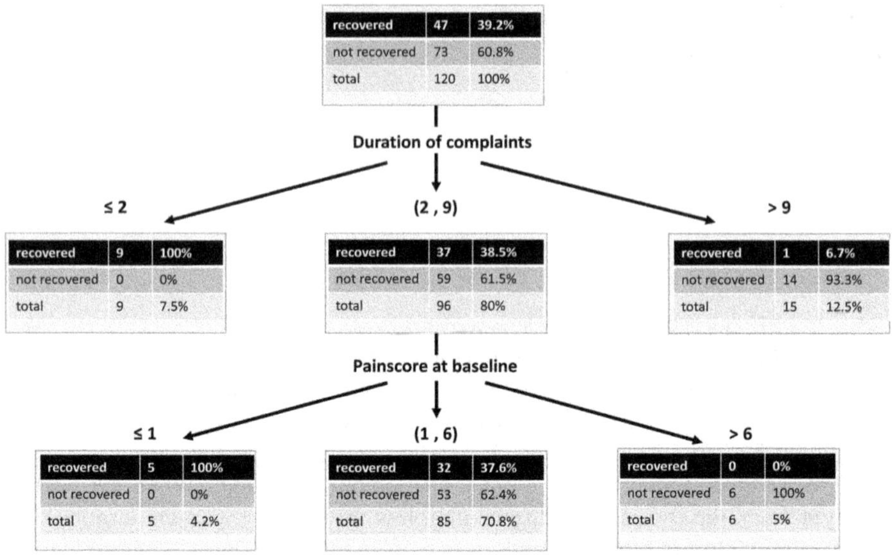

Fig. 8.1 Result of the classification tree analysis to predict recovery

are considered. Regarding these continuous independent variables, the best cut-off values for splitting the study population are determined and the study population is split into different parts according these cut-off values. Figure 8.1 shows the result of a classification tree analysis to predict recovery using the data from Example 7.2.

In Fig. 8.1 it can be seen that the first split in the classification tree is made for the independent variable duration of complaints. Because this is a continuous variable the split is made on two cut-off values. The two cut-off values are at 2 months and at 9 months duration of complaints. It can further be seen that when the duration of complaints is $\leq$2 months, the probability of recovery is very high. The nine patients that have a duration of complaints $\leq$2 months all recovered. When the duration of complaints is >9 month on the other hand, the probability of recovery is very low. From the 15 patients that have a duration of complaints >9 month, only 1 patient recovered. For the patients who have a duration of complaints between the two cut-off values, a second split is made, which is based on pain. Also for the pain score the split is made on two cut-off values. The first cut-off value is a pain score of 1 and the second cut-off value is a pain score of 6. In the classification tree it can be seen that the five patients with a duration of complaints between 2 and 9 months and a pain score ≤ 1, all recovered. On the other hand, the six patients with a duration of complaints between 2 and 9 months and a pain score > 6, all not recovered. For the patients with a duration of complaints between 2 and 9 months and a pain score between 1 and 6, there is sort of mixture with subjects recovered and not recovered. However, for this subgroup no further relevant split is found. So, the classification tree in the present example contains two so-called nodes; the first one defined by duration of complaints and the second one defined by pain. It should be noted that

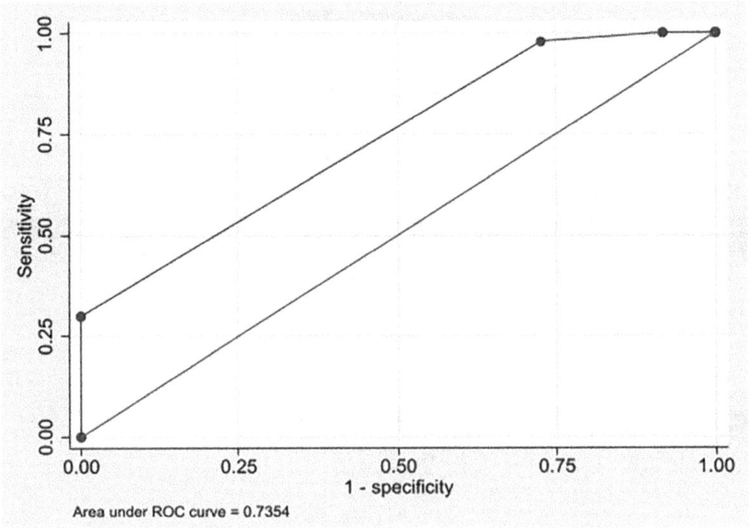

Fig. 8.2 ROC curve for the classification tree to predict recovery

these two independent variables are also present in the final logistic prediction model shown in Output 7.19 and these two independent variables have the lowest p-values of the final prediction model (see Sect. 7.4). The quality of the classification tree shown in Fig. 8.1 can also be determined by comparing the predicted probabilities derived from the classification tree with the observed values. For example, the C-statistic can be calculated (see Sect. 7.4.1). Figure 8.2 shows the ROC-curve and the C-statistic for the classification tree shown in Fig. 8.1.

Because the classification tree analysis only leads to five different probabilities, the ROC curve shown in Fig. 8.2 only shows five different combinations of sensitivity and 1 - specificity. The C-statistic for the final classification tree is 0.74, which is more or less the same as the C-statistic for the final logistic prediction model (see Sect. 7.4.1). In Fig. 8.2 it can be seen that especially in the extremities of the classification tree, the predictions are very good. However, in the middle of the classification tree, the predictions are not good. It is possible to perform an exhaustive classification tree analysis, in which also the patients with a duration of complaints between 2 and 9 months and a pain score between 1 and 6 are further divided into relevant subgroups. Figure 8.3 shows the result of the exhaustive classification tree analysis.

In Fig. 8.3 it can be seen that the first independent variable used to split the group of patients with a duration of complaints between 2 and 9 months and a pain score between 1 and 6 is age. Age is divided into 5 subgroups ($\leq$ 41.2; 41.2–44.3; 44.3–45.5; 45.5–46.6 and $>$ 46.6 years). It can further be seen that the subgroup with patients aged 41.2–44.3 is further divided into patients that use medication and patients that do not use medication. When the quality of the exhaustive classification tree is determined by the C-statistic, the value (i.e. 0.88) is much higher than the

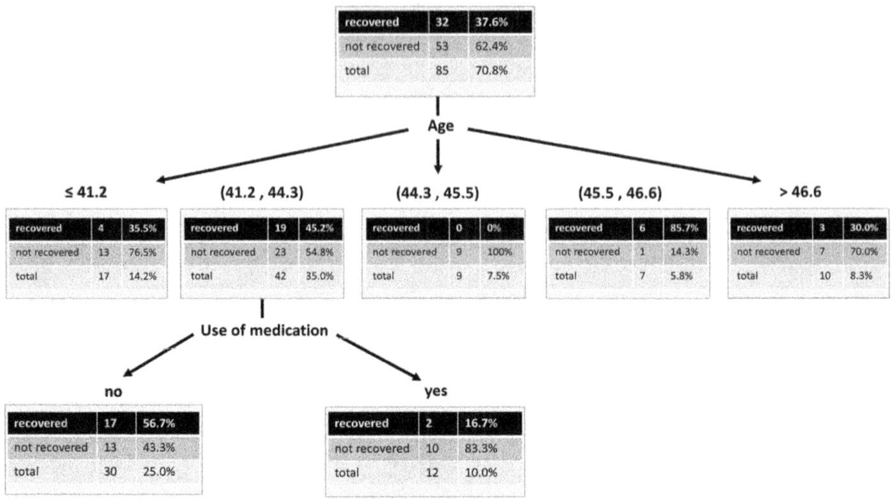

Fig. 8.3 Result of the exhaustive classification tree analysis to predict recovery

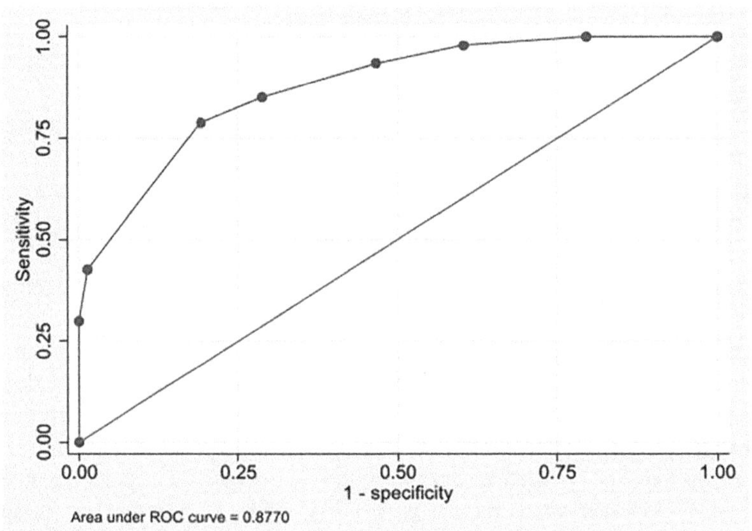

Fig. 8.4 ROC curve for the exhaustive classification tree to predict recovery

C-statistic for both the first classification tree and the final logistic prediction model (see Fig. 8.4).

In Fig. 8.4 it can nicely be seen that now, the predictions in the middle part of the curve are much better than in the ROC curve based on the first classification tree.

One of the advantages of classification tree analysis is that the final result can be interpreted very easily and that the way the classification tree is build mimics the way a prediction model is used in, especially, diagnostics. A disadvantage is, however, that the final model is highly data driven and that holds especially for the cut-off values used for splitting the population on continuous independent variables. It is therefore, often argued that a classification tree has a very high quality (i.e. a very high C-statistic), but a very low validity. In the present example, especially the exhaustive classification tree has a very high C-statistic, but especially because the classification tree is based on a lot of data driven cut-off values for continuous independent variables it is expected that the validity of the exhaustive classification tree will be low.

Classification tree analysis is used to predict a dichotomous outcome variable. However, the method can also be used to predict a continuous outcome variable. When a continuous outcome variable is used, the method is known as regression tree analysis.

8.2.2 *Regression Tree Analysis*

Regression tree analysis is basically the same as classification tree analysis. The only difference is that the outcome variable is continuous instead of dichotomous and that, therefore, linear regression analysis is used for building the tree. This means also that the mean value of the continuous outcome variable is predicted by the regression tree. Regression tree analysis is illustrated with Example 7.1 and the aim of the regression tree analysis is to predict cholesterol with independent variables, sex, age, body mass index, smoking, alcohol consumption and physical activity. Figure 8.5 shows the result of the regression tree analysis to predict cholesterol.

In Fig. 8.5 it can be seen that the first split is made for age and that three age groups are considered ($\leq$ 61 years of age, between 61 and 64 years of age and $>$ 64 years of age). It can also be seen that with increasing age, mean cholesterol is higher and that mean cholesterol is the highest in the oldest age group (i.e. 6.77). In the next step, the regression tree is further divided into subgroups, but only for the youngest and the oldest age groups. The middle age group is not divided any further. The youngest age group is further divided into males and females, while the oldest age group is divided into five subgroups based on body mass index. While the five body mass index groups are the final nodes, the males are further divided into two groups regarding physical activity (moderate and low physical activity versus high physical activity) and the females are divided into four subgroups regarding body mass index. So, body mass index is used twice as a splitting variable. Based on the regression tree, cholesterol can be predicted for each subject given the values of the independent variables in the model. When, for example, the data of the first subject of Example 7.1 (a subject with a body mass index of 27.41, 66 years of age, who is non-smoker and non-drinker) are entered into the regression tree, the predicted cholesterol is 7.10. This prediction is slightly better than the prediction based on the final linear regression prediction model (6.63), but still an underestimation of the observed cholesterol, which is 7.90 (see Sect. 7.3.2).

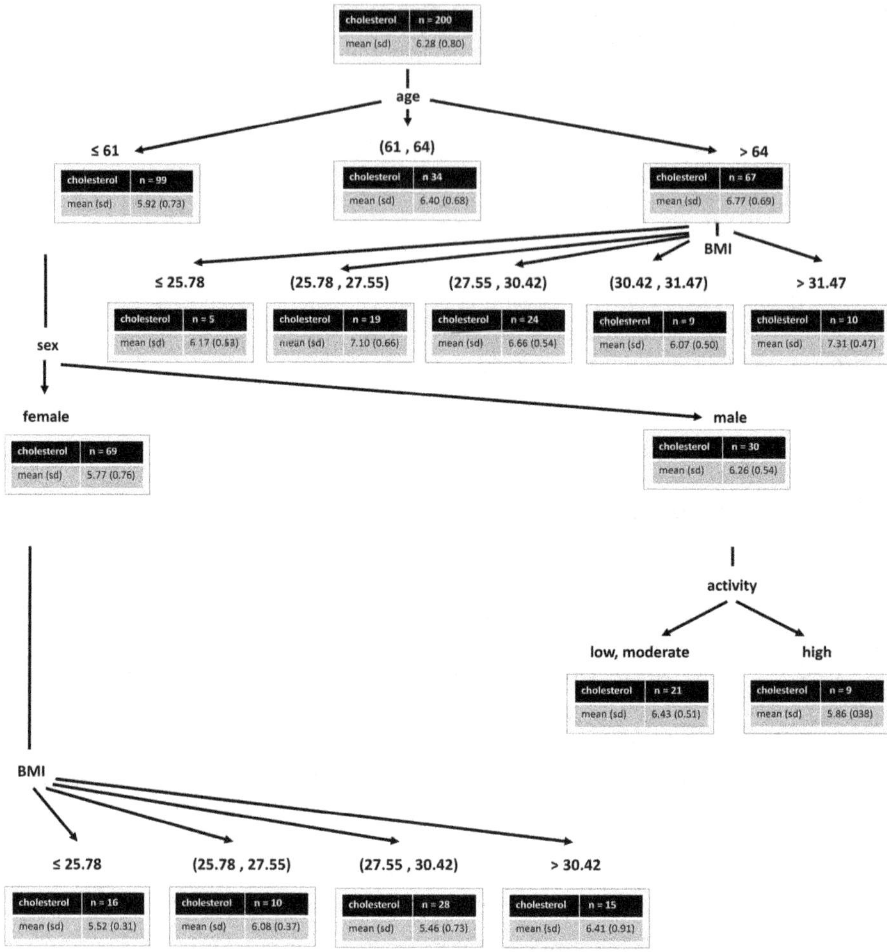

Fig. 8.5 Result of the regression tree analysis to predict cholesterol

After building the regression tree (as has been mentioned for the classification tree), the quality of the regression tree must be quantified. For a regression tree, which predicts a continuous outcome variable, the explained variance can be used. In this example the explained variance of the regression tree is 0.46. It should be noted that the explained variance is lower than the explained variance of the final linear regression prediction model (see Sect. 7.3.6). This is not expected, because regression trees are known to be very data driven, leading to a high quality of the model, but to a low validity of the model. Maybe the fact that the continuous independent variables are categorized in the regression tree analysis is the reason for the relative low quality of the regression tree. Categorization of continuous independent variables lead to information loss, which can lead to a lower quality of the model. It should also be noted that the variables included into the different prediction models are different. In both prediction models, age and body mass index are present, but smoking and alcohol consumption are present in the final linear regression prediction model, but not in the regression tree. Sex and physical activity on the other hand are present in the regression tree, but not in the final linear regression prediction model.

8.2.3 Bagging, Boosting and the Bias-Variance Trade-off

An extension of classification and regression tree analysis is random forest analysis. In a random forest analysis, multiple classification or regression trees are made on randomly chosen subsets of independent variables. By default the number of independent variables used in the subsets is equal to the (rounded) square root of the number of independent variables in the dataset. It should be noted that the random selection of independent variables is performed after each split, so at each split in the classification or regression tree analysis, different independent variables are used.

The result of a random forest analysis is the relative importance of a particular independent variable in the different classification or regression trees. The relative importance of a particular independent variable is calculated by the difference in quality between a classification or regression tree with the particular independent variable and one without the particular independent variable. It should be noted that random forest analysis is particularly useful when the number of independent variables is (very) large and it should also be noted that the interpretation of the result from a random forest analysis is much more difficult than the interpretation of the result from a single classification or regression tree analysis.

Random forest analysis is known as a bagging method. Bagging stands for bootstrap aggregating and means that many different trees are built in a parallel way. Boosting is more or less the same, but differs from bagging in such a way that many different trees are built in a sequential way. This means that information of the first tree is used for building the second tree and so forth and so on. Boosting is for example implemented in the machine learning method XGBoost (eXtreme Gradient Boosting).

Bagging and boosting are so-called ensemble methods, which means that information of (many) different trees are combined to obtain the best result. Because bagging is a parallel method it leads to a lower quality of the prediction model, while it leads to an increase in the validity of the prediction model. Boosting on the other hand, leads to a higher quality of the prediction model, but to a lower validity of the prediction model. An increase in the quality of the prediction model and a decrease in the validity of the prediction model is known as the bias-variance trade-off. Bias is the difference between the predicted values and the observed values (i.e. the quality of the model), while the variance is the difference between the prediction in the dataset used for building the model and the prediction in new, unseen data (i.e. the validity of the model). When a prediction model becomes more complex, the quality of the model will increase (i.e. the bias will decrease), but the validity of the model will decrease (i.e. the variance will increase). The other way round, when a prediction model becomes less complex, the quality of the model will decrease (i.e. the bias will increase), but the validity of the model will increase (i.e. the variance will decrease).

It should be realised that all ensemble methods have the same problem as a random forest analysis, i.e. the interpretation of the result is complicated and, therefore, the result is difficult to use in real life practice.

For both classification tree and regression tree analysis, the earlier mentioned bias-variance trade-off can be manipulated by choosing the depth of the tree (i.e. the maximum number of nodes) or the minimum number of subjects within a node. Decreasing the depth of the tree leads to an increase in bias but to a decrease in variance. Decreasing the minimum number of subjects in the final node of the tree on the other hand leads to a decrease in bias but to an increase in variance. For example, the regression tree (see Fig. 8.5) was built with a minimum number of five subjects in a final node of the tree. It should be noted that the final node of the tree, is also known as the leaf of the tree.

Regarding the bias-variance trade-off it should be noted that within classification and regression tree analysis and also for the related bagging and boosting methods, such as random forest analysis and XGBoost, mostly cross-validation is used to perform (internal) model validation. As has been mentioned before (see Sect. 7.5), within cross-validation the dataset is randomly divided into two groups. One part of the dataset is used to build the classification or regression tree while the other part of the dataset is used to validate the classification or regression tree. When the dataset is divided into two groups, the cross-validation method is known as two-fold cross-validation. However, mostly the dataset is divided into more groups and more cross-validations are used to validate the classification or regression tree. Mostly a five-fold cross-validation or a ten-fold cross-validation is used for validation.

It should be realized that also the rule of thumb for the maximum number of variables in a final prediction model (see Sect. 7.5.1) is related to the bias-variance trade-off. When more independent variables are added to the prediction model, the quality of the model will increase (i.e. the bias will decrease), but the validity of the model will decrease (i.e. the variance will increase).

8.3 Shrinkage Methods

As has been mentioned before, one of the problems of prediction models is that the validity of the prediction model is often low. Or in other words, because the prediction model is data driven, the performance of the prediction model in a new dataset is often poor. This phenomenon is also known as overfitting. Shrinkage methods, which are also known as regularization methods are developed to deal with this problem. It is assumed that when a shrinkage method is used, the validity of the prediction model will increase. Basically there are two methods used for shrinkage of prediction models, i.e. LASSO regression and ridge regression. LASSO stands for

Table 8.1 Regression coefficients obtained from logistic, LASSO and ridge regression analysis to predict recovery

	Logistic regression: Final model	LASSO	Logistic regression: Full model	Ridge
Sex		−0.36	−0.98	−0.53
Medication	−0.90	−0.54	−1.01	−0.60
Overweight			0.08	0.03
Pain	−0.38	−0.27	−0.40	−0.25
Function			−0.03	−0.02
Duration	−0.21	−0.15	−0.22	−0.14
Age			0.09	0.04

Least **A**bsolute **S**hrinkage and **S**election **O**perator and that describes exactly what the methods does. So, it is a selection method which uses shrinkage to increase the validity of the final prediction model. Ridge regression is more or less the same. i.e. it is a shrinkage method, but the difference with LASSO regression is that within ridge regression no selection is performed. Ridge regression was originally developed to detect collinearity in multiple regression models (see Sect. 11.1), but nowadays it is used as a shrinkage method. Both LASSO regression and ridge regression can be used for prediction models with a continuous outcome variable (i.e. to shrink the regression coefficients obtained from a linear regression analysis), but they are mostly used for prediction models with a dichotomous outcome variable (i.e. to shrink the regression coefficients obtained from a logistic regression analysis). It should be noted that there are different ways to estimate the optimal shrinkage factors for the different independent variables in the prediction model. The mostly used method is cross-validation (see Sect. 7.5). To illustrate the influence of using LASSO regression and ridge regression on the result of the prediction model built for recovery in Example 7.2, Table 8.1 shows the different regression coefficients calculated with logistic regression analysis and with the two shrinkage methods. Because in LASSO regression besides shrinkage also a selection is performed, the result of the LASSO regression analysis is compared to the result of the final logistic prediction model including the independent variables medication, duration and pain (see Output 7.19). The result of the ridge regression analysis is compared to the result of the logistic regression analysis including all independent variables (see Output 7.16).

In Table 8.1 it can be seen that with LASSO regression analysis, also sex is included in the final prediction model. This is different from the final logistic prediction model (see Sect. 7.4). However, within the backward selection, sex was the last variable that was removed from the prediction model, while the p-value for the regression coefficient for sex was very close to the predefined cut-off value of 0.10. Furthermore, sex was also included in the final prediction model when the AIC was used for selection (see Table 7.8).

In Table 8.1 it can also be seen that all regression coefficients obtained from the LASSO regression analysis are lower than the ones obtained from the logistic

Table 8.2 C-statistics and 95% confidence intervals for logistic, LASSO and ridge regression analysis to predict recovery

	C-statistic	95% confidence interval
Logistic regression analysis: Full model	0.75	0.66–0.84
Logistic regression analysis: Final model	0.73	0.64–0.82
Ridge regression	0.75	0.66–0.84
LASSO regression	0.75	0.65–0.84

regression analysis. This is not surprising, because LASSO regression analysis is a shrinkage method, which means that all regression coefficients are shrunken towards zero. The shrinkage is also observed in the result of the ridge regression, i.e. the regression coefficients obtained from the ridge regression analysis are all lower (closer to zero) than the ones obtained from the logistic regression analysis. However, compared to LASSO regression analysis, in ridge regression analysis no selection is performed.

It should be realized that also shrinkage is related to the bias-variance trade-off. In a prediction model the quality of the model will increase (i.e. the bias will decrease) with model complexity, whereas the variance of the model (i.e. the validity) will decrease with model complexity. Shrinkage is used to reduce the model complexity, which leads to an increase of the validity of the prediction model and in general to a decrease in the quality of the model. However, in the present example, the quality of the logistic prediction models including shrinkage is not lower compared to the quality of the logistic regression prediction models without shrinkage. To illustrate this, Table 8.2 shows the C-statistics of the different prediction models.

Before LASSO regression and ridge regression were commonly used as shrinkage methods, the problem of overfitting of a prediction model was already recognized. To deal with this overfitting, the so-called heuristic shrinkage factor was used to shrink the regression coefficients of a prediction model. The heuristic shrinkage factor can be calculated with Eq. 8.1.

$$shrinkage = \frac{X^2{}_{model} - df}{X^2{}_{model}} \tag{8.1}$$

where $X^2{}_{model}$= difference in −2 log likelihood between the model without independent variables and the final prediction model, and df = degrees of freedom, i.e. difference in number of parameters estimated by the model without independent variables and the final prediction model.

For the prediction model to predict recovery, for example, the difference in −2 log likelihood between the final prediction model and the model without independent variables is 20.185 and the number of degrees of freedom is three, because three independent variables are present in the final prediction model, so three additional parameters are estimated in the final prediction model. With these numbers, the heuristic shrinkage factor can be calculated.

$$shrinkage = \frac{20.187 - 3}{20.187} = 0.85$$

This shrinkage factor (0.85) is multiplied with the regression coefficients of the final logistic prediction model to obtain the (heuristic) shrunken regression coefficients of the final logistic prediction model, which is then adjusted for overfitting.

8.4 Other Methods

The machine learning methods discussed so far are all prediction models and all these methods belong to the so-called supervised machine learning methods. When the classification is not related to an outcome variable (e.g. methods such as K-means clustering or latent class analysis), the methods are known as unsupervised machine learning methods. Besides the machine learning methods described in this section, there are many other statistical methods available that belong to the group of machine learning methods. Most of them are mathematically complicated and are therefore beyond the scope of this book. However, all the more complicated machine learning methods are either classification methods or shrinkage methods. For example, elastic net analysis is a shrinkage method that combines LASSO regression and ridge regression. Support vector machine analysis and neural networks are complicated classification methods. Although the complicated machine learning methods are increasingly used in medical science, the results are very difficult to interpret and, therefore, they can hardly be used in real life practice. For detailed information about machine learning methods see for example Smola & Schölkopf, 2004; Maley et al., 2011; Hastie et al., 2017; Riley et al., 2021, and Wallace et al., 2023.

Chapter 9
Other Outcome Variables

Abstract In the first chapters of this book, the analysis of a continuous outcome variable, a dichotomous outcome variable and survival data was discussed. This chapter dealt with the analysis of other outcome variables, such as a categorical outcome variable, a count outcome variable, an outcome variable with a floor or ceiling effect and correlated outcome variables. It is shown that for the analysis of a categorical outcome variable, multinomial logistic regression analysis can be used, while for a count outcome variable, either Poisson regression analysis or negative binomial regression analysis can be used. For the analysis of an outcome variable with a floor or ceiling effect, it is possible to use tobit regression analysis. Regarding the analysis of correlated outcome variables, mixed model analysis and generalised estimating equations are briefly introduced. One of the important conclusions of this chapter is that all regression analyses are basically the same regarding the interpretation of the regression coefficients, the evaluation of linearity of the relationship with a continuous independent variable, the adjustment for confounding and the investigation of effect modification.

9.1 Introduction

In Chaps. 4, 5 and 6, the analysis of a continuous outcome variable, a dichotomous outcome variable and survival data has been discussed. While these three types of outcome variables are by far the most common in practice, there are other types of outcome variables as well, such as a categorical outcome variable, a count outcome variable or an outcome variable with a floor or ceiling effect.

J. W. R. Twisk, *Basic Principles of Applied Medical Statistics*,
https://doi.org/10.1007/978-3-031-86278-6_9

9.2 The Analysis of a Categorical Outcome Variable

9.2.1 Introduction

In Chap. 1 it was already mentioned that a categorical outcome variable consists of more than two groups and that a distinction can be made between ordinal and nominal categorical outcome variables (see Sect. 1.2). Regarding the analysis of a categorical outcome variable discussed in this section, it is not really important whether the categorical outcome variable is ordinal or nominal. Both can be analysed with the same methods. The analysis of a categorical outcome variable will be discussed using Example 9.1, a cross-sectional cohort study in which self-reported health of 100 subjects is measured. The categorical outcome variable self-reported health is divided into three groups: bad, not good/not bad, and good. The aim of the study is to investigate the relationship between self-reported health and a number of independent variables such as smoking, social class and age. Table 9.1 shows descriptive information of the variables used in this example.

9.2.2 Comparing Two Groups

The first question is whether there is a difference in self-reported health between smokers and non-smokers. Comparable to the analysis of a dichotomous outcome variable (see Sect. 5.1), the relationship between self-reported health and smoking can be shown by a cross table, i.e. a 3 × 2 table (see Table 9.2).

Table 9.1 Descriptive information of the variables used in Example 9.1

	Mean	Standard deviation		Number of subjects
Age (years)	47.4	15.5		
Self-reported health			Bad	33
			Not good/not bad	38
			Good	29
Smoking			Non-smoker	62
			Smoker	38
Social class			Low	42
			Middle	31
			High	27

Table 9.2 3 × 2 table for the relationship between self-reported health and smoking

	Self-reported health			
	Bad	Not good/not bad	Good	Total
Non-smoking	16	24	22	62
Smoking	17	14	7	38
Total	33	38	29	100

Output 9.1 Result of the Fisher exact test and the chi-square test for the relationship between self-reported health and smoking

	Value	df	Asymptotic p-value	Exact p-value (2-sided)
Fisher's exact test				0.09
Chi-square test	4.96	2	0.08	

Table 9.3 3 × 3 table for the relationship between self-reported health and social class

	Self-reported health			
Social class	Bad	Not good/not bad	Good	Total
Low	22	12	8	42
Middle	7	15	9	31
High	4	11	12	27
Total	33	38	29	100

In Sect. 5.3 the analysis of a dichotomous outcome variable with a categorical independent variable was discussed. Basically, the analysis of the relationship between a categorical outcome variable and a dichotomous independent variable is exactly the same. So the 3 × 2 table can be analysed with the Fisher exact test or the chi-square test (see Output 9.1).

The p-values reported in Output 9.1 have the same interpretation as always. The probability of finding the 3 × 2 table shown in Table 9.1 or more extreme away from the null-hypothesis, when the null-hypothesis is true, is 0.09 or 0.08. The null-hypothesis is that the proportion of smokers and non-smokers in the three groups of self-reported health are exactly the same. The magnitude of the relationship between self-reported health and smoking cannot be derived from the 3 × 2 table. To obtain effect estimates, for several 2 × 2 tables effect estimates can be calculated or a regression method can be used. For categorical outcome variables, the regression method that can be used is multinomial logistic regression analysis (see Sect. 9.2.4).

9.2.3 Comparing More than Two Groups

Using data from Example 9.1, comparing more than two groups with a categorical outcome variable will be illustrated by analysing the relationship between self-reported health and social class (see Table 9.3).

Although the interpretation of a cross table becomes increasingly difficult as the number of columns and/or rows increases, in Table 9.3 it can be seen that there seems to be a relationship between self-reported health and social class. Subjects with low social class mostly report bad health, while individuals with high social class mostly report good health. As for all other cross tables, also the 3 × 3 table can be analysed by the Fisher Exact test or the chi-square test (see Output 9.2).

In Output 9.2 it can be seen that there is a statistically significant association between self-reported health and social class (both p-values for the Fisher exact test and the chi-square test are ≤0.05). Without an interpretation of the numbers shown

Output 9.2 Result of the Fisher exact test and the chi-square test for the relationship between self-reported health and social class

	Value	df	Asymptotic p-value	Exact p-value (2-sided)
Fisher exact test				0.008
Chi-square test	14.08	4	0.007	

in the 3 × 3 table, the observed p-value does not say much. Therefore, when this p-value is reported, it must be accompanied by an interpretation of the numbers from the 3 × 3 table.

9.2.4 Multinomial Logistic Regression Analysis

In Sects. 9.2.2 and 9.2.3 the analysis of a categorical outcome variable with a dichotomous and a categorical independent variable was discussed using cross tables. However, when the relationship between a categorical outcome variable and a continuous independent variable is investigated, a cross table cannot be used. In previous chapters, it was mentioned that the relationship with continuous independent variables can be analysed with a linear regression analysis (when the outcome variable is continuous), logistic regression analysis (when the outcome variable is dichotomous) or Cox regression analysis (when the outcome variable is survival data). When the outcome variable is categorical, multinomial logistic regression analysis can be used. Multinomial logistic regression analysis is a method that is probably best characterized as a multivariate logistic regression analysis. Multivariate because multiple groups of the outcome variable are analysed at the same time, or in other words more than one logistic regression analysis is performed at the same time. The name of the method suggests that the method is suitable for categorical outcome variables which are nominal, but this is a misconception. Multinomial logistic regression analysis can be used to analyse both nominal and ordinal categorical outcome variables. The detailed (mathematical) background of multinomial logistic regression analysis will not be discussed in detail. However, the interpretation of the result of a multinomial logistic regression analysis will be discussed using Example 9.1. In this example the relationship between self-reported health and age is analysed. Output 9.3 shows the result of the multinomial logistic regression analysis.

In Output 9.3 it can be seen that two logistic regression analyses are simultaneously performed. In the first part of the output, the group with a bad self-reported health is compared to the group with a good self-reported health, which is the reference group in the analysis. In the second part of the output, the group with a not good/not bad self-reported health is compared to the group with a good self-reported health. In the first part of the output it can be seen that the regression coefficient for age is 0.081, which corresponds with an odds ratio of 1.08. The interpretation of this odds ratio is that with a 1 year difference in age, the odds of

Output 9.3 Result of the multinomial logistic regression analysis to analyse the relationship between self-reported health and age

							95% confidence interval	
	Coefficient	se	Wald	df	p-value	Odds ratio	Lower	Upper
Bad self-reported health								
Age	0.081	0.021	14.54	1	<0.001	1.08	1.04	1.13
Constant	−3.79	1.07	14.54	1	<0.001			
Not good/not bad self-reported health								
Age	0.021	0.018	1.34	1	0.25	1.02	0.99	1.06
Constant	−0.61	0.79	0.59	1	0.44			

se standard error, *df* degrees of freedom

Output 9.4 Result of the multinomial logistic regression analysis to analyse the relationship between self-reported health and smoking

							95% confidence interval	
	Coefficient	se	Wald	df	p-value	Odds ratio	Lower	Upper
Bad self-reported health								
Smoking	1.21	0.56	4.70	1	0.03	3.40	1.12	9.94
Constant	−3.18	0.33	0.94	1	0.33			
Not good/not bad self-reported health								
Smoking	0.61	0.55	1.22	1	0.27	1.83	0.63	5.38
Constant	0.09	0.30	0.09	1	0.77			

se standard error, *df* degrees of freedom

reporting bad health is 1.08 times higher than the odds of reporting good health. It can also be seen that the 95% confidence interval around the odds ratio of 1.08 ranges between 1.04 and 1.13 and that this odds ratio is statistically significant ($p < 0.001$). In the second part of the output, the regression coefficient for age is 0.021, which corresponds with an odds ratio of 1.02. The interpretation of the odds ratio of 1.02 is that with a one-year difference in age, the odds of reporting a not good/not bad health is 1.02 times higher than the odds of reporting good health. It can also be seen the 95% confidence interval around the odds ratio of 1.02 ranges between 0.99 and 1.06 and that this odds ratio is not statistically significant ($p = 0.25$).

It should be realized that multinomial logistic regression analysis is a regression analysis, so evaluation of effect modification, adjustment for confounding, and evaluation of the linearity of the relationship with continuous independent variables are exactly the same as has been discussed for the other regression methods.

Multinomial logistic regression analysis can also be used to compare a categorical outcome variable between two groups and to compare a categorical outcome variable between more than two groups. To illustrate this, Output 9.4 shows the result of a multinomial logistic regression analysis to analyse the relationship between self-reported health and smoking.

Table 9.4 Dummy coding for the variable social class

	Dummy 1	Dummy 2
Low	0	0
Middle	1	0
High	0	1

Output 9.5 Result of the multinomial logistic regression analysis to analyse the relationship between self-reported health and social class

							95% confidence interval	
	Coefficient	se	Wald	df	p-value	Odds ratio	Lower	Upper
Bad self-reported health								
Dummy 1	−1.26	0.65	3.76	1	0.05	0.28	0.08	1.01
Dummy 2	−2.11	0.71	8.84	1	0.003	0.12	0.03	0.49
Constant	1.01	0.41	6.00	1	0.01			
Not good/not bad self-reported health								
Dummy 1	0.11	0.62	0.03	1	0.87	1.11	0.33	3.76
Dummy 2	−0.49	0.62	0.63	1	0.43	0.61	0.18	2.05
Constant	0.41	0.46	0.79	1	0.37			

se standard error, *df* degrees of freedom

In the first part of Output 9.4 it can be seen that the regression coefficient for smoking is 1.21. The corresponding odds ratio of 3.40 indicates that the odds of reporting bad health compared to good health is 3.40 times higher for smokers than for non-smokers. The odds ratio shown in the second part of Output 9.4 (i.e. 1.83) indicates that the odds of reporting not good/not bad health compared to good health is 1.83 times higher for smokers than for non-smokers.

Regarding the comparison of a categorical outcome variable between more than two groups (i.e. social class) two dummy variables must be made to represent social class (see Table 9.4). Output 9.5 shows the result of a multinomial logistic regression analysis to analyse the relationship between self-reported health and social class.

Output 9.5 is slightly more difficult to interpret, because there is not only a categorical outcome variable but also a categorical independent variable. In the output, therefore, for each comparison two dummy variables appear for social class. Regarding the interpretation of the different odds ratios, for example, the odds ratio of 0.28, which belongs to the first dummy variable in the comparison between bad self-reported health and good self-reported health, indicates that the odds of reporting bad health compared to good health is 0.28 times higher for subjects with a middle social class than for subjects with a low social class. In general it can be seen that social class is mostly related to the difference between bad self-reported health and good self-reported health.

9.3 The Analysis of a Count Outcome Variable

A special kind of a categorical outcome variable is a count outcome variable. Count outcome variables are quite common in medical science, for example the number of side effects of a new medication, the number of epileptic seizures, the number of asthma attacks, the number of falls in elderly people, etc. A count outcome variable mostly has a Poisson distribution. A count outcome variable has a Poisson distribution when the distribution is skewed to the right and when the mean is more or less equal to the variance. When the outcome variable has a Poisson distribution, Poisson regression analysis can be used to analyse the outcome variables. Poisson regression analysis is the same as linear regression analysis, logistic regression analysis, Cox regression analysis and all other regression analyses; the only difference is that the outcome variable is different. Without explaining the mathematical background in detail, the outcome variable that is analysed is the natural logarithm of the count. Comparable to logistic regression analysis, and Cox regression analysis, the regression coefficient of a Poisson regression analysis can be transformed into an effect estimate, by taking the e-power of the regression coefficient. The effect estimate obtained from a Poisson regression analysis is a ratio of counts, which is better known as a rate ratio. To illustrate the use of Poisson regression analysis for the analysis of a count outcome variable, Example 9.2 is used. Example 9.2 contains data of a cross-sectional cohort study among 882 subjects in which four risk factors for cardiovascular disease (CVD) are measured. For each subject the number of CVD risk factors present is calculated which leads to a CVD risk cluster score ranging between 0 and 4. Besides the clustering of CVD risk factors, in the study also physical activity is measured. Physical activity is a continuous independent variable which can theoretically range between 0 and 10 and in this example, the relationship between the CVD risk cluster score and physical activity is analysed. Table 9.5 shows descriptive information of the variables used in this example.

In Table 9.5 it can be seen that the mean of the CVD risk cluster score is slightly higher than the variance. The variance is the standard deviation squared so, the variance is equal to $0.96 \times 0.96 = 0.92$ which is very close to the mean (0.97). From the number of subjects with a different number of risk factors it can also be seen that the distribution is skewed to the right. So the count outcome variable has more or less a Poisson distribution and, therefore, Poisson regression analysis is used to analyse

Table 9.5 Descriptive information of the variables used in Example 9.2

	Mean	Standard deviation		Number of subjects
Physical activity	2.82	0.95		
CVD risk cluster score	0.97	0.96	0 Risk factor	337
			1 Risk factor	309
			2 Risk factors	172
			3 Risk factors	55
			4 Risk factors	9

Output 9.6 Result of the Poisson regression analysis to analyse the relationship between the CVD risk cluster score and physical activity

							95% confidence interval	
	Coefficient	se	Wald	df	p-value	Rate ratio	Lower	Upper
Activity	−0.20	0.04	23.95	1	<0.001	0.82	0.76	0.89
Constant	0.51	0.11	20.34	1	<0.001			

se standard error, *df* degrees of freedom

Output 9.7 Result of the Poisson regression analysis to analyse the relationship between the CVD risk cluster score and physical activity including physical activity squared

							95% confidence interval	
	Coefficient	se	Wald	df	p-value	Rate ratio	Lower	Upper
Activity	−0.31	0.15	4.20	1	0.04	0.74	0.55	0.99
Activity squared	0.017	0.022	0.57	1	0.45	1.02	0.97	1.06
Constant	0.66	0.24	7.91	1	0.005			

se standard error, *df* degrees of freedom

the relationship between the CVD risk cluster score and physical activity. Output 9.6 shows the result of this Poisson regression analysis.

In Output 9.6 it can be seen that the regression coefficient for physical activity is −0.20. The interpretation of the regression coefficient is, again, exactly the same as the interpretation of the regression coefficient in all other regression analyses. A one unit difference in physical activity is related to a − 0.20 unit difference in the outcome variable, i.e. the natural logarithm of the CVD risk cluster score. As mentioned before, the regression coefficient has to be transformed into a rate ratio by taking the e-power of the regression coefficient. The rate ratio for physical activity (i.e. 0.82) indicates that for a one unit difference in physical activity the CVD risk cluster score is 0.82 times higher. So, the more physically active, the lower the CVD risk cluster score.

Like all other regression methods, Poisson regression analysis can also be used to compare two groups with each other and to compare more than two groups with each other. Furthermore, evaluation of effect modification, adjustment for confounding, and evaluation of the linearity of the relationship with continuous independent variables are exactly the same as has been discussed for the other regression methods. To illustrate one of the additional analyses, the linearity of the relationship between the CVD risk cluster score and physical activity is evaluated. First a different mathematical function (i.e. a quadratic relationship) is analysed. Output 9.7 shows the result of the Poisson regression analysis including physical activity and physical activity squared as independent variables.

The most interesting parts of Output 9.7 are the regression coefficient for activity squared and the corresponding p-value. Because this regression coefficient is not statistically significant it can be concluded that analysing a quadratic relationship between the CVD risk cluster score and physical activity is not better than analysing

Table 9.6 Dummy coding for the variable physical activity

	Dummy 1	Dummy 2	Dummy 3
Quartile 1	0	0	0
Quartile 2	1	0	0
Quartile 3	0	1	0
Quartile 4	0	0	1

Output 9.8 Result of the Poisson regression analysis to analyse the relationship between the CVD risk cluster score and physical activity as categorical variable

							95% confidence interval	
	Coefficient	se	Wald	df	p-value	Rate ratio	Lower	Upper
Dummy 1	0.03	0.09	0.08	1	0.78	1.03	0.86	1.23
Dummy 2	−0.23	0.10	5.76	1	0.016	0.79	0.66	0.96
Dummy 3	−0.31	0.10	9.72	1	0.002	0.73	0.61	0.89
Constant	0.09	0.06	1.81	1	0.18			

se standard error, *df* degrees of freedom

a linear relationship (see Sect. 4.4.4.1). A second possibility to evaluate whether the relationship between the CVD risk cluster score and physical activity is linear is to divide the continuous independent variable physical activity into groups. In the next step this categorical variable is represented by dummy variables and the relationship between the CVD risk cluster score and the dummy variables for physical activity is then analysed. In the example, physical activity is divided into four equally sized groups based on quartiles (see Table 9.6). Output 9.8 shows the result of the Poisson regression analysis.

In Output 9.8 it can be seen that there is no linear relationship between the CVD risk cluster score and physical activity. The difference in the outcome variable between subjects in the first and second quartile of physical activity is very small, leading to a regression coefficient of 0.03 and a corresponding rate ratio of 1.03, while the regression coefficients for the third and fourth quartile of physical activity are negative and much higher. These negative regression coefficients lead to rate ratios which were much lower than 1 (i.e. 0.79 and 0.73). The interpretation of these rate ratios is that subjects in the third quartile of physical activity have 0.79 times as much risk factors compared to subjects in the first quartile of physical activity. Subjects in the fourth quartile of physical activity have 0.73 times as much risk factors compared to subjects in the first quartile of physical activity. As has been discussed before, for a proper interpretation of the rate ratios reported in Output 9.8, they must be accompanied by the mean physical activity values of the four quartiles (see Table 9.7).

The third possibility to evaluate whether or not a linear relationship exist between a certain outcome variable and a continuous independent variable is the use of splines (see Sect. 4.4.4.1). As has been discussed before, the general idea of this method is that the independent variable is divided into separate parts in which a different relationship between the outcome variable and the independent variable is estimated. The most simple spline regression analysis that can be applied is a linear

Table 9.7 Physical activity values of the four quartiles used in the Poisson regression analysis

	Mean physical activity	Range in physical activity
Quartile 1	1.83	1.04—2.18
Quartile 2	2.41	2.18—2.65
Quartile 3	2.93	2.65—3.27
Quartile 4	4.09	3.27—8.99

Table 9.8 Part of the dataset that is used in the linear spline Poisson regression analysis to analyse the relationship between the CVD risk cluster score and physical activity

Id	Cluster score	Active	Active1	Active2
1	1	3.52	2.65	0.87
2	1	3.95	2.65	1.30
3	1	2.85	2.65	0.20
.				
5	0	2.19	2.19	0
6	0	1.85	1.85	0
.				
882	1	1.94	1.94	0

Output 9.9 Result of the linear spline Poisson regression analysis with one knot to analyse the relationship between the CVD risk cluster score and physical activity

							95% confidence interval	
	Coefficient	se	Wald	df	p-value	Rate ratio	Lower	Upper
Active1	−0.29	0.09	9.16	1	0.002	0.75	0.62	0.90
Active2	−0.15	0.06	5.90	1	0.015	0.86	0.76	0.97
Constant	0.70	0.21	10.58	1	0.001			

se standard error, *df* degrees of freedom

spline regression analysis with one knot, i.e. a linear spline regression analysis in which the continuous independent variable is divided into two parts and in which for both parts a different (linear) relationship between the outcome variable and the continuous independent variable is estimated. In the present example, the use of linear spline Poisson regression analysis is illustrated using one knot, for which the median value of physical activity is used. This median value is 2.65, so in the dataset two new physical activity variables are made based on the median value of 2.65. Table 9.8 shows part of the dataset that is used in the analysis and Output 9.9 shows the result of the linear spline Poisson regression analysis with one knot to analyse the relationship between the CVD risk cluster score and physical activity.

In Output 9.9 it can be seen that the regression coefficient for the first activity variable is −0.29. This regression coefficient indicates that a one unit difference in physical activity is related to a − 0.29 unit difference in the outcome variable, i.e. the natural logarithm of the number of CVD risk factors. However, this only holds for physical activity values ≤ the median value of 2.65. The rate ratio for a one unit difference in physical activity for physical activity values ≤2.65 is 0.75. For physical activity values >2.65 the regression coefficient and the rate ratio are slightly different (i.e. -0.15 and 0.86) indicating a slightly less strong effect. Regarding the evaluation of a linear relationship between the CVD risk cluster score and physical activity, based on the result shown in Output 9.9, it is difficult to conclude whether the relationship is linear or not (see Sect. 4.4.4.1).

That the negative relationship between the CVD risk cluster score and physical activity is stronger for physical activity values below the median is maybe a bit unexpected when this result is compared to the result of the Poisson regression analysis reported in Output 9.8, but is shows nicely that the different methods to evaluate whether or not a linear relationship exists can lead to a different result and a different conclusion and it also nicely shows that independent of the method used, the results of these analyses should be interpreted with caution.

9.3.1 Negative Binomial Regression Analysis

In Sect. 9.3 Poisson regression analysis was used to analyse a count outcome variable. One of the assumptions of using Poisson regression analysis is that the outcome variable has a Poisson distribution. A Poisson distribution is characterised by skewness to the right and the fact that the mean is more or less equal to the variance. It should be noted that very often the variance of the count outcome variable is (much) higher than the mean. This phenomenon is known as overdispersion and when there is a lot of overdispersion in the count outcome variable, Poisson regression analysis cannot be used anymore. To deal with overdispersion in a count outcome variable, negative binomial regression analysis is developed. The interpretation of the regression coefficients obtained from a negative binomial regression analysis is exactly the same as the interpretation of the regression coefficients obtained from a Poisson regression analysis. The regression coefficient obtained from a negative binomial regression analysis can also be transformed into a rate ratio by taking the e-power of the regression coefficient. To illustrate the use of a negative binomial regression analysis, Output 9.10 shows the result of the negative binomial regression analysis to analyse the relationship between the CVD risk cluster score and physical activity in which a linear relationship is assumed.

When the result shown in Output 9.10 is compared to the result shown in Output 9.6 in which the same analysis was performed, but with a Poisson regression

Output 9.10 Result of the negative binomial regression analysis to analyse the relationship between the CVD risk cluster score and physical activity

							95% confidence interval	
	Coefficient	se	Wald	df	p-value	Rate ratio	Lower	Upper
Activity	−0.19	0.05	12.90	1	<0.001	0.82	0.74	0.92
Constant	0.50	0.15	10.31	1	0.001			

se standard error, *df* degrees of freedom

analysis, it can be seen that the results are only slightly different. With a negative binomial regression analysis, the regression coefficient is slightly lower (−0.19 versus −0.20) and the standard error is slightly higher (0.05 versus 0.04), which leads to a slightly wider 95% confidence interval. However, the difference between the results of the two methods is very small. This is, of course, not surprising, because the outcome variable (i.e. the CVD risk cluster score) has a more or less Poisson distribution. Only in the situation when there is a lot of overdispersion in the count outcome variable, the results of the two methods will be different from each other. When there is a lot of overdispersion, it is advised to use negative binomial regression analysis instead of Poisson regression analysis.

9.4 The Analysis of an Outcome Variable with a Floor or Ceiling Effect

In medical science, outcome variables often suffer from floor or ceiling effects. For example, when patients receive effective treatment after a certain disease and the outcome variable is physical functioning with is measured by a functional ability instrument, it may result in reaching the limit of the instrument. When many patients reach this limit, it results in a skewed distribution of the outcome variable with an excess of the highest score on the instrument. A phenomenon which is known as a ceiling effect. Of course, it can also be the case that an outcome variable has a skewed distribution with an excess of the lowest score, which is mostly an excess of zeros. A phenomenon, which is known as a floor effect.

Sometimes the true outcome variable has a normal distribution, but values below (or above) a certain threshold are not possible to be measured. These floor or ceiling effects are also known as censoring. It should be noted that this censoring is different from censoring when survival data is analysed (see Sect. 6.2). A nice example of a measurement scale with a ceiling effect due to censoring is the Barthel Index. With the Barthel index, activities of daily living, such as going to the toilet, standing up from a chair or taking a shower are measured. The maximum score of the Barthel index is 20, which indicates that all activities of daily living can be performed sufficiently. The problem with the ceiling effect of the Barthel index is that subjects who have the maximal score of 20 should not be regarded as subjects that truly all have the same score. Some subjects with the maximal score of 20 have better functional ability than other subjects with the maximal score of 20. In other words, there is a certain variance between subjects at the limit of the measurement scale that cannot be measured.

Reviewing the medical literature, it is striking to see how outcome variables with either floor or ceiling effects due to censoring are analysed. Mostly the floor or ceiling effects are ignored and linear regression analysis is used to estimate the relationship with independent variables. Also non-parametric testing is sometimes used for outcome variables with floor or ceiling effects. However, with

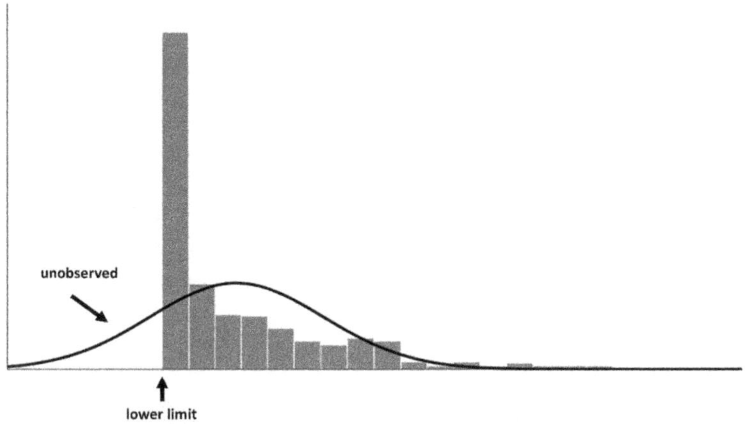

Fig. 9.1 The basic principle of tobit regression analysis with a floor effect

Table 9.9 Descriptive information of the variables used in Example 9.3

	Median	Interquartile range		Number of subjects
Barthel index	12	7—19		
Intervention			Usual care Intervention	96 96
Age			<= 60 years > 60 years	80 112

non-parametric testing it is not possible to obtain effect estimates and 95% confidence intervals, which is, therefore, not preferable. The good news is that a regression method is available to analyse an outcome variable with either a floor or ceiling effect due to censoring. This regression method is known as tobit regression analysis and assumes that there is a certain variation in the upper or lower limit in the scale of measurement of the outcome variable. Tobit regression analysis assumes a partly unobserved normally distributed outcome variable, where observations are censored when they are below or above a certain threshold. This enables the estimation of values outside the range of the observed values, which may better match the true variation in the outcome variable (see Fig. 9.1).

To illustrate the use of tobit regression analysis, Example 9.3 will be used. Example 9.3 consists of data from an intervention study on 192 patients who suffered from stroke. In this study the Barthel index is used to measure functional ability after the intervention and in the study the intervention is compared to usual care. Table 9.9 shows descriptive information of the variables used in the example and Fig. 9.2 shows the distribution of the outcome variable, i.e. the Barthel index.

Figure 9.2 nicely shows the skewed distribution with a ceiling effect of the Barthel index in which 38 patients score the maximal value of 20. Because of this distribution, a tobit regression analysis is performed to analyse the relationship

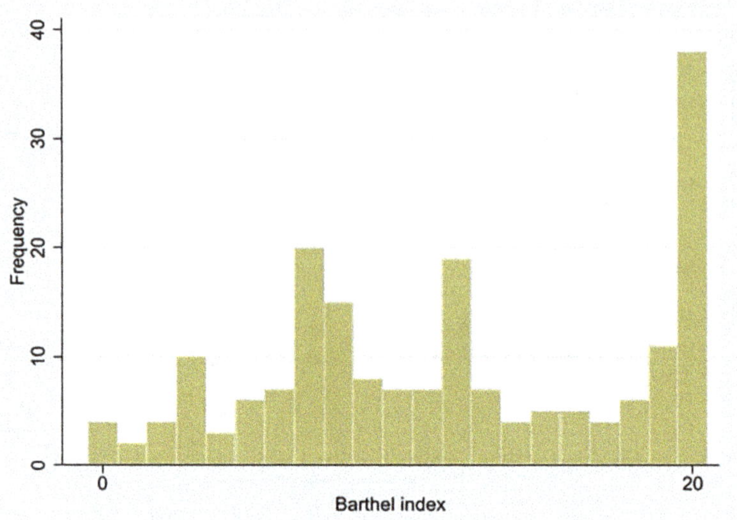

Fig. 9.2 Distribution of the Barthel index

Output 9.11 Result of the tobit regression analysis to analyse the relationship between the Barthel index and the intervention

					95% confidence interval	
	Coefficient	se	t-value	p-value	Lower	Upper
Intervention	1.92	1.07	1.79	0.08	−0.19	4.03
Constant	11.67	0.75	15.54	<0.001	10.19	13.15

se standard error

between the Barthel index and the intervention. Output 9.11 shows the results of this analysis.

Because tobit regression analysis assumes an underlying normal distribution, the interpretation of the regression coefficients is exactly the same as the interpretation of the regression coefficients obtained from a linear regression analysis. So the regression coefficient for the intervention shown in Output 9.11 indicates that the Barthel index for patients in the intervention group is 1.92 points higher than for patients in the usual care group. The 95% confidence interval around this difference ranges between −0.19 and 4.03 and the corresponding p-value is 0.08.

Again, it should be realized that tobit regression analyses is a regression analysis, so evaluation of effect modification, adjustment for confounding, and evaluation of the linearity of the relationship with continuous independent variables are exactly the same as has been discussed for the other regression methods. To illustrate one of the additional analysis, it is evaluated whether age is an effect modifier in the relationship between the Barthel index and the intervention. Output 9.12 shows the result of this analysis.

Output 9.12 Result of the tobit regression analysis to analyse the relationship between the Barthel index and the intervention including age and the interaction between the intervention and age

					95% confidence interval	
	Coefficient	se	t-value	p-value	Lower	Upper
Intervention	3.00	1.77	1.69	0.09	−0.50	6.50
Age	−0.64	1.70	−0.37	0.71	−3.98	2.71
Intervention*age	−3.05	2.28	−1.34	0.18	−7.55	1.44
Constant	12.13	1.47	8.26	<0.001	9.24	15.03

se standard error

Output 9.13 Result of the tobit regression analysis to analyse the relationship between the Barthel index and the intervention including age

					95% confidence interval	
	Coefficient	Se	t-value	p-value	Lower	Upper
Intervention	1.15	1.12	1.03	0.30	−1.05	3.36
Age	−2.33	1.14	−2.05	0.04	−4.57	−0.09
Constant	13.41	1.13	11.87	<0.001	11.18	15.63

se standard error

In Output 9.12 it can be seen that the p-value for the interaction term is not statistically significant ($p = 0.18$), which indicates there is no statistically significant effect modification with age. However, the difference in the effect estimate for the intervention between younger and older patients is quite big. For younger patients (<= 60 years) the effect of the intervention is 3.00, while the effect of the intervention for the older patients (> 60 years) is equal to 3.00–3.05 = −0.05. So, in the older patients, almost no difference between the intervention group and the usual care group in the Barthel index is observed, while in the younger patients, the difference in the Barthel index is 3 points, which is quite a relevant difference on a scale of 0 to 20. In this case it is maybe worthwhile to report the effect estimates for both age groups, even though the difference between the effect estimates is not statistically significant.

When the effect modification is ignored, it can be evaluated whether or not age is a relevant confounder in the relationship between the Barthel index and the intervention. To evaluate whether age is a relevant confounder, age can be added to the analysis which only includes the intervention variable. Output 9.13 shows the result of this analysis.

To evaluate whether age is a relevant confounder in the relationship between the Barthel index and the intervention, the regression coefficient for the intervention has to be compared between the unadjusted analysis (the analysis with only the intervention variable; see Output 9.11) and the adjusted analysis (see Output 9.13). The two regression coefficients are respectively 1.92 and 1.15. So, part of the relationship between the Barthel index and the intervention is due to age differences between the intervention group and the usual care group, i.e. in the intervention group there are

Table 9.10 2 × 2 table with the number of younger and older patients in both groups

	<= 60 year	> 60 year	Total
Intervention	56	40	96
Usual care	24	72	96
Total	80	112	192

more younger patients (<= 60 year), while in the usual care group there are more older patients (> 60 year) (see Table 9.10).

9.5 The Analysis of Correlated Outcome Variables

9.5.1 Repeated Measurements

In all regression methods discussed so far, it is assumed that the observations are independent of each other. However, in some studies this assumption is violated and, therefore, the regular regression methods cannot be used. In these studies, an alternative regression method must be used, in which the possible dependency of the observations is taken into account. For example, in Sect. 6.9, Cox regression analysis for recurrent events was briefly discussed. This method can be seen as a Cox regression analysis which takes into account the fact that multiple observations are performed on the same subject, i.e. that multiple observations are correlated within a subject. One of the designs in which multiple observations are performed in the same subjects is the longitudinal study design. In longitudinal studies, the same subjects are repeatedly measured over time, and when analysing longitudinal data it has to be taken into account that the repeated observations within a subject are not independent of each other.

The most simple example of a longitudinal study is Example 4.1 (see Sect. 4.1). In this example, cholesterol is measured in 100 subjects twice with a time interval of 6 months. The dependency of the two repeated observations was taken into account in the analysis by analysing the change between the two measurements (i.e. using the paired t-test). When more than two repeated observations are performed on the same subject, a paired t-test cannot be used. In that situation a generalized linear model (GLM) for repeated measures can be used. Within GLM for repeated measures two approaches can be applied. The multivariate approach, which can be seen as a multivariate extension of a paired t-test and the univariate approach, which can be seen as an extension of analysis of variance (see Sect. 4.3). GLM for repeated measures is limited because it can only be applied for continuous outcome variables, it can only handle dichotomous and categorical independent variables that do not change over time and the method is based on statistical testing rather than on effect estimation. To deal with these limitations, other methods for longitudinal data analysis are developed. The two mostly used methods are mixed model analysis and Generalised Estimating Equations (GEE analysis). Basically the two methods are regression methods that take into account the dependency of the observations within the subject. The most important difference between the two methods is that they perform the adjustment for the dependency of the repeated observations within the subject in a slightly different way. Within mixed model analysis (which is also known as multilevel analysis) the adjustment for the dependency of the observations is performed by modelling the differences between the subjects, while within GEE analysis the adjustment for the dependency of the observations is performed by directly modelling the correlations within the subject. A detailed discussion of both methods is beyond the scope of this book, but a reference can be made to Twisk (2023). Most important is that both methods are regression methods and that both methods can be applied to all kinds of outcome variables. Because they are both regression methods, the interpretation of the regression coefficients is the same as has been discussed for the regular regression methods assuming independent observations. Furthermore, evaluation of effect modification, adjustment for confounding, and evaluation of the linearity of the relationship with continuous independent variables are exactly the same as has been discussed for the regular regression methods.

9.5.2 Other Correlated Outcome Variables

In Sect. 9.5.1 it was mentioned that mixed model analysis can be used for the analysis of longitudinal data. However mixed model analysis can be used in many more situations where correlated outcome variables occur. The method, which was developed by Goldstein in the early 1980s, was originally intended for analysing research data collected within education (Goldstein, 2003). When analysing the academic performance of students, the performance of students from the same class is more similar than the performance of students from other classes. In other words, there are correlated observations of students within a class, which have to be taken into account when this kind of data is analysed. In medical science, comparable correlated observations are, for example, found in multicentre studies in which patients from different hospitals are included in the study. Because patients from a certain hospital are more alike patients from the same hospital than they are alike patients from other hospitals, the observations of patients within the same hospital are correlated and when analysing data from these patients these correlations should be taken into account. As has been mentioned before, within mixed model analysis this adjustment is performed by modelling the differences between, in this case, the hospitals. The reason why mixed model analysis is also known as multilevel analysis has to do with the fact that within the data, different levels can be distinguished (see Fig. 9.3).

A detailed discussion of the use of mixed model analysis in different situations is beyond the scope of this book, but a reference can be made to Twisk (2017). Again, most important is that mixed model analysis is a regression method, which means that the interpretation of the regression coefficients is the same as has been discussed for the regular regression methods assuming independent observations and that

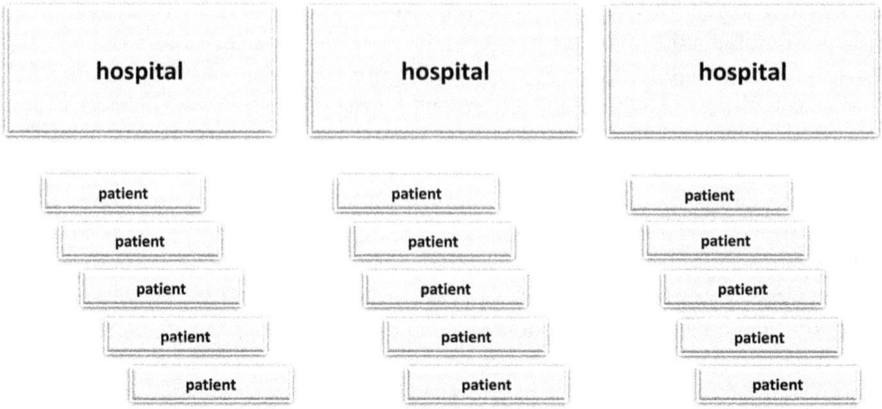

Fig. 9.3 Illustration of a multilevel data structure. Patients are clustered within hospitals

evaluation of effect modification, adjustment for confounding, and evaluation of the linearity of the relationship with continuous independent variables are exactly the same as has been discussed for the regular regression methods.

Chapter 10
Missing Data

Abstract It is important to realise that in most studies not for every subject, all data is available. In other words, in almost every study there will be missing data. Regarding missing data a distinction can be made between missing completely at random (MCAR), missing at random (MAR) and missing not at random (MNAR). In this chapter it is discussed how it can be explored which missing data mechanism occurs and how to deal with missing data. In light of this, multiple imputation is briefly discussed. Finally, the chapter contains an advise in which situation imputation should be used or should not be used.

10.1 Introduction

In most of the examples used in the foregoing chapters, the dataset was complete, i.e. all variables were measured for every subject in the dataset. It should be realised that in most studies not for every subject, all data will be available. In other words, in almost every study there will be some missing data. Because ignoring missing data in statistical analysis can lead to results of the statistical analysis that are not valid, it is important to discuss missing data mechanisms and to discuss the methods that are available to deal with missing data.

10.2 Missing Data Mechanisms

Rubin (1976) was the first to develop a framework of different types of missing data (missing data mechanisms), which is important to determine the next steps in missing data handling. The three missing data mechanisms are missing completely at random (MCAR), missing at random (MAR) and missing not at random (MNAR). MCAR means that missing values are randomly distributed over the data. The reason for missing data is not related to the outcome variable or the relevant independent variables. For example, suppose a study in which subjects with familial hypertension are invited to come to the research centre where blood pressure and several

J. W. R. Twisk, *Basic Principles of Applied Medical Statistics*,
https://doi.org/10.1007/978-3-031-86278-6_10

independent variables are measured in order to investigate which independent variables are related to blood pressure in this particular population. When data on blood pressures are missing, because some subjects randomly forgot to come to the research centre, these missing data are MCAR. Missing at random (MAR) means that the probability of missing is related to other variables. For example when more data on blood pressure are missing from subjects with high body mass index these missing data are MAR. Missing not at random (MNAR) means that the probability of missing is dependent on the values of the variable itself (i.e. dependent on data which is not observed). This is the case when, in the example, subjects with relative high values for blood pressure do not visit the research centre. This latter situation is problematic because it is never known whether this is the case or not. When missing data is MNAR, there is no statistical method available to produce valid results. It should be realised that the missing data mechanism is variable dependent, i.e. in one study, missing data on some of the variables can be MCAR, while for other variables missing data can be MAR or MNAR. Regarding the missing data mechanism, it does not matter whether the particular variable with missing data is the outcome variable or one of the independent variables.

10.3 Exploring Missing Data

It should be realized that by definition, it is not possible to evaluate when missing data are MAR or MNAR. The difference between the two is that when missing data are MNAR, missing data are (also) related to unobserved data. Because the data are unobserved and therefore unknown, it is impossible to evaluate whether the unobserved data are related to the missing data. There are, however, several possibilities to explore whether or not the missing data are MCAR or not MCAR. An independent t-test (see Sect. 4.2) or a logistic regression analysis (see Sect. 5.5) can be used to evaluate whether there is a relationship between missing data and either the outcome variable or the independent variables. For this analysis a missing data variable must be made, which is coded 0 when the particular variable is observed and coded 1 when the particular variable is missing. When this missing data variable is used as group variable in an independent t-test, or as outcome variable in a logistic regression analysis, the relationship with other variables can be analysed. To illustrate this, Example 10.1 is used. The example contains data from a cross-sectional cohort study among 400 subjects in which the relationship between depression and a few independent demographic variables (i.e. sex, age, social class and marital status) is investigated. The continuous outcome variable depression contains 30% missing data, while the independent variables are measured for all 400 subjects (see Table 10.1 for descriptive information of the dataset).

To explore whether missing data on depression are related to any of the demographic independent variables, a logistic regression analysis is performed between the dichotomous outcome variable missing depression (yes or no) and the independent variables sex, age, social class and marital status. Regarding age, a linear

Table 10.1 Descriptive information of the variables used in Example 10.1

	Mean	Standard deviation		Number of subjects
Depression	14.4	11.1		
Age	63.6	11.0		
Sex			Females Males	224 176
Social class			Low High	196 204
Marital status			Single Not-single	192 208

Output 10.1 Result of the logistic regression analysis to analyse the relationship between missing depression and demographic independent variables

							95% confidence interval	
	Coefficient	se	Wald	df	p-value	Odds ratio	Lower	Upper
Sex	−0.31	0.24	1.61	1	0.20	0.73	0.46	1.18
Social class	−0.90	0.24	14.84	1	<0.001	0.41	0.26	0.64
Marital	0.15	0.24	0.40	1	0.53	1.16	0.73	1.84
Age	0.029	0.011	7.44	1	0.006	1.029	1.008	1.051
Constant	−2.22	0.68	10.56	1	0.01			

se standard error, *marital* marital status

relationship with the missing data variable is assumed. Output 10.1 shows the result of this logistic regression analysis.

In Output 10.1 it can be seen that two demographic independent variables are statistically significant associated with missing depression. The odds ratio for social class (i.e. 0.41) indicates that subjects with high social class have a 0.41 times higher odds for being missing for depression compared to subjects with low social class. The other way round, it means that subjects with low social class have a $1/0.41 = 2.44$ times higher odds to be missing for depression compared to subjects with high social class. It can further be seen that subjects with a 1 year higher age have a 1.029 times higher odds to be missing for depression. Based on this analysis it can be concluded that the missing data are not MCAR, because missing data for depression seems to be related to (especially) social class and age. Again, whether missing data are MAR or MNAR cannot be evaluated. It can be concluded that missing data for depression are related to observed data, but it is never known whether missing data on depression are (also) related to non-observed data. It should be noted that in exploring missing data, statistical significance plays an important role, although the concept of statistical significance testing is highly debatable (Twisk, 2024a).

10.4 Methods to Deal with Missing Data

There are different methods available to deal with missing data. A method that is still commonly used is complete-case analysis (CCA), where all subjects with missing data on one (or more) variable(s) are excluded from the analysis. CCA has a lot of drawbacks and should be avoided in general. However, when missing data are MCAR, a complete case analysis lead to valid results. Furthermore, in longitudinal data analyses, when the outcome variable is missing in some of the repeated measures, an analysis on the available data will also provide valid results (Twisk et al., 2013).

One of the mostly used methods to deal with missing data is imputation (replacement of missing data by real values). There are several imputation methods available. Mean imputation indicates that the mean value of the variable with missing data is imputed for all subjects with missing data. Regarding the example, mean depression can be imputed for the cases with missing depression. A slightly more complicated method is the hot-deck method, in which not the mean value of all subjects is imputed, but the mean value of subjects who are comparable to the subject with missing data. For example, for all males with missing depression data, the mean depression for males can be imputed, while the mean depression for females can be imputed for the missing depression data for females. It is also possible to use a multiple regression model including more independent variables to predict depression and impute the predicted values, obtained from the multiple regression model, for the missing depression data. For longitudinal data, last value (last observation) carried forward is available. In this method a missing value at a certain time-point is imputed with the last available value for that particular subject measured one (or more) time-point(s) earlier. Most of these methods impute a sort of mean value which has the disadvantage that imputation leads to an artificial decreased standard deviation in the variables to be analysed and, therefore, result in too small standard errors and too low p-values. This problem can be partly solved by, for example, not imputing the predicted value of a multiple regression analysis, but by taking a random draw from a distribution made around the predicted value. This distribution can, for example, be based on the 95% confidence interval around the predicted value.

The imputation methods discussed so far are so-called single imputation methods. However, the recommended method for imputing missing data, nowadays, is multiple imputation (van Buuren, 2018; Rubin, 1987). Multiple imputation is based on the earlier mentioned multiple regression analysis, taking a random draw from a distribution around the predicted value. The difference, however, is that the imputation is done multiple times.

One of the problems using a random draw from a distribution around the predicted value is that sometimes unrealistic or impossible values are imputed. It is, for example, possible that in the example, negative values for depression are imputed. An alternative way to obtain a value based on the predicted values is

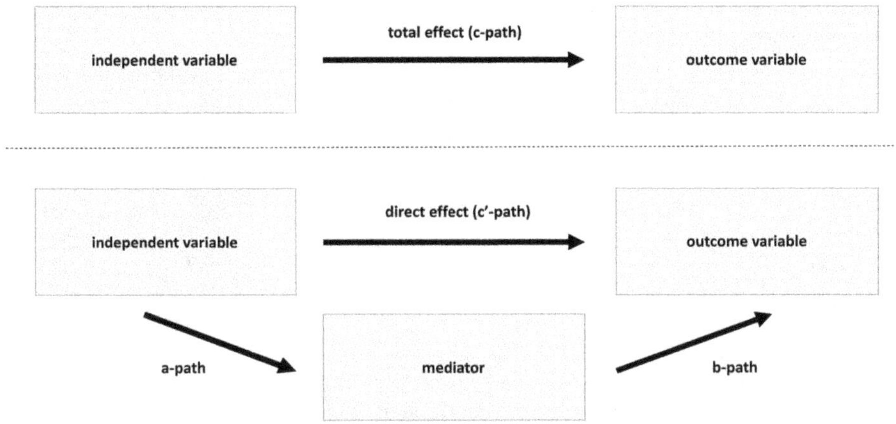

Fig. 10.1 The three phases of multiple imputation

predictive mean matching (PMM) (Moons et al., 2006). PMM uses observed values to impute missing data based on closest matches (nearest-neighbour) and because PMM prevents against imputing unrealistic or impossible values, PMM is the preferred method for (multiple) imputation.

Multiple imputation consists of three phases: imputation, analysis and pooling (see Fig. 10.1). In the imputation phase, each missing value is replaced by several different values, which leads to multiple imputed datasets. As has been mentioned before, the values used for imputation are obtained from a multiple regression analysis. Although several methods are available for generating the imputed values, the Multivariate Imputation by Chained Equations (MICE) method is mostly used and is implemented in most statistical software. The MICE method is mathematically complicated and a detailed explanation is, therefore, beyond the scope of this book (see for details, for example, Buuren, 2018). In the analysis phase, the different datasets are analysed with the appropriate statistical method and in the pooling phase, the results of the statistical analyses are summarized into one final effect estimate according to Rubin's Rule. The general idea of Rubin's Rule is that in the pooling phase, the pooled regression coefficient is the mean of the estimated regression coefficients of the analyses performed on the imputed datasets. The standard error of the pooled regression coefficient consist of two parts; the first part is the mean of the estimated standard errors of the analyses performed on the imputed datasets. The second part is based on the variance of the regression coefficients of the analyses performed on the imputed datasets. So, the standard error of the pooled result is increased with the uncertainty due to the imputation. The increased standard error makes a lot of sense, because the analysis on an imputed dataset includes artificial data, which are more or less uncertain.

Output 10.2 Result of the linear regression analysis to analyse the relationship between depression and demographic independent variables on the complete cases

					95% confidence interval	
	Coefficient	se	t-value	p-value	Lower	Upper
Sex	−3.71	1.18	−3.15	0.002	−6.02	−1.39
Social class	1.46	1.14	1.28	0.20	−0.79	3.70
Marital	−3.23	1.13	−2.86	0.005	−5.46	−1.01
Age	0.58	0.06	10.29	<0.001	0.47	0.69
Constant	−19.53	3.44	−5.68	<0.001	−26.30	−12.75

se standard error, *marital* marital status

Output 10.3 Pooled result of the linear regression analysis to analyse the relationship between depression and demographic independent variables on the multiple imputed data

					95% confidence interval	
	Coefficient	se	t-value	p-value	Lower	Upper
Sex	−3.60	1.25	−2.89	0.004	−6.05	−1.14
Social class	1.19	1.24	0.96	0.34	−1.25	3.64
Marital	−3.25	1.32	−2.47	0.02	−5.85	−0.65
Age	0.58	0.08	7.35	<0.001	0.42	0.73
Constant	−18.95	4.43	−4.28	<0.001	−27.76	−10.14

se standard error, *marital* marital status

When performing multiple imputation, it is important to realize how many imputed datasets must be created. In the earlier days, it was assumed that five imputed datasets are enough to obtain valid results. However, when multiple imputation became available in most statistical software, the advised number of imputations has increased to the percentage of missing data observed. So, in the example with 30% missing depression data it is advised to perform at least 30 imputations. Therefore, in the example, 30 imputations are performed with an imputation model including all variables in the dataset. The final analysis is a multiple linear regression analysis to analyse the relationship between depression and the demographic independent variables, sex, age, social class and marital status. To illustrate the influence of using multiple imputation, Output 10.2 shows the result of the linear regression analysis on the complete cases without imputation, while Output 10.3 shows the pooled result of the multiple imputed linear regression analysis.

Comparing the result of the analysis on the complete cases with the pooled result of the analyses performed on the multiple imputed data, it is clear that the regression coefficients for the four independent variables are only slightly different. Furthermore, it can be seen that the pooled standard errors obtained from the analyses performed on the multiple imputed data are slightly higher than the ones obtained from the analysis on the complete cases.

It should be realised that the pooled result of the analysis on multiple imputed datasets is not a stable result. When the multiple imputation is performed for the second time, the pooled regression coefficients will be different from the ones obtained from the first analyses on the multiple imputed datasets. And when the multiple imputation is performed for the third time, the result will be different again.

10.5 To Impute or Not to Impute

Table 10.2 shows an overview of handling missing data, i.e. it shows when imputation is necessary and which imputation method should be used. First of all, it should be realized that when missing data are MCAR, complete case analysis is a valid way to analyse the data. It is sometimes argued that also in MCAR situations, imputation should be used to increase the power of the analysis. That is a bad argument and should not be used to perform missing data imputation. As in all statistical methods, there are some guidelines about the percentage of missing data above which imputation is necessary. Mostly a missing data percentage of 5% is mentioned as a cut-off value. When the missing data percentage is lower than 5%, imputation does not seem to be necessary and a complete case analysis can be performed. It is, furthermore, suggested that multiple imputation can be used (or has to be used) even in datasets with, for example, more than 50% missing data. However, when 50% or more of a particular variable is missing, it is highly questionable whether the available data of that particular variable is valid and/or reliable. In situations like that, it is probably better to leave that particular variable out of the analysis. That does not have to be a big problem, because in all studies some important variables are not measured at all.

Of course, there is much more to discuss about missing data, but that is beyond the scope of this book. For a detailed discussion about missing data, one is referred to other literature (for example van Buuren, 2018).

Table 10.2 An overview of handling missing data

Missing data mechanism	Analysis	Imputation
MCAR	Complete case analysis	No imputation necessary
MAR	No complete case analysis	Single imputation methods not valid Multiple imputation needed
MNAR	No complete case analysis	All imputation methods not valid

Chapter 11
Pitfalls in (Multiple) Regression Analysis

Abstract In this chapter, two important pitfalls in (multiple) regression analysis are discussed. Collinearity occurs when two independent variables are highly correlated with each other. This can lead to huge standard errors and sometimes to a so-called sign switch. Mediation analysis is an important tool to investigate causal mechanisms. Within mediation analysis, a distinction is made between the total effect, the direct effect and the indirect effect. The problem with mediation analysis is that it is basically the same as the analysis of confounding. The only difference is the interpretation of the results of the analysis. It is also shown, that there is a pitfall within the pitfall of mediation analysis, i.e. the estimation of the standard error of the indirect effect.

11.1 Collinearity

Collinearity means that two independent variables are so strongly related to each other that, when they are both analysed in a multiple regression analysis, the results can no longer be interpreted properly. The pitfall of collinearity will be illustrated using Example 11.1, a cross-sectional cohort study among 167 subjects. The aim of the study is to investigate the relationship between high density lipoprotein (hdl) cholesterol and body fat measured at different locations of the body, i.e. trunk fat mass, peripheral fat mass and total fat mass. Table 11.1 shows descriptive information of the variables used in the example and Table 11.2 shows the Pearson correlation coefficients (see Sect. 4.4.5) between the three body fat indicators.

In Table 11.2 it can be seen that there is strong collinearity between total fat mass and trunk fat mass and between total fat mass and peripheral fat mass and that there is marginal collinearity between trunk fat mass and peripheral fat mass. To illustrate the influence of this collinearity on the result of a multiple regression analysis, several regression analyses are performed. Because hdl-cholesterol is a continuous outcome variable, the relationships between hdl-cholesterol and the three body fat indicators are analysed with linear regression analyses. Output 11.1 shows the result of the three separate linear regression analyses. In all analyses, a linear relationship is assumed between hdl-cholesterol and the three body fat indicators.

J. W. R. Twisk, *Basic Principles of Applied Medical Statistics*,
https://doi.org/10.1007/978-3-031-86278-6_11

Table 11.1 Descriptive information of the variables used in Example 11.1

	Mean	Standard deviation
Hdl-cholesterol (mmol/l)	1.22	0.29
Trunk fat mass (10 kg)	0.83	0.45
Peripheral fat mass (10 kg)	0.77	0.25
Total fat mass (10 kg)	1.82	0.71

Table 11.2 Pearson correlation coefficients between three body fat indicators

	Trunk fat mass	Peripheral fat mass	Total fat mass
Trunk fat mass	1.00		
Peripheral fat mass	0.77	1.00	
Total fat mass	0.97	0.90	1.00

Output 11.1 Result of separate linear regression analyses to analyse the relationship between hdl-cholesterol and three body fat indicators

					95% confidence interval	
	Coefficient	se	t-value	p-value	Lower	Upper
Trunk fat	−0.25	0.05	−5.42	<0.001	−0.34	−0.16
Constant	1.43	0.04	33.08	<0.001	1.34	1.51
					95% confidence interval	
	Coefficient	se	t-value	p-value	Lower	Upper
Peripheral fat	−0.24	0.09	−2.74	<0.001	−0.41	−0.07
Constant	1.41	0.07	19.71	<0.001	1.27	1.55
					95% confidence interval	
	Coefficient	se	t-value	p-value	Lower	Upper
Total fat	−0.14	0.03	−4.63	<0.001	−0.20	−0.08
Constant	1.47	0.06	25.37	<0.001	1.36	1.59

In Output 11.1 it can be seen that all three body fat indicators have a negative relationship with hdl-cholesterol. Furthermore, it can be seen that all three negative relationships are statistically significant. Next, multiple linear regression analyses are performed in which the relationship between hdl-cholesterol and two body fat indicators is analysed in one multiple linear regression analysis. Output 11.2 shows the result of the three analyses.

Output 11.2 shows an interesting phenomenon, which is related to collinearity. It can be seen that the relationship between hdl-cholesterol and trunk fat remains negative and becomes a bit stronger, while the relationship between hdl-cholesterol and the other two body fat indicators in the analysis together with trunk fat becomes positive. This phenomenon is known as the sign switch due to collinearity. Surprisingly the sign switch not only occurs when trunk fat and total fat are analysed together, but also when trunk fat and peripheral fat are analysed together. Surprisingly, because the Pearson correlation coefficient between trunk fat and peripheral fat is only 0.77. The same sign switch occurs when peripheral fat and total fat are analysed together. In this analysis the regression coefficient for

Output 11.2 Result of three multiple linear regression analyses to analyse the relationship between hdl-cholesterol and three body fat indicators

					95% confidence interval	
	Coefficient	se	t-value	p-value	Lower	Upper
Trunk fat	−0.36	0.07	−5.02	<0.001	−0.50	−0.22
Peripheral fat	0.25	0.13	1.99	0.048	0.002	0.51
Constant	1.32	0.07	19.12	<0.001	1.18	1.46

					95% confidence interval	
	Coefficient	se	t-value	p-value	Lower	Upper
Trunk fat	−0.61	0.18	−3.39	0.001	−0.97	−0.25
Total fat	0.24	0.11	2.08	0.04	0.01	0.46
Constant	1.29	0.08	16.80	<0.001	1.14	1.45

					95% confidence interval	
	Coefficient	se	t-value	p-value	Lower	Upper
Peripheral fat	0.61	0.19	3.18	0.002	0.23	0.99
Total fat	−0.33	0.07	−4.91	<0.001	−0.46	−0.20
Constant	1.35	0.07	19.94	<0.001	1.22	1.49

peripheral fat becomes positive, while the regression coefficient for total fat remains negative and becomes stronger. It can, furthermore, be seen that the standard errors in the multiple linear regression analyses are much higher than the standard errors in the univariable linear regression analyses. In general, when a sign switch occurs in a multiple regression analysis, the regression coefficient for the independent variable with the strongest univariable relationship keeps the same sign and becomes stronger. The regression coefficient for the other independent variable shows a sign switch. For both independent variables, the standard errors are higher with an amount that depends on the magnitude of the Pearson correlation coefficient between the two independent variables. It should be noted that in all three analyses shown in Output 11.2 the regression coefficients for the independent variables with the sign switch are statistically significant. The fact that these regression coefficients are statistically significant is often used as an argument that the multiple regression analysis is valid and, therefore, also the regression coefficient with the sign switch can be reported and interpreted in the usual way. However, a sign switch is an indicator for a problem in the regression analysis. In other words, a sign switch is an indicator for an ill-conditioned regression analysis, which is due to collinearity and should, therefore, be interpreted with caution or not be interpreted at all.

In many situations, collinearity diagnostics are calculated after performing a multiple linear regression analysis in order to evaluate whether or not collinearity is a problem in the analysis performed. The two mostly used collinearity diagnostics are the variance inflation factor and the tolerance. The variance inflation factor is calculated as: 1/(1−Pearson correlation coefficient squared), while the tolerance is calculated as: 1−Pearson correlation coefficient squared. So, basically the two collinearity diagnostics are based on the observed Pearson correlation coefficient between the two independent variables. Regarding the variance inflation factor, it is

Table 11.3 Collinearity diagnostics for the multiple regression analyses to analyse the relationship between hdl-cholesterol and three body fat indicators

	Variance inflation factor	Tolerance
Trunk fat and peripheral fat	2.5	0.41
Trunk fat and total fat	15.8	0.06
Peripheral fat and total fat	5.4	0.19

Output 11.3 Result of the multiple linear regression analysis to analyse the relationship between hdl-cholesterol and three body fat indicators

					95% confidence interval	
	Coefficient	se	t-value	p-value	Lower	Upper
Trunk fat	−0.83	0.70	−1.19	0.23	−2.21	0.54
Peripheral fat	−0.24	0.74	−0.33	0.74	−1.70	1.21
Total fat	0.45	0.66	0.69	0.49	−0.85	1.76
Constant	1.28	0.09	13.73	<0.001	1.09	1.46

assumed that values below 5 indicate no collinearity, values between 5 and 10 indicate moderate collinearity, while values above 10 indicate high collinearity. A variance inflation factor above 10 corresponds with a Pearson correlation coefficient of about 0.95, so only really high Pearson correlation coefficients are considered to be a problem. Like for any other cut-off value, the cut-off values for collinearity are arbitrary and should, therefore, be interpreted with caution. To illustrate the problem of the use of collinearity diagnostics, Table 11.3 shows the collinearity diagnostics for the three multiple regression analyses shown in Output 11.2.

Table 11.3 shows that based on the collinearity diagnostics, only the multiple linear regression analysis including trunk fat mass and total fat mass is ill-conditioned, while the other multiple linear regression analyses are not or only slightly ill-conditioned. This nicely shows the limitations of only using collinearity diagnostics without evaluating the results of the different regression analyses. Based on the sign switch and increased standard errors of the regression coefficients, all three multiple regression analyses are ill-conditioned, while based on the collinearity diagnostics, only the multiple regression analysis including trunk fat mass and total fat mass is considered to be ill-conditioned. It should also be realized that collinearity diagnostics are based on Pearson correlation coefficients, so these diagnostics are difficult to interpret when dichotomous or categorical independent variables are involved. It is, therefore, recommended not to use the collinearity diagnostics as the only tool to evaluate collinearity.

To expand the discussion on collinearity a bit further an analysis is performed in which hdl-cholesterol is related to all three body fat indicators together. Output 11.3 shows the result of this analysis.

In Output 11.3 it can be seen that the sign switch only occurred for total fat mass, but it can also be seen that the standard errors for the regression coefficients of the three body fat indicators have increased enormously compared to the earlier performed analyses. This huge increase in standard error indicates a highly

Table 11.4 Collinearity diagnostics for the multiple regression analysis to analyse the relationship between hdl-cholesterol and three body fat indicators

	Variance inflation factor	Tolerance
Trunk fat	236.1	0.004
Peripheral fat	80.9	0.012
Total fat	521.4	0.002

ill-conditioned regression analysis. In this case, it is also confirmed by the collinearity diagnostics (see Table 11.4).

Of course, the problem of collinearity is not limited to linear regression analysis. Collinearity can also be a problem in multiple regression analysis with other outcome variables. However, in most statistical software, collinearity diagnostics are only provided when a multiple linear regression analysis is performed. So, when collinearity diagnostics are not provided, it is even more important to evaluate the results of the different analyses to determine whether or not the regression analysis is ill-conditioned due to collinearity.

When collinearity between two independent variables is present, the most obvious solution to avoid collinearity is to make a choice between the two collinear independent variables and to include only one of them in the statistical analysis. Sometimes a combination of the two independent variables is analysed. For example, when diastolic and systolic blood pressure are both considered as independent variables, there is collinearity between the two blood pressure measurements. To avoid collinearity in the regression analysis, mostly the two blood pressure measurements are combined into one independent variable, i.e. the mean arterial pressure.

A sign switch is not always an indication of an ill-conditioned regression analysis. An interpretable sign switch is known as Simpson's paradox. Figure 11.1a,b illustrate Simpson's paradox. In the example the relationship between a continuous outcome variable and a continuous independent variable is analysed. In Figure 11.1a it can be seen that in the unadjusted analysis (which is also known as the crude analysis), a positive relationship between the two variables is observed. It can also be seen that in the population there are two subgroups. In the subgroup coded 0, both the outcome variable and the independent variable are lower than the values in the subgroup coded 1. Figure 11.1b shows that, when an adjustment is made for the group variable, the regression coefficient for the independent variable becomes negative. It can also be seen that this sign switch is not the result of an ill-conditioned regression analysis. The negative relationship between the outcome variable and the independent variable nicely indicates the relationship between the outcome variable and the independent variable observed within the two subgroups.

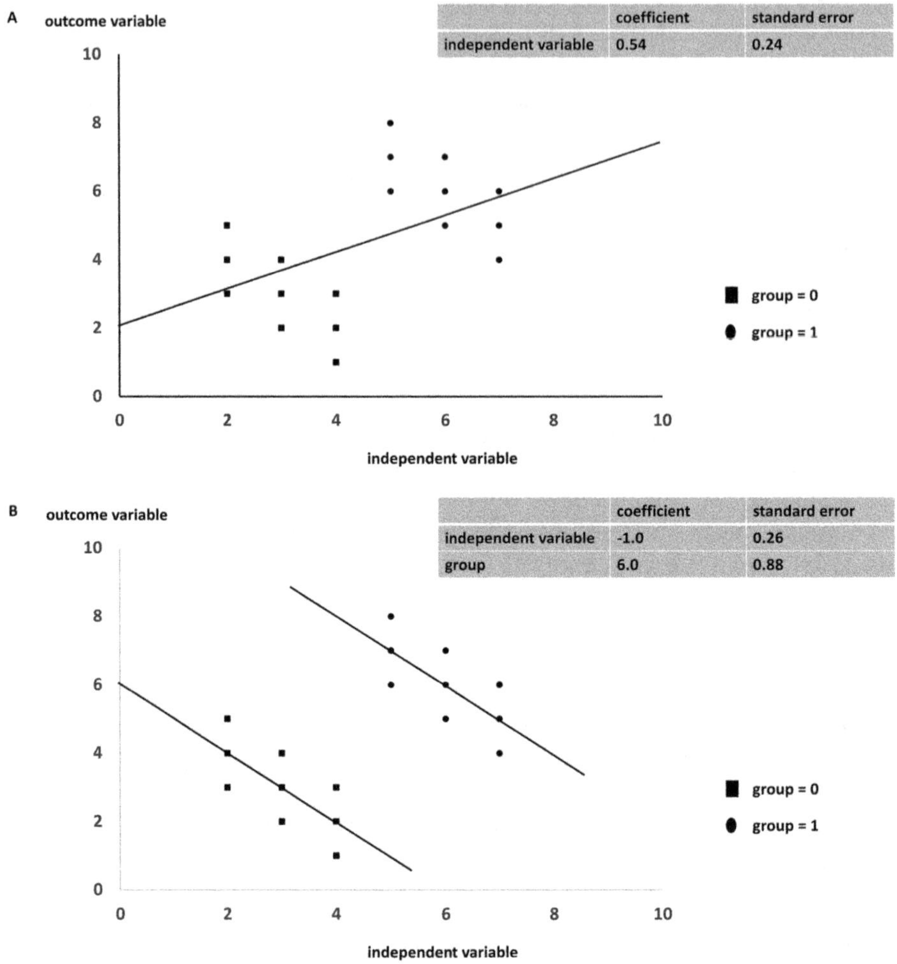

Fig. 11.1 Illustration of Simpson's paradox

11.2 Mediation Analysis

Mediation analysis is increasingly being applied in medical research in order to investigate possible causal pathways. The general idea of mediation analysis is to decompose the relationship between an outcome variable and an independent variable into a direct effect and an indirect effect, through a mediator variable. For example, mediation analysis can be used to investigate body mass index as a mediator in the relationship between systolic blood pressure and physical inactivity or to investigate systolic blood pressure as a mediator in the relationship between having a myocardial infarction and smoking. Throughout the years, various methods for mediation analysis have been described in the literature. From these, the

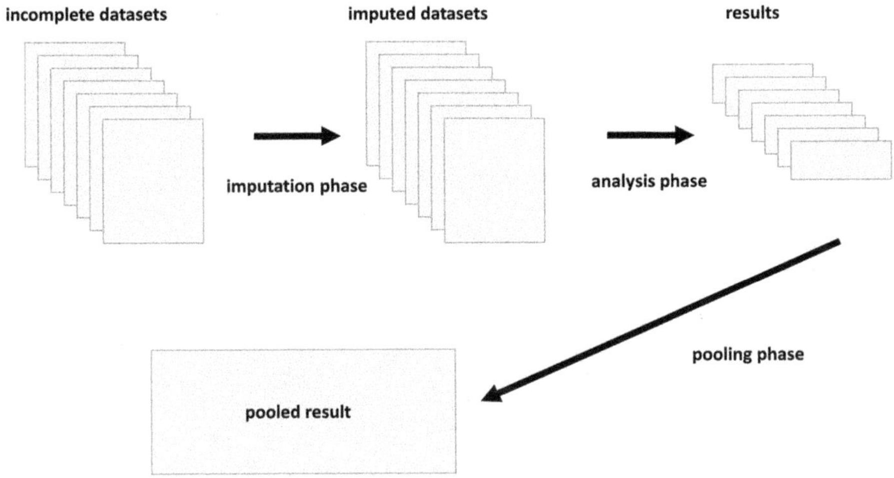

Fig. 11.2 General idea of mediation analysis

Table 11.5 Descriptive information of the variables used in Example 11.2

	Mean	Standard deviation		Number of subjects
Inactivity			No	211
			Yes	209
Systolic blood pressure (mmHg)	130.6	12.6		
Body mass index	25.5	3.1		

product-of-coefficients method and the difference-in-coefficients method are most often used to determine the presence of a mediated effect (McKinnon, 2008). The product-of-coefficients method is based on the estimation of the relationship between the mediator and the independent variable (the a-path) and between the outcome variable and the mediator (the b-path). Multiplying the regression coefficients of the a-path and the b-path provides an estimate of the indirect effect. The difference-in-coefficients method is based on the estimation of the relationship between the outcome variable and the independent variable (the c-path, i.e. the total effect) and the estimation of the same relationship adjusted for the mediator (the c'-path, i.e. the direct effect). The difference between the regression coefficients of the c-path and the c'-path provides an estimate of the indirect effect (see Fig. 11.2).

The statistical methods used for mediation analysis will be illustrated with Example 11.2, i.e. an observational cohort study among 420 subjects to investigate the relationship between systolic blood pressure and physical inactivity. Table 11.5 shows descriptive information of the variables used in the example.

In the example, the aim of the analysis is to analyse the mediating effect of body mass index in the relationship between systolic blood pressure and inactivity.

Output 11.4 Result of the linear regression analysis to analyse the relationship between systolic blood pressure and inactivity

					95% confidence interval	
	Coefficient	se	t-value	p-value	Lower	Upper
Inactivity	2.86	1.23	2.33	0.020	0.45	5.27
Constant	129.12	0.87	149.25	<0.001	127.42	130.82

se standard error

Output 11.5 Result of the linear regression analysis to analyse the relationship between systolic blood pressure and inactivity including body mass index

					95% confidence interval	
	Coefficient	se	t-value	p-value	Lower	Upper
Inactivity	1.28	1.29	1.00	0.32	−1.25	3.81
bmi	0.76	0.21	3.60	<0.001	0.34	1.17
Constant	110.62	5.22	21.21	<0.001	100.37	120.87

se standard error, *bmi* body mass index

The first step in the analysis is to investigate the relationship between systolic blood pressure and inactivity. Because systolic blood pressure is a continuous outcome variable, a linear regression analysis is performed to analyse this relationship. Output 11.4 shows the result of this analysis.

In Output 11.4 it can be seen that there is a positive relationship between systolic blood pressure and inactivity. The regression coefficient for inactivity (2.86) indicates that subjects who are inactive have 2.86 higher systolic blood pressure than subjects who are not inactive. In the next step of the analysis, body mass index is added to the model. Output 11.5 shows the result of this analysis.

In Output 11.5 it can be seen that the regression coefficient for inactivity is much lower than the one reported in Output 11.4. The difference between the two regression coefficients is equal to $2.86 - 1.28 = 1.58$. In mediation terminology this means that the total effect of inactivity on systolic blood pressure is 2.86, the direct effect of inactivity on systolic blood pressure is 1.28 and the indirect effect of inactivity on systolic blood pressure going through body mass index is 1.58. In Sect. 4.5 more or less the same analysis was performed (comparing an unadjusted analysis with an adjusted analysis), but in Sect. 4.5 the difference between the two regression coefficients for the independent variable of interest was interpreted as confounding. In mediation analysis the same difference between the two regression coefficients is interpreted as mediation. Basically a mediator is in the causal pathway between the outcome variable and the independent variable, while a confounder is not in the causal pathway. Sometimes that distinction is easy to make. Sex for example is never in the causal pathway and should therefore always be interpreted as confounder. For other variables, it is not that easy. In the present example, body mass index is considered to be in the causal pathway between systolic blood pressure and inactivity, but in a cross-sectional study that is not as straightforward as it seems. Anyway, interpreting the two analyses in light of a mediation analysis, it can be concluded that

Output 11.6 Result of the linear regression analysis to analyse the relationship between body mass index and inactivity

					95% confidence interval	
	Coefficient	se	t-value	p-value	Lower	Upper
Inactivity	2.09	0.28	7.42	<0.001	1.53	2.64
Constant	24.43	0.20	123.31	<0.001	24.04	24.82

se standard error

more than 50% of the relationship between systolic blood pressure and inactivity is mediated by body mass index.

The same mediation effect can be obtained by performing the product-of-coefficients method. To perform that method, first the a-path has to be estimated. The a-path is the relationship between the mediator and the independent variable, i.e. the relationship between body mass index and inactivity. Output 11.6 shows the result of this analysis.

The regression coefficient for inactivity in Output 11.6 (i.e. 2.09) is the a-path of the product-of-coefficients method. This coefficient has to be multiplied with the b-path, which is the regression coefficient for the mediator variable obtained from a linear regression analysis to analyse the relationship between systolic blood pressure and body mass index, adjusted for inactivity. This coefficient can be found in Output 11.5 and is 0.76. The multiplication of the two regression coefficients ($2.09 \times 0.76 = 1.59$) can be interpreted as the indirect effect of inactivity on systolic blood pressure mediated by body mass index. Due to rounding, the two indirect effect estimates obtained from the difference-in-coefficients method and the product-of-coefficients method are slightly different, but basically they are exactly the same. So, it does not matter which is of the two methods is used for the estimation of mediation effects. The reason why most researchers prefer the product-of-coefficients method is that based on the a-path and the b-path the standard error of the indirect effect can be calculated. With the standard error, a 95% confidence interval around the indirect effect can be calculated and a p-value can be obtained. Equation 11.1 shows how to calculate the standard error of the indirect effect based on the a-path and the b-path. This equation is known as the Sobel equation.

$$se_{ab} = \sqrt{a^2 \times se_b^2 + b^2 \times se_a^2} \tag{11.1}$$

where se_{ab} = standard error of the indirect effect, a = regression coefficient of the a-path, b = regression coefficient of the b-path, se_a = standard error of the regression coefficient of the a-path and se_b = standard error of the regression coefficient of the b-path.

Entering the results shown in Outputs 11.5 and 11.6 into Eq. 11.1, the standard error of the indirect effect is 0.49.

Table 11.6 Descriptive information of the variables used in Example 11.3

	Mean	Standard deviation		Number of subjects
Myocardial infarction			No Yes	210 210
Smoking			No Yes	328 92
Systolic blood pressure (mmHg)	130.6	12.6		

$$se_{ab} = \sqrt{2.09^2 \times 0.21^2 + 0.76^2 \times 0.28^2} = 0.49$$

With this standard error the 95% confidence interval around the indirect effect can be calculated. The 95% confidence interval ranges between 0.63 (1.59 − 1.96 × 0.49) and 2.55 (1.59 + 1.96 × 0.49). The corresponding p-value is <0.001, which is based on a z-value of 3.24 (1.59/0.49 = 3.24) (see Table 3.8).

Although one of the advantages of using the product-of-coefficients method is that a standard error of the indirect effect can be calculated it should be realised that the calculation of the standard error of the indirect effect is highly debatable (Twisk, 2024b). It is even advised not to use this standard error and therefore, also not to test the indirect effect for statistical significance. Instead of testing the indirect effect for statistical significance it is advised to evaluate the magnitude of the indirect effect only by its clinical relevance.

So, when both the mediator and the outcome variable are continuous. i.e. when linear regression analyses are used for the estimations, the results obtained from the difference in coefficients method and the product-of-coefficients method are exactly the same. However, when the outcome variable, for example, is dichotomous and the mediator is continuous, the product-of-coefficients method cannot be used. This is due to the fact that for the a-path a linear regression analysis has to be used, while for the b-path a logistic regression analysis has to be used. The difference in coefficients method, however, can always be used.

To illustrate a mediation analysis using logistic regression analysis (i.e. when the outcome variable is dichotomous) Example 11.3 will be used, i.e. a case-control study among 420 subjects to investigate the relationship between having a myocardial infarction and smoking. Table 11.6 shows descriptive information of the variables used in the example.

The aim of the analysis is to investigate the mediating effect of systolic blood pressure in the relationship between having a myocardial infarction and smoking. In the mediation analysis first the relationship between having a myocardial infarction and smoking is analysed. Output 11.7 shows the result of the logistic regression analysis to analyse this relationship.

In Output 11.7 the regression coefficient for smoking (i.e. 0.80) indicates the difference in the natural logarithm of the odds for having a myocardial infarction between smokers and non-smokers. This regression coefficient can be transformed into an odds ratio by taking the e-power of the regression coefficient. The odds ratio for smoking compared to non-smoking to have a myocardial infarction is 2.23. In the

Output 11.7 Result of the logistic regression analysis to analyse the relationship between having a myocardial infarction and smoking

							95% confidence interval	
	Coefficient	se	Wald	df	p-value	Odds ratio	Lower	Upper
Smoking	0.80	0.25	10.63	1	0.001	2.23	1.38	3.60
Constant	−0.17	0.11	2.38	1	0.12			

se standard error

Output 11.8 Result of the logistic regression analysis to analyse the relationship between having a myocardial infarction and smoking including systolic blood pressure

							95% confidence interval	
	Coefficient	se	Wald	df	p-value	Odds ratio	Lower	Upper
Smoking	0.69	0.25	7.60	1	0.006	1.99	1.22	3.25
Systolic	0.026	0.008	10.08	1	0.002	1.03	1.01	1.04
Constant	−3.58	1.08	10.99	1	<0.001			

se standard error, *systolic* systolic blood pressure

next step the mediation effect of systolic blood pressure is investigated by adding systolic blood pressure to the logistic regression analysis. Output 11.8 shows the result of this analysis.

In Output 11.8 it can be seen that the regression coefficient for smoking is reduced from 0.80 to 0.69, which indicates a mediation effect of 0.11. When this number is represented as a percentage of the total effect of 0.80 it can be seen that about 14% of the effect of smoking on having a myocardial infarction is mediated by systolic blood pressure.

Besides the difference-in-coefficients method and the product-of-coefficients method, which are known as the more traditional methods for mediation analysis, in the last decade, causal mediation analysis has gained popularity. A detailed discussion of causal mediation analysis is beyond the scope of this book, but it should be noted that causal mediation analysis mostly provides the same results as the traditional methods for mediation analysis (Rijnhart et al., 2017, 2021).

It has already been mentioned that the estimation of the standard error of the indirect effect is problematic. This is true for the estimation of the standard error with the Sobel equation, but also for other methods to estimate the uncertainty of the estimated indirect effect. One of the mostly used methods for estimating the uncertainty of the indirect effect is bootstrapping. Bootstrapping is a method that is used for all kinds of purposes and one of them was already discussed in Chap. 7,i.e. for the validation of a prediction model (see Sect. 7.5). With bootstrapping a new dataset is created by randomly drawing the same number of observations as the original dataset, but with replacement. So, the difference between the original dataset and the new dataset is that in the new dataset, certain observations can occur more than once. Then the mediation analysis is performed on the bootstrap sample which leads to an estimation of the indirect effect. The bootstrap procedure is repeated many times (e.g. 1000), which leads to many different estimates of the indirect effect. Based on these estimates, the (empirical) 95% confidence interval can be calculated. The bootstrap method to obtain a 95% confidence interval is very popular, especially when the distributions of the variables are skewed. Because it is assumed that the distribution of the indirect effect is somewhat skewed it is often argued that bootstrapping should be used for the estimation of the uncertainty of the indirect effect instead of the Sobel equation (Rijnhart et al., 2017). However, it does not matter what method is used for the estimation of the uncertainty of the indirect effect, all estimations are problematic, so it is highly advised not to use the standard error of the indirect effect and also to refrain from statistical testing for the indirect effect. Instead, the importance of mediation should be evaluated based on its clinical relevance (Twisk, 2024b).

Chapter 12
Miscellaneous

Abstract In the last content-related chapter of the book, two miscellaneous topics are discussed. Regarding the first one, i.e. sample size calculation, the chapter not only contains some equations that can be used for sample size calculation, it also contains a critical discussion of the use of sample size calculations. The second miscellaneous topic is the estimation of the reliability of measurements. In light of this, methods such as a Bland-Altman plot and the kappa statistic are discussed.

12.1 Sample Size Calculation

12.1.1 Introduction

Before performing a study, it is necessary to determine how many subjects have to be included in the study. This is mostly done by performing a sample size calculation. In fact, a sample size calculation is found to be so important that in all grant application forms a section is included in which the sample size calculation must be given. Medical ethics committees only allow a study to be performed when a sample-size calculation can be provided. In addition, in the so-called CONSORT statement, a statement that specifies how a scientific paper that reports the results of an intervention study must be written in order to be published in a scientific journal, it is stated that a sample size calculation must be included in the paper. Because all major medical journals (New England Journal of Medicine, JAMA, Lancet, British Medical Journal, etc.) endorse this CONSORT statement, it is more or less mandatory to include a sample size calculation in the scientific paper reporting the results of an intervention study.

Sample-size calculations are initially set up to determine the number of subjects that has to be included in an intervention study. The idea of a sample size calculation is to calculate how many subjects should be included in both the intervention group and the control group in order for a predetermined effect (i.e. the difference between the two groups) to be statistically significant. For a sample size calculation, many statistical software is available. However, a sample size calculation is basically very simple and can be easily calculated by hand.

J. W. R. Twisk, *Basic Principles of Applied Medical Statistics*,
https://doi.org/10.1007/978-3-031-86278-6_12

12.1.2 A Continuous Outcome Variable

Equation 12.1 shows how to calculate the number of subjects needed in an intervention study with a continuous outcome variable.

$$n_1 = n_2 = \frac{\left(Z_{(1-\alpha/2)} + Z_{(1-\beta)}\right)^2 \times sd^2 \times 2}{v^2} \tag{12.1}$$

where n_1, n_2= number of subjects in both groups, $Z_{(1-\alpha/2)} = (1-\alpha/2)$ percentile point of the standard normal distribution, $Z_{(1-\beta)} = (1-\beta)$ percentile point of the standard normal distribution, sd = standard deviation of the outcome variable and v = difference in mean value of the outcome variable between the groups.

In the equation to calculate the number of subjects, the significance (α) and the power ($1-\beta$) play an important role. So, a sample size calculation is based on testing theory (see Sect. 3.3.1). Furthermore, the standard deviation of the outcome variable is important. This is not surprising, because the standard deviation of the outcome variable is an important component of the uncertainty of the effect estimate. Finally, of course, the magnitude of the effect, i.e. the magnitude of the difference in outcome variable between the two groups, is important in the calculation of the number of subjects that has to be included. The smaller the difference between the two groups, the more subjects are needed to make that difference statistically significant.

So, assume that an intervention study is performed to estimate the effect of a new drug to lower systolic blood pressure. In the sample size calculation a few relatively arbitrary numbers have to be entered. First of all, the magnitude of the expected difference between the groups has to be determined. In most cases, the clinical relevant difference is used. Next, the standard deviation of the outcome variable has to be chosen. This is rather arbitrary, because it is not known which standard deviation will be observed when the study is performed. Sometimes a small pilot study is performed to find an acceptable value of the standard deviation or existing literature is used. Finally, a choice has to be made for the significance level and the power of the statistical test (see Sect. 3.3.1). In general, the significance level is set at 0.05 and the power is set at either 0.80 or 0.90.

With a power of 0.90 and a significance level of 0.05, the first part of Eq. 12.1 looks as follows (the numbers 1.96 and 1.28 are derived from Table 3.8):

$$\left(Z_{(1-\alpha/2)} + Z_{(1-\beta)}\right)^2 = (1.96 + 1.28)^2 = 10.51$$

With a power of 0.80 instead of 0.90, the number is a bit lower.

$$\left(Z_{(1-\alpha/2)}+Z_{(1-\beta)}\right)^2=(1.96+0.84)^2=7.84$$

Now suppose that a difference of 3 is found to be a clinically relevant difference, and that it is assumed that a standard deviation of 8 will be observed in the upcoming study. Assuming further a significance level of 0.05 and a power of 0.90, it can be calculated that around 150 subjects are needed in both groups.

$$n_1=n_2=\frac{10.51\times 8^2\times 2}{3^2}=149.5$$

So, around 150 subjects must be included in both groups to make a difference of 3 between the intervention group and the control group statistically significant with a power of 0.90, assuming a standard deviation of 8.

With a power of 0.80, of course, less subjects are needed, i.e. around 112 subjects in both groups.

$$n_1=n_2=\frac{7.84\times 8^2\times 2}{3^2}=111.5$$

When the standard deviation is assumed to be a bit lower, e.g. 6, the required sample size becomes even smaller and only around 63 subjects are needed in both groups.

$$n_1=n_2=\frac{7.84\times 6^2\times 2}{3^2}=62.7$$

When then also the magnitude of the clinically relevant difference between the intervention and control group is slightly increased from 3 to 5, only around 23 subjects are needed in both groups.

$$n_1=n_2=\frac{7.84\times 6^2\times 2}{5^2}=22.6$$

The example nicely shows that with a few small realistic changes in the numbers entered into the equation, the required number of subjects can change remarkably. Instead of 150 subjects per group, only 23 subjects per group are needed.

In the above example, it has been assumed that the intervention group and the control group have the same number of subjects. Although this is the most efficient way to divide the study population into two groups, sometimes it is, however, decided to randomize more subjects in the intervention group than in the control group, or the other way round. When the ratio of the number of subjects in the two groups is different than 1: 1, the equation to calculate the number of subjects is slightly different (see Eq. 12.2).

$$n_1 = \frac{\left(Z_{(1-\alpha/2)} + Z_{(1-\beta)}\right)^2 \times sd^2 \times (r+1)}{v^2 \times r} \quad (12.2)$$

where r = ratio of the number of subjects in both groups.

Going back to the example where a standard deviation of 6 was assumed with an expected relevant difference of 3. With a significance level of 0.05 and a power of 0.80, it was calculated that 62.7 subjects are needed in both groups. Suppose now that twice as many subjects will be included in the intervention group as in the control group. Using Eq. 12.2, it can be calculated that 94 subjects are needed in the intervention group and half of them in the control group.

$$n_1 = \frac{(1.96 + 0.84)^2 \times 6^2 \times (1/2 + 1)}{3^2 \times 1/2} = 94$$

$$n_2 = \frac{(1.96 + 0.84)^2 \times 6^2 \times (2 + 1)}{3^2 \times 2} = 47$$

When twice as much subjects are included in the intervention group compared to the control group (or the other way round) a total of 141 (94 + 47) subjects have to be included in the study. It was earlier calculated that with the same number of subjects in both groups, 126 (63 + 63) subjects have to be included. This illustrates that an equal number of subjects in the intervention group and in the control group is the most efficient way to divide the study population into two groups.

12.1.3 A Dichotomous Outcome Variable

When a dichotomous outcome variable is analysed, the equation to calculate the number of subjects is slightly different (see Eqs. 12.3a and 12.3b).

$$n_1 = n_2 = \frac{\left(Z_{(1-\alpha/2)} + Z_{(1-\beta)}\right)^2 \times \overline{p}(1-\overline{p}) \times (r+1)}{(p_1 - p_2)^2 \times r} \quad (12.3a)$$

$$\overline{p} = \frac{p_1 + (r \times p_2)}{1 + r} \quad (12.3b)$$

where n_1, n_2= number of subjects in both groups, $Z_{(1-\alpha/2)}$ = $(1-\alpha/2)$ percentile point of the standard normal distribution, $Z_{(1-\beta)} = (1-\beta)$ percentile point of the standard normal distribution, $\overline{p}$ = mean value of $p_1$and p_2, p_1 = proportion of subjects with the dichotomous outcome in the intervention group, p_2 = proportion of subjects with the dichotomous outcome in the control group and r = ratio of numbers in both groups.

In Eqs. 12.3a and 12.3b, $\overline{p}(1-\overline{p})$ is an indicator of the variance of the average proportion (see also Sect. 5.1.2).

To illustrate the use of Eqs. 12.3a and 12.3b suppose an intervention study is performed in patients with low back pain. In this study a new intervention program is compared to usual care and the outcome variable is recovery. Previous research has shown that a recovery proportion of 0.30 can be expected with usual care. Suppose that a clinical relevant effect of the intervention is defined as a difference in recovery proportion of 0.10. This means that a recovery proportion of 0.40 is expected in the intervention group. Assuming a significance level of 0.05, a power of 0.80 and equal numbers in both groups, it can be calculated that around 357 patients are needed in both groups.

$$n_1 = \frac{(1.96+0.84)^2 \times 0.35(1-0.35) \times (1+1)}{(0.40-0.30)^2 \times 1} = 356.7$$

As has been discussed for a sample size calculation for a continuous outcome variable, of course, a change in the numbers entered into the equation leads to a different number of subjects and by changing the ratio between the number of subjects in the intervention group and the usual care group, also a different number of subjects is calculated.

12.1.4 Remarks

In the foregoing sections it was illustrated that a few small realistic changes in the numbers entered into the sample size calculation can lead to a highly different number of subjects to be included in the study. It should be noted that in practice the sample size calculation is usually adapted to the possibilities. Suppose, for example, that it is not possible for logistic, ethical or financial reasons to include more than 100 subjects in the study. It is quite simple to produce a sample-size calculation that leads to a slightly lower number of subjects than 100. A slightly lower number makes sense, because there are always subjects who drop out during the study. So, when a sample size of 90 subjects is calculated, it can be argued that 100 subjects have to be included in the study to take into account possible drop-outs. One of the main criticisms of using a sample size calculation is that (more or less) arbitrary numbers have to be used for the calculation and that only a small change in the numbers entered into the equation can lead to a large difference in the calculated number of subjects. It should further be realized that nobody knows what the numbers will be in the upcoming study. So, basically, each sample size calculation will be a (wild) guess, even when some of the numbers used are taken from a pilot study or from existing literature.

Another point of criticism is the prominent role that testing theory plays in a sample size calculation. In an era in which less importance is attached to testing theory, this is rather strange. In fact, the prominent role of the testing theory implies that a study with a number of subjects that is too small to find a statistically significant result should not be performed. In practice, however, decisions about, for example, the implementation of new interventions are never based on individual studies. Within evidence-based medicine, conclusions and decisions about implementation of new interventions are only made on the basis of well performed meta-analyses, in which small studies can also play an important role.

It is important that the number of subjects should not be limited based on statistical (i.e. test theory) arguments. In fact, the number of subjects that are included in a study should depend much more on logistic, financial, and ethical considerations. Based on these considerations, one should aim for the largest possible number of subjects in each study. Whether or not a statistically significant result is found, is of secondary (or maybe even of no) importance (Twisk, 2024a, c).

12.2 Reliability of Measurements

The reliability of measurements plays an important role in medical research. There are basically two important aspects of reliability, i.e. reproducibility and validity. Reproducibility concerns, for example, test-retest reliability; when a measuring instrument is used twice on the same subject, then approximately the same value should be measured. Test-retest reliability is more or less the same as intra-observer reliability. When the same researcher uses the same measurement twice on the same subject, then approximately the same value should be measured. Reproducibility can also concern inter-observer reliability; when two researchers use the same measuring instrument on the same subject, then they should measure approximately the same value. Validity, on the other hand, is a different issue. Validity has to do with comparing the result of one measuring instrument with the result of another measuring instrument. Preferably, one of these instruments is the so-called golden standard, but that does not necessarily have to be the case. When a new measuring instrument is compared to a golden standard, the comparison is mostly between a relatively simple measuring instrument against a more complex golden standard. When the relatively simple measuring instrument is valid compared to the complicated (and usually more expensive) golden standard, then the new measuring instrument is a good alternative to use. This chapter will not focus on the theoretical aspects of the reliability of measurements (see for theoretical details for example de Vet et al., 2011), it will focus on the statistical methods that can be used to assess reproducibility and/or validity of measurements.

In Example 12.1, physical activity is measured on 50 subjects with both a questionnaire and an accelerometer. In the study it is important to define whether a subject is active or inactive. Whether a subject is classified as active, is defined according the guideline for healthy physical activity, i.e. at least 30 minutes of moderate physical activity per day. Because the accelerometer is considered to be the golden standard, this study deals with validity. The most simple way to evaluate

Table 12.1 2 × 2 table with the number of subjects active and inactive measured in two ways

	Accelerometer		
Questionnaire	Active	Inactive	Total
Active	15	5	20
Inactive	10	20	30
Total	25	25	50

the validity of the physical activity questionnaire is to make a 2 × 2 table (see Table 12.1).

In Table 12.1 it can be seen that for 35 subjects the two instruments provide the same result and for 15 subjects the result is different.

One of the statistical estimates that can be derived from this 2 × 2 table is the proportion of agreement between the two instruments, which in this case is 0.35/0.50 = 0.70. The problem with this approach is that dividing the 50 subjects randomly over the 2 × 2 table leads to a proportion of agreement of 0.50. The proportion of agreement that can be expected due to chance corresponds to the numbers in the cells that are expected when there is no association between the two instruments (see also Sect. 5.1.3). To take into account the proportion of agreement due to chance, kappa can be used (see Eq. 12.4).

$$\kappa = \frac{\overline{p} - \widehat{p}}{1 - \widehat{p}} \tag{12.4}$$

where κ = kappa, $\overline{p}$ = observed proportion of agreement and $\widehat{p}$ = expected proportion of agreement due to chance.

When the numbers from Table 12.1 are entered into Eq. 12.1, kappa is 0.40.

$$\kappa = \frac{0.70 - 0.50}{1 - 0.50} = 0.40$$

Based on either the proportion of agreement or kappa, it is difficult to indicate whether the validity of the activity questionnaire is acceptable or not acceptable. In the literature it is sometimes indicated that a kappa <0.4 indicates that the agreement (i.e. the validity) is moderate to poor, a kappa between 0.4 and 0.7 indicates a reasonable agreement, and a kappa >0.7 indicates a good agreement. Although this guideline provides some guidance, (as with all guidelines and cut-off values used in statistics) it should be interpreted with caution. When kappa is estimated by statistical software, also the standard error of kappa and the result of a statistical test for kappa is provided. The null-hypothesis of this statistical test is that kappa is 0. The problem with this test is that some researchers use (or better misuse) the result of this statistical test to conclude whether the agreement between two measurements is good or not good. Regarding the degree of agreement, the statistical test, which provides a p-value whether kappa differs statistically significant from 0, is not informative and, therefore, irrelevant. The standard error of kappa, on the other hand, can be used as in indicator of uncertainty of the estimate and in light of this,

Table 12.2 Descriptive information of systolic blood pressure measured by two observers

	Number of subjects	Minimum	Maximum	Mean	Standard deviation
Observer 1	50	116	143	128.30	6.52
Observer 2	50	118	143	130.38	4.94

also a 95% confidence interval can be calculated around kappa (i.e. kappa ±1.96 times the standard error). In practice, however, the 95% confidence interval around kappa is not much reported.

In addition to the fact that the proportion of agreement and kappa can be used for dichotomous outcome variables, both statistical measures are also suitable for categorical (both nominal and ordinal) outcome variables. Furthermore, in the example, the proportion of agreement and kappa are used to evaluate the validity of a new measuring instrument. Of course, both are also suitable for investigating test-retest reliability or intra- or inter-observer reliability. However, when a continuous outcome variable is measured, both the proportion of agreement and kappa cannot be used.

In Example 12.2 inter-observer reliability of the measurement of systolic blood pressure is evaluated. In the study, systolic blood pressure is measured by two observers. Table 12.2 shows descriptive information of the variables used in the example.

In Table 12.2 it can be seen that the mean systolic blood pressure measured by observer 2 is slightly higher than the mean systolic blood pressure measured by observer 1 and it can also be seen that the standard deviation in the systolic blood pressure values for observer 1 is slightly higher than for observer 2. Although the descriptive information already gives an impression of the inter-observer reliability, there are a few statistical methods available to quantify the inter-observer reliability when a continuous outcome variable is measured. Mostly the Pearson correlation coefficient (see Sect. 4.4.5) is used as an indicator for the inter-observer reliability. Besides that, the scatterplot is mostly given (see Fig. 12.1). The Pearson correlation coefficient in this example is 0.91.

Although the Pearson correlation coefficient is quite high, in Fig. 12.1 it can be seen that there is a difference between the two observers which is most pronounced when the systolic blood pressure is relatively low. An alternative, widely used way of representing the agreement between two observers is the Bland-Altman plot (Bland & Altman, 1986). The x-axis of the Bland-Altman plot shows the mean systolic blood pressure measured by the two observers and the y-axis shows the difference in systolic blood pressure between the two observers. Figure 12.2 shows the Bland-Altman plot for the inter-observer reliability of the systolic blood pressure measurement. Regarding the difference, the systolic blood pressure measured by observer 1 is subtracted from the systolic blood pressure measured by observer 2.

The advantage of the Bland-Altman plot is that it can directly be seen (better than with the scatter plot) how the pattern of the differences between the two observers is related to the mean systolic blood pressure. In the Bland-Altman plot it can be seen that the difference between the two observers is especially found when the systolic

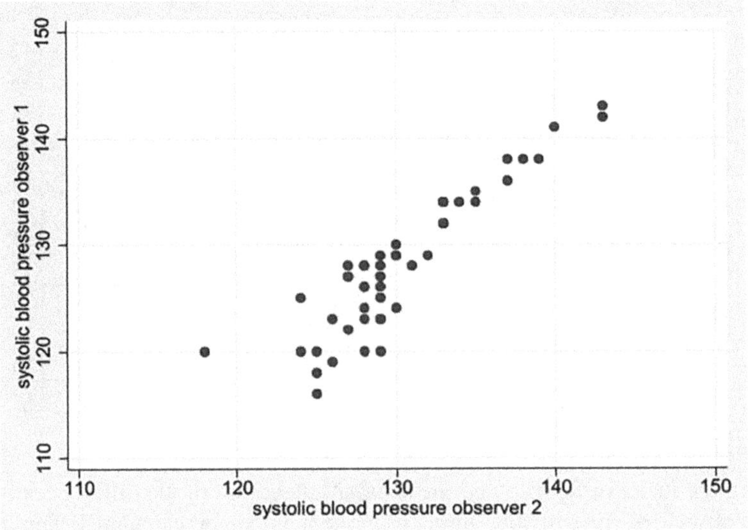

Fig. 12.1 Scatterplot to compare systolic blood pressure measurements between two observers

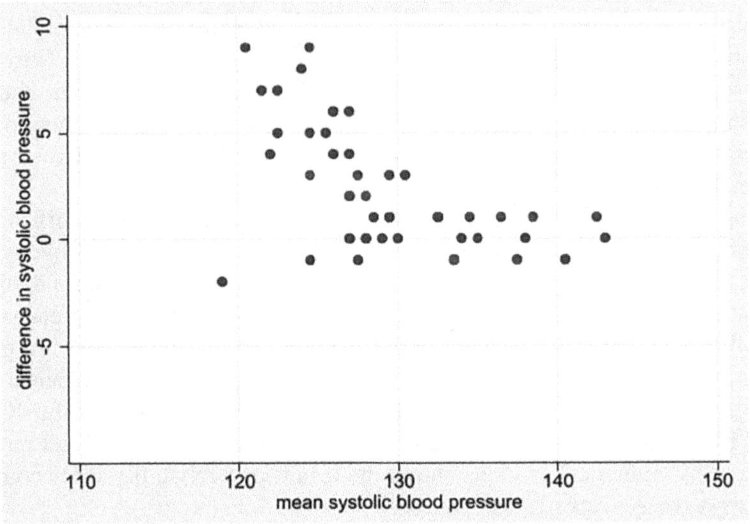

Fig. 12.2 Bland-Altman plot to compare systolic blood pressure measurements between two observers

blood pressure is relatively low. Furthermore, it can be seen that when there is a difference between the two observers, observer 2 mostly measures a higher systolic blood pressure than observer 1, especially at these relatively low systolic blood pressures.

Table 12.3 Numerical example to compare two observers

Id	Observer 1	Observer 2
1	10	12
2	11	13
3	11	13
4	12	14
5	12	14
6	12	14
7	13	15
8	13	15
9	13	15
10	14	16
11	14	16
12	15	17

Using the mean difference and the standard deviation of the differences between the two observers, the so-called limits of agreement can be calculated. The limits of agreement are defined as the mean difference ± 1.96 times the standard deviation of the differences between the two observers. The mean difference between the two observers in this example is 2.08 and the limits of agreement are −3.56 and 7.72. The idea behind the limits of agreement is that (based on the properties of the normal distribution; see Sect. 2.4) it can be stated that 95% of the differences between the two observers are between −3.56 and 7.72. The limits of agreement should be interpreted with caution because they are based on a normal distribution of the differences. In the present example, for example, the differences between the two observers are not really normally distributed.

Earlier in this section it was indicated that the Pearson correlation coefficient is an indicator for the agreement between two observers. One of the problems of the Pearson correlation coefficient is that when, for example, the second observer systematically measures 5 units higher than the first observer, the correlation coefficient will be 1, which suggests a non-existing perfect agreement. A possible solution for this problem is the use of the intraclass correlation coefficient (ICC). Although there are many different methods available to calculate the ICC, the general idea of the ICC is fairly simple and will be illustrated by a small numerical example. This numerical example shows the results of a reliability study comparing two observers (see Table 12.3).

Table 12.3 shows that there is a systematic difference of 2 points between the two observers; the second observer measures 2 points higher than the first observer for each subject in the dataset. When these data are displayed in a scatterplot then all points are on a straight line and the Pearson correlation coefficient is 1.

Because the ICC does take the systematic difference into account, the ICC in this example will be lower than 1. The idea behind the calculation of the ICC is that the data can be divided into different variances, i.e. different sum of squares. A sum of squares is the squared difference between the observations and the mean value (see

Table 12.4 Simple numerical example to compare two observers including mean values

Id	Observer 1	Observer 2	Mean
1	10	12	11
2	11	13	12
3	11	13	12
4	12	14	13
5	12	14	13
6	12	14	13
7	13	15	14
8	13	15	14
9	13	15	14
10	14	16	15
11	14	16	15
12	15	17	16
Mean	12.5	14.5	

also Sect. 4.3). When two observers are compared to each other, two variances (i.e. two sum of squares) can be calculated, i.e. the between subject sum of squares and the within subject sum of squares (see Eqs. 12.5a and 12.5b).

$$SS_b = \sum_{i=1}^{n} \sum_{j=1}^{J} \left(y_{ij} - \overline{y}_j\right)^2 \tag{12.5a}$$

$$SS_w = \sum_{i=1}^{n} \sum_{j=1}^{J} \left(y_{ij} - \overline{y}_i\right)^2 \tag{12.5b}$$

where SS_b = between subject sum of squares, SS_w = within subject sum of squares, J = number of observers, n = number of subjects, y_{ij} = observation of subject i for observer j, $\overline{y}_i$ = mean value of subject i and $\overline{y}_j$ = mean value of observer j.

In order to calculate the between subject sum of squares and the within subject sum of squares, Table 12.3 is extended with some additional information (see Table 12.4).

Entering the numbers shown in Table 12.4 into Eq. 12.5a and 12.5b, the between subject sum of squares (SS_b) is equal to: $(10-12.5)^2 + (11-12.5)^2 + \dots + (17-14.5)^2 = 46$ and the within subject sum of squares (SS_w) is equal to: $(10-11)^2 + (12-11)^2 + (11-12)^2 + \dots + (17-16)^2 = 24$.

Using Eq. 12.6 the ICC can be calculated.

$$ICC = \frac{SS_b}{SS_b + SS_w} \tag{12.6}$$

When the between and within subject sum of squares derived from Table 12.4 are entered into Eq. 12.6, the ICC is 0.66.

Table 12.5 Between and within subject sum of squares and the ICC for the measurement of systolic blood pressure between two observers

Between subject sum of squares	3074.4
Within subject sum of squares	312.0
ICC	0.91

$$ICC = \frac{46}{46 + 24} = 0.66$$

So, in the simple example where a relatively large systematic difference occurs between two observers, the Pearson correlation coefficient is 1, while the ICC is 0.66.

In Example 12.2 it is of course also possible to calculate the ICC. It has already been mentioned that the Pearson correlation coefficient between the two observers in this example is 0.91. Table 12.5 shows the between subject sum of squares, the within subject sum of squares and the ICC for the measurement of systolic blood pressure between two observers. In Table 12.5 it can be seen that in Example 12.2 the ICC is exactly the same as the Pearson correlation coefficient.

It has already been mentioned that the ICC can be calculated in many different ways and it is known from the literature that different calculation methods can lead to different ICC's (Müller & Büttner, 1994). A discussion of all possible methods to calculate an ICC is beyond the scope of this book, but when they are used in the present example, comparing systolic blood pressure between two observers, the ICC's calculated with different methods range between 0.83 and 0.92. Although the ICC is currently the standard indicator for quantifying the agreement between observers, within observers and between different instruments, it is advised to interpret the ICC with caution.

Chapter 13
Overview

Abstract This chapter shows an overview of the different statistical methods that can be used for the different outcome variables and when they can be used.

Table 13.1 shows an overview of the different statistical methods that can be used for the different outcome variables and when they can be used.

J. W. R. Twisk, *Basic Principles of Applied Medical Statistics*,
https://doi.org/10.1007/978-3-031-86278-6_13

Table 13.1 Overview of the different statistical methods that can be used in the analysis of different outcome variables

Comparison	Statistical method	Effect estimate
Continuous outcome variables		
Within a group	Paired t-test Wilcoxon rank sign test[a]	Change None
Between two groups	Independent t-test Mann-Whitney U test[a]	Difference between means None
Between > two groups	Analysis of variance Kruskal-Wallis test[a]	Difference between means[b] None
Between variables	Linear regression analysis	Regression coefficient Pearson correlation Spearman correlation[a]
Dichotomous outcome variables		
Within a group	McNemar test	Difference between proportions
Between two groups	Fisher exact test Chi-square test	Relative risk/risk difference/odds ratio
Between > two groups	Fisher exact test Chi-square test	Relative risk/risk difference/odds ratio[c]
Between variables	Logistic regression analysis	Odds ratio
Survival data		
Between two groups	Log rank test	None
Between > two groups	Log rank test	None
Between variables	Cox regression analysis	Hazard ratio
Categorical outcome variables		
Between two groups	Fisher exact test Chi-square test	Relative risk/risk difference/odds ratio[c]
Between > two groups	Fisher exact test Chi-square test	Relative risk/risk difference/odds ratio[c]
Between variables	Multinomial logistic regression analysis	Odds ratio
Poisson distributed outcome variables		
Between variables	Poisson regression analysis Negative binomial regression analysis[d]	Rate ratio
Outcome variables with floor or ceiling effects		
Between variables	Tobit regression analysis	Regression coefficient

[a] Non-parametric methods; in the case of non-normally distributed residuals, always try to apply a transformation first and use non-parametric methods only in small study populations

[b] When comparing more than two groups, post-hoc procedures should be used to estimate the difference of means

[c] Separate 2 × 2 tables should be used for effect estimation

[d] When there is overdispersion

Chapter 14
Example Datasets

Abstract This chapter shows the example datasets that are used in this book.

In this book the following example datasets are used:

Example 2.1
Design: observational cross-sectional cohort study
Sample size: 100 subjects
Outcome variable: cholesterol
Independent variables: age, alcohol consumption, smoking
Dataset: example 2_1

Example 4.1
Design: observational prospective cohort study
Sample size: 100 subjects
Outcome variable: cholesterol
Independent variables: none
Repeated measurements: 2
Time interval: 6 months
Dataset: example 4_1

Example 4.2
Design: observational cross-sectional cohort study
Sample size: 100 subjects
Outcome variable: cholesterol
Independent variables: social class, age, alcohol consumption, smoking
Dataset: example 4_2

Example 4.3
Design: observational cross-sectional cohort study
Sample size: 100 subjects
Outcome variable: triglyceride
Independent variables: overweight
Dataset: example 4_3

J. W. R. Twisk, *Basic Principles of Applied Medical Statistics*,
https://doi.org/10.1007/978-3-031-86278-6_14

Example 4.4
Design: small intervention study
Sample size: 12 subjects
Outcome variable: decrease in systolic blood pressure
Independent variables: intervention, overweight
Dataset: example 4_4

Example 5.1
Design: RCT
Study population: patients with low back pain
Study population size: 100 in both groups
Outcome variable: perceived recovery (yes/no)
Independent variable: activity program versus usual care, sex
Dataset: example 5.1

Example 5.1a
Design: RCT
Study population: patients with low back pain
Study population size: 100 in both groups
Outcome variable: perceived recovery (yes/no)
Independent variable: activity program, activity program + behavioural therapy versus usual care
Dataset: example 5.1a

Example 5.2
Design: cross-over trial
Study population size: 50 patients
Outcome variable: improvement in pain
Independent variable: drug A versus drug B
Dataset: example 5_2

Example 5.3
Design: case-control study
Study population size: 100 cases, 100 controls
Outcome variable: myocardial infarction (yes/no)
Independent variables: smoking, alcohol consumption, body mass index
Dataset: example 5_3

Example 6.1
Design: RCT
Study population: patients with low back pain
Study population size: 100 in the intervention group, 100 in the control group
Outcome variable: perceived recovery (yes/no) and time to recovery
Independent variable: activity program versus usual care
Dataset: example 6_1

Example 6.1a
Design: RCT
Study population: patients with low back pain
Study population size: 100 in both intervention groups, 100 in the control group
Outcome variable: perceived recovery (yes/no) and time to recovery
Independent variable: activity program, activity program + behavioural therapy versus usual care
Dataset: example 6_1a

Example 6.2
Design: observational cohort study
Study population size: 288 subjects
Outcome variable: stroke (yes/no) and time to stroke
Independent variables: cholesterol, age, sex
Dataset: example 6_1

Example 6.3
Design: observational cohort study
Study population size: 42 patients
Outcome variable: mortality and time to mortality
Independent variable: intervention
Dataset: example 6_3

Example 7.1
Design: observational cross-sectional cohort study
Sample size: 200 subjects
Outcome variable: cholesterol
Independent variables: body mass index, age, sex, smoking, alcohol consumption, physical activity
Dataset: example 7_1

Example 7.2
Design: intervention study without control condition
Sample size: 120 patients with low back pain
Outcome variable: recovery
Independent variables: sex, medication use, overweight, pain, function score, duration of complaints, age
Dataset: example 7_2

Example 9.1
Design: cross-sectional cohort study
Study population size: 100
Outcome variable: perceived health (bad, not good/not bad, good)
Independent variables: smoking, social class, age
Dataset: example 9_1

Example 9.2
Design: cross-sectional cohort study
Study population size: 882
Outcome variable: CVD risk cluster score
Independent variable: physical activity
Dataset: example 9_2

Example 9.3
Design: RCT
Study population: patients suffering from stroke
Study population size: 96 patients in the both groups
Outcome variable: Barthel index
Independent variable: intervention versus usual care, age
Dataset: example 9_3

Example 10.1
Design: cross-sectional cohort study
Sample size: 400 subjects
Outcome variable: depression
Independent variables: age, sex, social class, marital status
Dataset: example 10_1

Example 11.1
Design: cross-sectional cohort study
Sample size: 167 subjects
Outcome variable: hdl-cholesterol
Independent variables: trunk fat mass, peripheral fat mass, total fat mass
Dataset: example 11_1

Example 11.2
Design: observational cohort study
Sample size: 420 subjects
Outcome variable: systolic blood pressure
Independent variables: inactivity, body mass index
Dataset: example 11_2

Example 11.3
Design: case-control study
Sample size: 420 subjects
Outcome variable: myocardial infarction
Independent variables: smoking, systolic blood pressures
Dataset: example 11_3

Example 12.1
Design: observational cross-sectional study
Sample size: 50 subjects
Outcome variable: physical activity measured in two ways
Dataset: example 12_1

Example 12.2
Design: observational cross-sectional study
Sample size: 50 subjects
Outcome variable: systolic blood pressure measured by two observers
Dataset: example 12_2

References

Bland, J. M., & Altman, D. G. (1986). Statistical methods for assessing agreement between two methods of clinical measurement. *Lancet, 1*(8476), 307–310.

Buuren, S. van (2018). Flexible imputation of missing data. In *Provides practical information and R code of the application of the multivariate imputation by chained equations (MICE) procedure* (2nd ed.). Chapman and Hall/CRC.

de Vet, H. C. W., Terwee, C. B., Mokkink, L. B., & Knol, D. (2011). *Measurement in medicine. A practical guide*. Cambridge University Press.

Goldstein, H. (2003). *Multilevel statistical models*. Edward Arnold.

Harrell, J., & Frank, E. (2015). *Regression modeling strategies with applications to linear models, logistic and ordinal regression, and survival analysis* (2nd ed.). Springer.

Hastie, T., Tibshirani, R., & Friedman, J. (2017). *The elements of statistical learning. Data mining, inference and prediction* (2nd ed.). Springer Series in Statistics.

Kirkwood, B. R., & Sterne, A. C. (2003). *Essential medical statistics*. Blackwell Publishing.

Kleinbaum, D. C. (1996). Survival analysis: A self learning text. In *Statistics in the health sciences*. Springer.

MacKinnon, D. P. (2008). *Introduction to statistical mediation analysis*. Erlbaum.

Maley, J. D., Malley, K. G., & Pajevic, S. (2011). *Statistical learning for biomedical data*. Cambridge University Press.

Moons, K. G., Donders, R. A., Stijnen, T., & Harrell, F. E., Jr. (2006). Using the outcome for imputation of missing predictor values was preferred. *Journal of Clinical Epidemiology, 59*(10), 1092–1101.

Müller, R., & Büttner, P. (1994). A critical discussion of intraclass correlation coefficients. *Statistics in Medicine, 13*(23–24), 2465–2476.

Rijnhart, J. J. M., Twisk, J. W. R., Chinapaw, M. J. M., de Boer, M. R., & Heymans, M. W. (2017). Comparison of methods for the analysis of relatively simple mediation models. *Contemporary Clinical Trials Communications, 7*, 130–135.

Rijnhart, J. J. M., Lamp, S. J., Valente, M. J., MacKinnon, D. P., Twisk, J. W. R., & Heymans, M. W. (2021). Mediation analysis methods used in observational research: A scoping review and recommendations. *BMC Medical Research Methodology, 21*, 226.

Riley, R. D., Snell, K. I. E., Martin, G. P., Whittle, R., Archer, L., Sperrin, M., & Collins, G. S. (2021). Penalization and shrinkage methods produced unreliable clinical prediction models especially when sample size was small. *Journal of Clinical Epidemiology, 132*, 88–96.

Rothman, K. J. (2002). *Epidemiology. An introduction*. Oxford University Press.

Rubin, D. B. (1976). Inference and missing data. *Biometrika, 63*(3), 581–592.

J. W. R. Twisk, *Basic Principles of Applied Medical Statistics*,
https://doi.org/10.1007/978-3-031-86278-6

Rubin, D. B. (1987). *Multiple imputation for nonresponse in surveys*. Wiley.

Schuster, N. A., Hoogendijk, E. O., Almar, A. L., Kok, A. A. L., JWR, T., & Heymans, M. W. (2020). Ignoring competing events in the analysis of survival data may lead to biased results: A nonmathematical illustration of competing risk analysis. *Journal of Clinical Epidemiology, 122*, 42e48.

Schuster, N. A., Rijnhart, J. J. M., Twisk, J. W. R., & Heymans, M. W. (2022). Modeling non-linear relationships in epidemiological data: The application and interpretation of spline models. *Frontiers in Epidemiology, 2*, 975380. https://doi.org/10.3389/fepid.2022.975380

Smola, A. J., & Schölkopf, B. (2004). A tutorial on support vector regression. *Statistics and Computing, 14*, 199–222.

Steyerberg, E. W. (2019). *Clinical prediction models. A practical approach to development, validation, and updating*. Springer.

Twisk, J. W. R. (2017). *Applied mixed model analysis: A practical guide*. Cambridge University Press.

Twisk, J. W. R. (2023). *Applied longitudinal data analysis for medical science: A practical guide* (3rd ed.). Cambridge University Press.

Twisk, J. W. R. (2024a). Refrain from statistical testing in medical research; it does more harm than good. *Annals of Epidemiology, 2*(3), 000540.

Twisk, J. W. R. (2024b). Indirect effects in mediation analyses should not be tested for statistical significance. *Journal of Clinical Epidemiology, 13*(171), 111393.

Twisk, J. W. R. (2024c). Sample size calculations are a waste of time, money and energy and should be replaced by sample size considerations. *Annals of Epidemiology, 2*, 1–3.

Twisk, J. W. R., Smidt, N., & de Vente, W. (2005). Applied analysis of recurrent events: A practical overview. *Journal of Epidemiology and Community Health, 59*(8), 706–710.

Twisk, J., de Boer, M., de Vente, W., & Heymans, M. (2013). Multiple imputation of missing values was not necessary before performing a longitudinal mixed-model analysis. *Journal of Clinical Epidemiology, 66*(9), 1022–1028.

Wallace, M. L., Mentch, L., Wheeler, B. J., Tapia, A. L., Richards, M., Zhou, S., Yi, L., Redline, S., & Buysse, D. J. (2023). Use and misuse of random forest variable importance metrics in medicine: Demonstrations through incident stroke prediction. *BMC Medical Research Methodology, 23*, 144.

GPSR Compliance
The European Union's (EU) General Product Safety Regulation (GPSR) is a set of rules that requires consumer products to be safe and our obligations to ensure this.

If you have any concerns about our products, you can contact us on

ProductSafety@springernature.com

In case Publisher is established outside the EU, the EU authorized representative is:

Springer Nature Customer Service Center GmbH
Europaplatz 3
69115 Heidelberg, Germany

www.ingramcontent.com/pod-product-compliance
Lightning Source LLC
Chambersburg PA
CBHW070352180625
PP16652000001B/25
* 9 7 8 3 0 3 1 8 6 2 7 7 9 *